The Essential Guide to Holistic and Complementary Therapy

HAIRDRESSING AND BEAUTY INDUSTRY AUTHORITY SERIES – RELATED TITLES

HAIRDRESSING

Mahogany Hairdressing: Steps to Cutting, Colouring and Finishing Hair *Martin Gannon and Richard Thompson*
Mahogany Hairdressing: Advanced Looks *Richard Thompson and Martin Gannon*
Essensuals, Next Generation Toni & Guy: Step by Step
Professional Men's Hairdressing *Guy Kemer and Jacki Wadeson*
The Art of Dressing Long Hair *Guy Kemer and Jacki Wadeson*
Patrick Cameron: Dressing Long Hair *Patrick Cameron and Jacki Wadeson*
Patrick Cameron: Dressing Long Hair Book 2 *Patrick Cameron*
Bridal Hair *Pat Dixon and Jacki Wadeson*
Trevor Sorbie: Visions in Hair *Kris Sorbie and Jacki Wadeson*
The Total Look: The Style Guide for Hair and Make-up Professionals *Ian Mistlin*
Art of Hair Colouring *David Adams and Jacki Wadeson*
Begin Hairdressing: The Official Guide to Level 1 *Martin Green*
Hairdressing – The Foundations: The Official Guide to Level 2 *Leo Palladino* (contribution Jane Farr)
Professional Hairdressing: The Official Guide to Level 3 4e *Martin Green, Lesley Kimber and Leo Palladino*
Men's Hairdressing: Traditional and Modern Barbering 2e *Maurice Lister*
African-Caribbean Hairdressing 2e *Sandra Gittens*
Salon Management *Martin Green*
eXtensions: The Official Guide to Hair Extensions *Theresa Bullock*

BEAUTY THERAPY

Beauty Therapy – The Foundations: The Official Guide to Level 2 *Lorraine Nordmann*
Beauty Basics – The Official Guide to Level 1 *Lorraine Nordmann*
Professional Beauty Therapy: The Official Guide to Level 3 *Lorraine Nordmann, Lorraine Williamson, Jo Crowder and Pamela Linforth*
Aromatherapy for the Beauty Therapist *Valerie Ann Worwood*
Indian Head Massage *Muriel Burnham-Airey and Adele O'Keefe*
The Official Guide to Body Massage *Adele O'Keefe*
An Holistic Guide to Anatomy and Physiology *Tina Parsons*
The Encyclopedia of Nails *Jacqui Jefford and Anne Swain*
Nail Artistry *Jacqui Jefford, Sue Marsh and Anne Swain*
The Complete Nail Technician *Marian Newman*
The World of Skin Care: A Scientific Companion *Dr John Gray*
Safety in the Salon *Elaine Almond*
An Holistic Guide to Reflexology *Tina Parsons*
Nutrition: A Practical Approach *Suzanne Le Quesne*
An Holistic Guide to Massage *Tina Parsons*

The Essential Guide to Holistic and Complementary Therapy

Helen Beckmann and
Suzanne Le Quesne

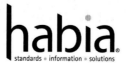

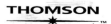

Australia • Canada • Mexico • Singapore • Spain • United Kingdom • United States

THOMSON
TM

The Essential Guide to Holistic and Complementary Therapy – first edition

British Library Cataloguing-in-Publication Data
A catalogue record for this book is available from the British Library.

ISBN 978-1-84480-026-1

First edition published 2005 by Thomson Learning

Reprinted 2006 by Thomson Learning

Typeset by Graphicraft Limited, Hong Kong

Printed in Croatia by Zrinski d.d.

Dedication

To my husband Howard, my children Connor and Alex, and my Mum and Dad. And, of course,
to all those who have developed and expanded my knowledge over the years. *Helen Beckmann*

To my husband Barry, who has looked after me and given me so much encouragement during
the writing of this book. *Suzanne Le Quesne*

Contents

Foreword x
Preface xi
Acknowledgements xii

1 Health and safety 1

Health and safety legislation 2
Personal hygiene and appearance 12
Knowledge review 13

2 Foundations of chemistry 14

Atoms and molecules 15
Elements 15
Compounds 15
Chemical reactions and chemical bonds 16
Transfer of substances – how do molecules move? 18
The pH scale – potential of hydrogen 18
Knowledge review 19

3 Understanding energy 20

Yin and yang 21
Meridians 21
Chakras 30
Ayurvedic influences 34
Knowledge review 36

4 Anatomy and physiology 37

Terminology 38
Organization of the body 38
The integumentary system 43
The circulatory system 61
The lymphatic/immune system 71
The skeletal system 76
The muscular system 85
The respiratory system 91
The digestive system 95
The nervous system 100
The special senses 108
The ear 111
The endocrine system 111
The genito-urinary system 116
Knowledge review 122

5

Client care 123

First impressions   124
Interpersonal skills   125
Counselling skills and the therapist   131
Protecting yourself   132
Preparing for a treatment   133
Consultation techniques   134
Contra indications   137
After care and advice   141
Knowledge review   145

6

Nutrition 146

The macro-nutrients – carbohydrates, proteins and lipids   147
Anti-nutrients, enzymes and water   154
The micro-nutrients – vitamins, minerals and trace minerals   156
A balanced diet   164
The nutrition consultation   165
Contra indications for nutritional therapy   165
Establishing weight parameters   166
Knowledge review   168

7

7 Posture and figure analysis 169

The process of a figure analysis   170
Body shapes   171
Posture and postural faults/weaknesses   172
Examination of muscular condition   178
Simple postural exercises   179
Concluding a figure analysis   182
Knowledge review 182

8

Classification of massage techniques 183

The benefits and effects of massage   184
Classic massage techniques   186
Preparation for massage   192
Additional massage techniques   192
Other massage therapies   194
Knowledge review   197

9

Body massage 198

A brief overview of the history of massage   199
Preparation for a massage treatment   199
A sample massage routine   202
Muscle stretching and energizing techniques   207
After care for massage   210
Adaptations to massage   210
General adaptations   212
Pre-heating treatments (heat therapy)   214
Knowledge review   218

10

Aromatherapy 219

A brief history of aromatherapy   220
What is aromatherapy?   220
What is an essential oil?   220

The physiology of aromatherapy 222
Safety issues 223
Clinical aromatherapy 225
The aromatherapy treatment 231
After care 238
Knowledge review 240

11 Chemistry and essential oils directory 241

Classification of essential oils 241
Chemotypes 243
Categories of essential oils 244
Synergy 244
Harmony 244
Directory of essential oils 244
Knowledge review 282

12 Holistic facial 283

What is an holistic facial? 284
Skin types 284
Skin care products 286
Preparing for an holistic facial 288
Carrying out a skin analysis 290
Basic face reading 291
Cleansing 292
Facial massage 294
Adaptation to massage 299
Masks 300
Contra actions and after care 301
Knowledge review 302

13 Indian head massage 303

A history of Indian head massage 304
Contra indications to Indian head massage 304
Preparation of therapist, client and treatment room 304
Physical and psychological benefits of Indian head massage 305
Oils used in Indian head massage 306
The massage routine 307
Adapting the massage for different individuals 314
After care advice for Indian head massage 315
Knowledge review 315

14 Reflexology 316

A brief history of reflexology 317
What is reflexology and how does it work? 317
Mapping the feet 320
Preparing for the treatment 321
Contra indications to reflexology treatment 323
Reading the feet 323
A reflexology treatment 325
Treatment techniques 327
Treatment adaptations 337
Contra actions and after care 337
Working the hands 338
Knowledge review 339

15 Stress management 341

What is stress? 342
Environmental, emotional, chemical and nutritional stress 342
The causes of stress 343
The symptoms of stress 344
The stress response (stressed out/burnt out) 345
How to reduce and/or manage stress 348
Knowledge review 356

16 Crystal therapy 357

A history of crystal therapy 358
What are crystals? 358
Grounding 359
Recommendations for a basic set of crystals 363
Types of crystal 366
Self-treatment 367
Chakra balancing 368
Using crystals with other therapies 370
Specific after care advice for crystal therapy 371
Knowledge review 372

17 Colour therapy 373

A brief history of colour therapy 374
The electromagnetic spectrum 374
How colour therapy works 375
Consultation for colour therapy 376
Colour therapy treatments 376
Ascertaining colour needs 379
Colour in our environment 380
Colours used in colour therapy 381
Contra indications to colour therapy 385
Specific after care advice 385
Knowledge review 386

18 Thermal auricular therapy 387

A history of ear candling 388
Contra indications and contra actions to ear candling 388
The manufacture and composition of candles 389
How do ear candles actually work? 389
The benefits and effects of ear candling 390
Ear candling treatment 390
After care advice 393
Essential anatomy for ear candling 393
Medical terms explained 396
Knowledge review 397

19 Reiki 398

What is Reiki? 399
Intent 399
The benefits and effects of Reiki 399
Reiki precepts and principles 400
Understanding Reiki attunements 401
Contra indications and contra actions to Reiki treatments 402
Reiki self-healing 403
How to give a Reiki treatment to others 404
The meaning of the Reiki symbols 412

Using Reiki with other treatments   413
Causes of *dis*-harmony and *dis*-ease   413
Knowledge review   416

20 Hot stone massage   417

A history of stone therapy   418
Hot basalt stones   418
Cold marine stones   419
Standard set of stones   419
Contra indications and contra actions to stone therapy   420
Massage treatment   422
Specific after care advice for hot stone massage   424
Knowledge review   424

21 Managing and marketing   425

Choosing premises   426
Business planning   430
Stock   432
Accounts and your accountant   433
Time management   433
Effective marketing   434
Knowledge review   439

Glossary   440
Appendix 1   First aid box   449
Appendix 2   Muscles table   453
Index   461

Foreword

The more I travel, the greater opportunity I get to learn about the different perceptions of health and beauty that people have. Japan is one place where it is considered that your spirit of beauty emanates from within just as much as how you look on the outside. But it is not just Japan that believes in this approach. The remarkable Helen Beckmann and the outstanding Suzanne Le Quesne are the inspirational author team for this stimulating and uplifting addition to the HABIA/Thomson Learning partnership.

The scope of alternative therapies and the depth of knowledge of therapies that are detailed here astound me, as does the way the authors have combined their specialist knowledge to enlighten us and lead us to discover new ways to revitalise, provide balance in mind and body, aid relaxation and promote a sense of well being in a busy world.

Helen is a renowned holistic therapy specialist; her dedication to continuing professional development shows a wealth of experience, knowledge and understanding which, when coupled with Suzanne's skills and passion for well-being, really makes this book come alive.

The Essential Guide to Holistic and Complementary Therapy is informative and comprehensive, and will become an invaluable source of guidance as you learn to appreciate the benefits alternative therapies can offer.

Let the authors inspire you as they did me.

Alan Goldsbro
Chief Executive Officer
HABIA

Preface

With 40 years' combined experience, Helen Beckmann and Suzanne Le Quesne are holistic therapy practitioners, teachers/lecturers of holistic studies and health/education writers. The combination of their skills has culminated in this comprehensive text on holistic and complementary therapies. They have combined their practical experience and skills in most aspects of complementary therapy with their extensive knowledge, teaching and training abilities to produce this invaluable book for all students of complementary and holistic therapies. Throughout their careers Helen and Suzanne have maintained their hands-on experience by managing their own holistic and beauty therapy salons while, at the same time, continuing their own professional development training, and teaching and lecturing to students in Further Education and Private colleges. Helen and Suzanne are both experienced assessors and verifiers for City and Guilds and VTCT, and their vast experience comes through clearly in the pages of this exciting book.

Over recent years there has been a substantial increase in the popularity of holistic therapies. With the upsurge of spa centres opening up across the country, clients have come to expect a variety of treatments to be available under one roof. This has resulted in employers needing staff trained in more than one discipline and more students wanting to be, and needing to be, multi-faceted when it comes to the variety of treatments they can offer. The more disciplines you are qualified in, the more employable you become. However, the message here is not to be a 'jack of all trades and master of none'! Training to National Vocational standards is essential and the level and standard of training is improving all the time.

With the continuing upsurge of interest in complementary therapies, many awarding bodies now offer qualifications in the lesser known of the holistic therapies, such as colour and crystal therapy, meditation and visualisation, thermal auricular therapy (ear candling) and Reiki, alongside the more well known holistic therapies, such as aromatherapy, reflexology, stress management and Indian head massage, which have become household names.

This book covers not only the most popular and the newest holistic therapies but also anatomy and physiology, energy, chemistry, salon management and marketing, and health and hygiene. The book is full of interesting facts and tips and offers practical step-by-step instructions to the therapies accompanied by excellent illustrations.

One of the main aims of the book is to provide an understanding of the word 'holistic' and an understanding of how the mind, body and spirit are all connected.

Acknowledgements

We would like to thank enormously:

Jeff Richards B.Sc. (Hons) Ost Med, D.O. (Hons)

Melanie Waite (Ideal Consultants)

Michaela Hudson (Lecturer in Holistic Therapies at Farnborough college)

For their time, invaluable advice and support.

Mary Wiles (Head of Department Crawley College). For the push in the right direction!

Barry Le Quesne for demonstrating the Indian Head Massage.

Dennis Prior for his expert assistance with the photography for the Indian Head Massage chapter.

Emma Louise Gibson for her patience as our model for the Indian Head Massage chapter.

All our many friends and colleagues for their continued support and encouragement.

Visit the *Essential Guide to Holistic and Complementary Therapy* companion website at www.thomsonlearning.co.uk/hairandbeauty/beckmann to find further teaching and learning material including:

For Students

- Chapter overviews to give you an indication of the coverage of the book.
- True/false and multiple choice questions to test your understanding of each chapter.
- Activities to help you become more familiar with the concepts outlined in the text.
- Web references to guide you towards further study.
- Answers to knowledge review exercises so that you can check your progress as you work through the text.

For Teachers

- Lecturer's notes to help you teach the course.
- A complete set of downloadable PowerPoint slides.

Health and safety

Learning objectives

This chapter covers the following:

- **health and safety legislation**
- **your expected duties, legal responsibilities and key contacts for health and safety at your place of work**
- **salon security**
- **personal hygiene and appearance**

Legislation and industry codes of practice requirements are of great importance to everyone working in the health and beauty industry. There are, at the time of writing, 18 Acts and regulations affecting hair and beauty salons, and you need an understanding of these regulations, as many aspects will feature in your day-to-day work. It is not only the employer who is responsible for health and safety in your working environment; *you* have *your* part to play in helping your manager/employer to maintain a healthy and safe working environment for yourself, your work colleagues and other business customers and visitors.

Health and safety legislation

This section will provide you with an outline of the main health and safety regulations that affect beauty and holistic therapists and their work. The Health and Safety at Work Act 1974 is the legislation that covers a variety of safe working practices and associated regulations. You do not need to know the full contents of the Act in detail, but you should at least be aware of the existence of relevant regulations made under its provisions that directly concern you and your work.

- Management of Health and Safety at Work Regulations 1999
- Workplace (Health, Safety and Welfare) Regulations 1992
- Personal Protective Equipment at Work (PPE) Regulations 1992
- Control of Substances Hazardous to Health (COSHH) Regulations 1999
- Electricity at Work Regulations 1989
- Health and Safety (First Aid) Regulations 1981
- Reporting of Injuries, Diseases and Dangerous Occurrences Regulations (RIDDOR) 1995
- Fire Precautions Act 1971 and Amendment Regulations 1999
- Health and Safety (Display Screen Equipment) Regulations 1999
- Manual Handling Operations Regulations 1992
- Provision of Use of Work Equipment (PUWER) Regulations 1998
- Health and Safety (Information for Employees) Regulations 1989.

Management of Health and Safety at Work Regulations 1999

The main regulation requires the employer to appoint competent personnel to conduct risk assessments for the health and safety of all staff employed or otherwise and other visitors to the business premises. Staff must be adequately trained to take appropriate action, eliminate or minimize any risks. Other regulations cover the necessity to set up procedures for emergency situations, reviewing the risk assessment process. In salons where five or more people are employed, there is the added obligation to set up a system for monitoring health surveillance, should the risk assessments identify a need. Main requirements for the management of health and safety are as follows:

- identification of any potential hazards
- assessment of the risks that could arise from these hazards
- identifying who is at risk
- eliminating or minimizing the risks
- training staff to identify and control risks
- regular review of the assessment processes.

Risk assessment

There is also a requirement to carry out a risk assessment for young people. Any staff member who is under school-leaving age must have a personalized risk assessment kept on file. This would be applicable to those on work experience or Saturday staff.

1 Take a walk around the salon looking for any hazards, i.e. anything with the potential to cause harm. Your salon should have risk assessment forms for recording any findings.

2 Decide what the risk is and who could be harmed by those hazards. A loose carpet in reception is a hazard to all clients and staff, whereas a poorly fitted plug on a kettle in the staff room would only affect the staff.

3 For each of the listed hazards decide what level of risk exists, e.g. low, medium or high. Then, looking at each entry, ask yourself if the risk can be eliminated or reduced. A loose carpet in reception is a hazard to everyone; if it were replaced the hazard would be eliminated. You must inform your staff of the assessment findings and give them necessary training to minimize the risks.

4 Write down the findings of your risk assessment (salons with less than five employees do not have to record these findings). However, you may get a visit from Environmental Health and physical records will prove that the assessments have been made.

5 Review your risk assessment at regular intervals. The introduction of new equipment, different product ranges or chemical processes will potentially create new hazards. Setting a review date within the assessment process will ensure that your salon is kept up to date in the future.

Workplace (Health, Safety and Welfare) Regulations 1992

This act covers the health and safety of the actual workplace, the effects of which will have an impact on the welfare of staff. Key points are:

- maintenance of the workplace and the equipment in it
- ventilation, temperature and lighting
- cleanliness
- sanitary and washing facilities
- drinking water supply
- resting, eating and changing facilities

COSHH risk assessment form for beauty salons

Date   Staff member responsible for assessment   Review date

Hazard	*What is the risk*	*Who is at risk*	*Degree of risk*	*Action*
Basalt and marine stones left on flat-topped trolley	These are very heavy and could easily fall off if the trolley were moved and could cause injury	*Everyone*: beauty therapists, juniors, trainees and clients, if walking past trolley	High	Move to a safe place. Advise staff that when not being used, stones should be stored on a towel, on the bottom shelf of cupboard. Alternatively, keep stones in the heating unit ready for use
Aromatherapy oils	Essential oils are flammable and could cause harm if taken internally	*Everyone*: beauty therapists, juniors, trainees and clients	High	Move essential oils to a locked or secure cupboard. Store in a cool dark place, away from reach of children. Keep in original bottles, which will be well labelled

- storage of clothing
- glazing
- traffic routes
- work space.

Amendments and additions to this Act provide new requirements for employers with particular attention focused on glazed areas such as windows and doors. Any transparent and translucent partitions must be made of safe materials, and if they could cause injury to anyone they should be appropriately marked. (Note that narrow panes of glass up to 250mm are excluded from this Act.)

Other amendments have particular rules for rest rooms and rest areas. These must include a suitable alternative arrangements to protect non-smokers from the effects caused by tobacco smoke and suitable rest facilities to be provided for any person at work who is either pregnant or a nursing mother.

Personal Protective Equipment at Work (PPE) Regulations 1992

The PPE Regulations 1992 require managers to make an assessment of the processes and activities carried out at work and to identify where and when special items of clothing should be worn. In beauty salon environments the potential hazards and dangers revolve around the tasks of providing certain beauty services – that is, in general, the application of beauty products. Potentially hazardous substances used by beauticians and/or holistic therapists include:

- products used in waxing – hot wax, warm wax, sugaring products
- vapours and dyeing compounds found in eyelash tints
- essential oils used in aromatherapy
- flammable liquids and products used in applying nail enhancements.

There are also potentially hazardous items of equipment and their individual applications, for example:

- electrical appliances
- heated/heating instruments
- sharp cutting tools – used in manicure/pedicure/nail enhancements, etc.

Control of Substances Hazardous to Health (COSHH) Regulations 1999

Beauty salon employers are required by law to make an assessment of the exposure to all the substances used in their salons that are potentially hazardous to themselves, their employees and other salon visitors, who may be affected by the work activity. The purpose of COSHH Regulations is to make sure that people are working in the safest possible environment and conditions. A substance is considered to be hazardous if it can cause harm to the body. It only presents a risk if it is:

- in contact with the skin or eyes
- absorbed through the skin or via the eyes (either directly or from contact with contaminated surfaces or clothing)

- inhaled, i.e. breathing in substances in the atmosphere
- ingested via contaminated food or fingers
- injected
- introduced into the body via cuts and abrasions.

Beauty products must comply with stringent UK cosmetics products safety regulations. The regulations detail how ingredients such as hydrogen peroxide and other chemicals can be used. Under new legislation introduced in the EU manufacturers have to list on the label all the ingredients that are used in their products. Therefore employers must make an assessment to find out the following:

- what products are used
- what is the potential of a product for causing harm
- what is the chance of exposure
- how much people are exposed to, for how long and how often
- whether the exposure be prevented, and if not, how can it be adequately controlled.

Wherever safer products are available they should be used; where not, the exposure should be controlled. Exposure can be controlled by:

- providing good ventilation
- using the product only in recommended concentrations
- clearing up spillages or splashes immediately
- resealing containers immediately after use
- providing safe storage
- using personal protective equipment.

Electricity at Work Regulations 1989

The Electricity at Work Regulations 1989 covers the installation, maintenance and use of electrical equipment and systems in the workplace. A qualified electrician must adequately check equipment on a yearly basis. An electrical testing record should be kept for each piece of equipment, which should clearly show:

- the electrician's/contractor's name, address and contact details
- an itemized list of salon electrical equipment along with the serial number (for individual identification)
- date of inspection
- date of purchase/disposal.

Health and Safety (First Aid) Regulations 1981

The Health and Safety (First Aid) Regulations 1981 require employers to provide equipment and facilities which are adequate and appropriate in the circumstances for administering first aid to their employees. Remember that any first aid materials used from the kit must be replaced as soon as possible. All accidents and emergency aid given within the salon must be documented in an accident book. The contents of the first aid box increases with the number of employees and regular assessment checks should be made to ensure there is a full kit. All accidents, no matter how minor they may seem, must be recorded in the accident book. The recording system should always be kept readily available for use and inspection. When you are recording accidents, you will need to document the following details:

- date, time and place of incident or treatment
- name and job of injured or ill person
- details of the injury/ill person and the treatment given
- details of what happened to the person immediately afterwards (home, hospital, etc.)
- name and signature of the person providing the treatment and entry.

Find out who the first aid person is in your salon and if there isn't one, why don't you consider taking an appropriate course? St John Ambulance, Red Cross, and hairdressing and beauty therapy awarding bodies all put on general first aid courses. You will find it very rewarding and may even save someone's life.

Reporting of Injuries, Diseases and Dangerous Occurrences Regulations (RIDDOR) 1995

Under these regulations there are certain diseases and groups of infections that if sustained at work are noticeable by law. So if any employees suffer a personal injury at work which results in either

- death
- major injury
- more than 24 hours in hospital
- an incapacity to work for more than three calendar days

you must report them to the incident contact centre. In addition to this, if a member of the public or salon visitor is injured within the salon and taken to hospital, this also must be reported.

Fire Precautions Act 1971 and the Amendment Regulations 1999

Fires occurring in salons would be most likely to arise from an electrical fault, a gas leak or smoking. Staff cooking facilities need to be closely monitored to prevent the gas being left on, whether lit or not. Smoking can cause fires when lit cigarettes are dropped, discarded or left unattended to smoulder in ashtrays. Your salon will have established fire safety procedures, which must always be followed.

Under the regulations a fire certificate is required for business premises if:

- more than 20 people are employed on one floor at any one time
- more than 10 people are employed on different floors at any one time.

Where premises are shared with other businesses, employers must include everyone collectively. All premises must be provided with an adequate means of escape in case of fire as well as a means of fighting fire, whether or not a fire certificate is required. All fire exits need to be clearly marked with the appropriate signs and all doors must be capable of being opened easily and immediately from the inside.

Every employer must carry out a fire risk assessment covering the premises. This should address the following key aspects.

- Assessment of fire risks within the premises as required under the Management of Health and Safety at Work Regulations 1999.
- The installation of suitable fire detection equipment, e.g. smoke alarms.
- The installation of a suitable warning system (this could be an automatic fire alarm system).
- Checks that everyone can get away safely from the premises in the event of fire and that all means of escape, including passageways, stairwells, etc., are kept clear of obstructions at all times. Where necessary adequate emergency lighting should be installed.
- The provision of adequate fire fighting equipment.
- The provision of adequate training for employees so that everyone knows what to do in the event of fire.
- Regular checks and maintenance of all fire safety equipment.
- Regular reviews of the fire safety arrangements.

Raising the alarm

In the event of fire breaking out, your main priorities are as follows.

- Raise the alarm – staff and customers must be warned and the premises must be evacuated.
- Call the fire brigade. Do this even if you believe that someone else has already phoned. Dial 999, ask the operator for the fire service and give the telephone number from where you are calling. Wait for the transfer to the fire service, then tell them your name and the address of the premises that are on fire.

Fire fighting

If the fire is small, you may tackle it with an extinguisher or fire blanket. Under the Fire Precautions Act 1971, all premises are required to have fire fighting equipment, which must be suitable and maintained in good working order. Different types of fire require different types of fire extinguisher.

There are four classifications of fire:

1. *Class A* fires involve solid material, i.e. paper, wood, hair, etc.
2. *Class B* fires involve liquids such as petrol, paraffin, etc.
3. *Class C* fires involve gases, i.e. propane, butane, etc.
4. *Class D* fires involve metals.

There are four types of fire extinguisher:

1. *Water*. These are *red* with a label to indicate type. They can only be used for Class A fires. The standard size is 9 litres (2 gallons). The main problem with this type of extinguisher is the subsequent damage caused by the water and that it cannot be used on electrical fires.
2. *Foam*. These used to be cream/buff, but are now *red* with a *cream/buff* label. They are used for Class B fires and small Class A fires. The standard capacity is 9 litres (2 gallons). This type of extinguisher has the same problems as water extinguishers.
3. *Carbon dioxide (CO_2)*. These used to be black, but are now *red* with a *black* label. They can be used on all fires but are particularly suitable for Class B and electrical fires. They are available in a range of sizes depending on the weight of CO_2 contained in the extinguisher.

4 *Dry powder*. These used to be blue, but are now *red* with a *blue* label. They can be used on all classes of fire, but are particularly suitable for Class B, C and electrical fires. They are available in a range of sizes from 0.75kg to 4kg. The main disadvantage is that the residual powder has to be cleaned up and can cause damage to electronic equipment.

Escape from fire

All premises must have a designated means of escape from fire. This route must be kept clear of obstructions at all times, and during working hours the fire doors must remain unlocked. The escape route must be easily identifiable, with clearly visible signs. In buildings with fire certificates, emergency lighting must be installed. These lighting systems automatically illuminate the escape route in the event of a power failure and are operated by independent battery back up.

Training is given to new members of staff during their induction period. This training must be regularly updated for all staff and fire drills must be held at regular intervals.

Health and Safety (Display Screen Equipment) Regulations 1999

These regulations cover the use of computers and similar equipment in the workplace. Although not generally a high risk, prolonged use of computers can lead to eyestrain, mental stress and possible muscular pain. As more salons now use information technology it is becoming a major consideration for employees.

It is the employer's duty to assess display screen equipment and reduce any risks discovered. They will need to plan the scheduling of work so that there are regular breaks or changes in activity and provide information training for the equipment users. Computer users will also be entitled to eyesight tests paid for by the employer.

Manual Handling Operations Regulations 1992

These regulations apply in all occupations where manual lifting occurs. They require employers to carry out a risk assessment of the work processes and activities that involve lifting. The risk assessment should address detailed aspects:

- any risk of injury
- the manual movement that is involved in the task
- the physical constraints that the loads incur
- the work environmental constraints that are incurred
- the worker's individual capabilities
- steps and/or remedial action to take in order to minimize the risk.

Provision of Use of Work Equipment Regulations (PUWER) 1998

These regulations refer to the regular maintenance and monitoring of work equipment. Any equipment, new or second hand, must be suitable for the

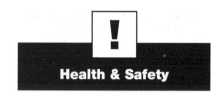

Fire safety training
It is essential for staff to know the following fire procedures:

- fire prevention
- raising the alarm
- evacuation during a fire
- assembly points following evacuation.

purposes for which it is intended. In addition to this the regulations require that anyone using this equipment must be adequately trained.

Health and Safety (Information for Employees) Regulations 1989

These regulations require the employer to make available to all employees, leaflets, notices and posters covering the acts and regulations for the relevant profession. These are available from:

> Health & Safety Executive (HSE) Books
> Box 1999
> Sudbury
> Suffolk CO16 6FS
> Tel. 01787 881165.

Your expected duties, legal responsibilities and key contacts for health and safety at your place of work

You share the responsibility with your employer for the safety of all the people in the salon. You need to be aware of the following:

1   Environmental hazards such as:
      • wet or slippery floors
      • cluttered passageways or corridors
      • rearranged furniture
      • electrical flexes.

2   Hazards to do with equipment and materials such as:
      • worn or faulty electrical equipment
      • incorrectly labelled substances such as cleaning fluids, aromatherapy oils, leaking or damaged containers.

3   Hazards connected with people such as:
      • visitors to the salon
      • handling procedures
      • intruders.

Simply being aware of potential hazards is not enough. You also have a responsibility to contribute to a safe working environment, so you must take steps to check and deal with any sources of risk. You can fulfil your role in two ways.

1   Deal directly with the hazard, which means that you have taken individual responsibility. This will probably apply to obvious hazards such as:
      • trailing flexes – roll them up and store them safely
      • cluttered doorways and corridors – remove objects and store them safely or dispose of them appropriately
      • fire – follow the correct procedures to raise the alarm and assist with evacuation.

2   Inform your manager or supervisor, which means that it becomes an organizational responsibility. This applies to hazards that are beyond your responsibility to deal with, e.g.:

- faulty equipment – kettles, electric heaters, computers, heating cabinet for hot stones, hot cabinet for towels, thermostats on any electrical equipment
- worn floor coverings or broken tiles
- loose or damaged fittings – mirrors, shelves, showers
- obstructions too heavy for you to move safely
- fire.

No matter how small or large your place of work is, you have a duty to your employer and your colleagues to keep the working environment safe. You need to be alert, spotting potential hazards and preventing accidents, thus helping to avoid emergency situations arising. Be responsible – do not leave it for someone else to do.

Obstructions

It is dangerous to obstruct areas used as thoroughfares such as doorways, corridors, stairs and fire exits. In an emergency people might have to leave the salon, or part of it, in a hurry, perhaps even in the dark. It could be disastrous if someone injured themselves or fell in these circumstances. Always be on the lookout for any obstruction in these areas. If you see something that could present a risk, move it away as quickly as you can.

Salon equipment

Each client must have a fresh, clean towel and gown, if treatment requires them. Couch covers should be replaced every day, assuming ample couch roll has been used over the couch cover, or replaced after each client. Towels and covers should be washed on a hot cycle with plenty of washing powder to remove soiling or staining and to prevent the spread of infection by killing any bacteria. Towelling gowns are large items to wash, however, never be tempted to use the same gown twice.

Preventing infection

A warm, humid salon can offer a perfect home for disease-carrying bacteria. If they can find food in the form of dust and dirt, they may reproduce rapidly. Good ventilation provides a circulating air current that will help to prevent their growth. This is why it is important to keep the salon clean, dry and well aired at all times. This includes clothing, work areas, tools and all equipment.

Some salons use sterilizing devices as a means of providing hygienically safe work implements. Sterilization means the complete eradication of living organisms. Different devices use different sterilization methods, which may be based on the use of heat, radiation or chemicals.

Ultra violet (UV) radiation

UV radiation provides an alternative sterilizing option. The items for sterilization are placed in wall or worktop-mounted cabinets fitted with UV-emitting light bulbs and exposed to the radiation for at least 15 minutes. Penetration of UV radiation is low, so sterilization by this method is not guaranteed.

Chemical sterilization

Chemical sterilization should be handled only with suitable personal protective equipment as many of the solutions used are hazardous to health and should not come into contact with the skin. The most effective form of sterilization is achieved by total immersion of the contaminated implements into a bath of fluid. This principle is widely used in the sterilization of babies' feeding utensils.

Disinfectants reduce the probability of infection and are widely used in general day-to-day hygienic salon maintenance. Antiseptics are used specifically for treating wounds. Many pre-packaged first aid dressings are impregnated with antiseptic fluids.

Salon security

Effective salon security is essential and your employer is required by law to provide secure business premises. Moreover, insurance companies would either refuse to insure a salon where adequate precautions were not taken, or would demand premiums so high that no salon could afford them. In order for your employer to establish and maintain the security of people and their belongings, money, equipment and premises, set procedures will have been laid down and put into action. The potential threats to salon security come from either external or internal sources, both in and out of business hours.

External provisions

No salon can make its premises totally burglar proof, but steps may be taken to deter entry by unauthorized people and to minimize any damage they might do. As long as reasonable measures have been taken, insurance will not be withheld. Security devices should be fitted such as:

- five-lever mortise locks (deadlocks) for all external doors – these locks are rebated into (cut out of both the door and the frame), not surface-mounted like latch locks, and require keys both to lock and unlock them
- locking catches or bolts on all external opening windows
- security bars or grilles on potentially vulnerable points of entry
- burglar alarms that sound in the event of forced intrusion or damage.

During the hours of normal business, be alert to the following risks:

- people in areas without the relevant authority
- unauthorized people asking for private or business information
- security of details relating to customers and staff.

Internal provisions

Unfortunately, outside intruders are not the only threat to salon security. Pilfering by staff and clients is also a possibility. Don't let yourself think that taking the occasional product home is a 'perk' of the job. Unless it has been paid for or you have permission, it is theft. Your salon may have its own policy in respect to staff purchases. Always ask. Theft at work is defined as an act of gross misconduct. A thief faces instant dismissal if an employer exercises their disciplinary rights. Your employer will have taken preventative steps to minimize the risk of theft. Procedures will be set in place to monitor till transactions, stock movements and personal items and valuables.

Money missing from the till will show up during the daily cashing up and book-keeping exercises. Shortfalls will be noticed when the number of clients attended, services and treatments provided and retail items sold do not tally with the available money and cash equivalents, the till rolls and the expected cumulative totals, daily reports and transaction breakdowns.

Missing items of stock will be noticed during normal stock control procedures, in routine situations where stock is not available as expected, and during spot checks and searches.

Personal possessions of both clients and staff also need protecting from theft. Make sure that these are kept safely away from risk situations. Clients' handbags, jewellery and any other valuables should remain with them at all times. Valuable items of money belonging to staff should be stored securely during working hours. Alternatively, staff should be encouraged to leave valuable items at home.

Security checklist

- Don't leave valuables in the salon overnight
- Don't leave money in the till overnight
- Leave the till drawer open overnight
- Lock all doors, windows and cupboards
- Secure all data/information relating to staff and clients.

Personal hygiene and appearance

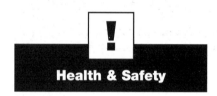

Health & Safety

Nail enamel
Remember: a small percentage of people are allergic to the chemicals in nail enamel and skin reaction commonly occurs around the eyes (face) rather than the fingers.

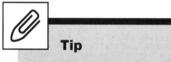

Tip

Use a fob watch or strategically placed clock for checking time rather than wearing a wristwatch.

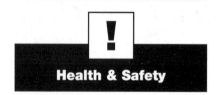

Health & Safety

Working in bare feet
Many therapists like to work in bare feet, and whilst this may give good grounding, in many establishments it is not hygienic and may constitute a health and safety hazard.

Therapists offering beauty and holistic treatments should be seen to practise what they preach. Clients will often judge your personal and professional standards by the way in which you present yourself. Remember that beauty and health belong to an image-conscious industry.

Hands and nails

Your hands should always be perfectly clean. Dirt on your hands and under your nails will harbour bacteria. Your hands need washing before and after every treatment. Where hands regularly come into contact with a client's skin and hair as in massage, aromatherapy, reflexology, Indian head massage, etc. it is paramount that you protect yourself by the thorough cleansing of hands. Long nails may look attractive but are not practical for body therapy work. They not only trap dirt, but can also cause discomfort to clients by inadvertently scratching and damaging the skin. Keeping nails short and neat can prevent the risk of spreading infection and disease. Clean, well-manicured nails without splits or tears are hygienic and safe.

Body

Taking a daily shower/bath is necessary to remove the build up of sweat, dead skin cells and surface bacteria. Skin in areas such as the armpits, feet and genitals have more sweat glands than elsewhere and the warm, moist conditions provide an idea breeding ground for bacteria. Regular washing is therefore essential if body odour (BO) is to be prevented.

Mouth

Unpleasant breath is offensive to clients. Bad breath (halitosis) is the result of particles decaying within spaces between the teeth. You need to brush your teeth after every meal. Bad breath can also result from digestive troubles, stomach upsets, smoking and strong foods such as onions, garlic and some cheeses.

Personal appearance

In addition to personal cleanliness, your personal appearance is an important factor. The effort you put into getting ready for work reflects your pride in the job. It is all right for you to have your own individual look, provided that you appreciate and accept that there are professional standards of dress and appearance that must be followed – a sort of personal code of practice. Work wear should be clean and well ironed. Shoes should be clean and have low heels. They should be smart, comfortable and made of materials suitable for wearing for long periods of time. Shoes should not be 'noisy' as you walk around the treatment room. Hair should be clean and tied back securely if long, and only the minimum of jewellery should be worn.

Knowledge review

1   What is the main requirement of the Management of Health & Safety at Work Regulations 1999?

2   What are the regulations covered by the Workplace (Health, Safety and Welfare) Regulations 1992 regarding non-smoking members of staff?

3   What do the PPE Regulations require?

4   What is the main purpose of the COSHH Regulations?

5   What are the requirements for a substance to be labelled 'hazardous'?

6   Give four examples of how exposure to hazardous substances can be controlled.

7   Under the Electricity at Work Regulations 1989, how often must a qualified electrician check equipment?

8   What do the Health and Safety (First Aid) Regulations 1981 specify?

9   What does RIDDOR stand for and what do these regulations state?

10 Under the Fire Precautions Act 1971, when is a fire certificate required?

11 There are four classifications of fire – what are these?

12 There are four classifications of fire extinguisher – what are these?

13 Under what circumstances can employees be entitled to free eyesight tests from their employers?

14 When do the Manual Handling Operations Regulations 1992 apply?

15 What does PUWER stand for and to what do the regulations refer?

16 State four security measures you can take to protect the salon when closed.

17 State three general ways in which you can help prevent infection.

18 What consideration should be given to work-wear shoes?

19 Where can you obtain leaflets, notices and posters covering all the Acts and Regulations of your profession?

2 Foundations of chemistry

Learning objectives

This chapter covers the following:

- **atoms and molecules**
- **elements**
- **compounds**
- **chemical reactions and chemical bonds**
- **transfer of substances**
- **the pH scale**

To understand the many mysteries surrounding holistic therapies the therapist needs to have an understanding of the basic principles of chemistry and the building blocks of life. This chapter will provide this knowledge. The mysteries in part will become more explicable, however, developments in science still have along way to go before we fully understand some aspects of our work.

Atoms and molecules

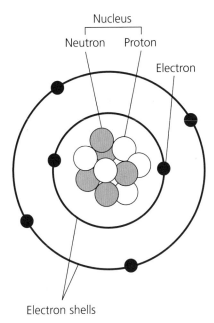

Nucleus

Neutron Proton

Electron

Electron shells

Simple atomic structure of a carbon atom

Atoms

All matter is made up of a collection of individual particles called atoms.

- At the centre of an atom is a core; this is called the nucleus.
- The nucleus is made up of particles called protons, which have a positive electrical charge, and neutrons, which are uncharged, i.e. neutral.
- Around this central cluster of particles is a successive layer of electron particles, which are negatively charged.
- These electrons circle very fast and form a cloud around the central nucleus, which is called a *shell*.
- The number of electrons is the same as the number of protons and so there is no overall charge as they complement each other.

An atom is given an atomic number and this represents the number of protons it contains.

Molecules

A molecule consists of two or more atoms.

Elements

Elements are defined as substances that contain only one type of atom, e.g. carbon or oxygen. Variants occur among elements due to a slight variation in the number of neutrons. These variants are called isotopes, e.g. isotope carbon –14, has 14 neutrons; isotope carbon –12 has 12 neutrons.

There are 109 known elements, 90 of which can be found in nature, and these make the building blocks of life.

Atoms can gain or lose electrons. This leaves them with a negative, or a positive charge; these are called ions. Negative ions are known as anions and are given a minus sign, e.g. Cl– (chlorine); positive ions are cations and are given a positive sign, e.g. Na+ (sodium).

Compounds

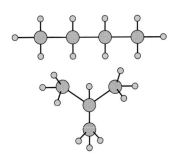

Isomers

Elements are not commonly found in their pure state but form stable interactions with other elements to form compounds, e.g. H_2O is water, which is made of two hydrogen molecules and one oxygen molecule.

Isomers are compounds which have the same chemical formula but the atoms of which are linked in a different way. The difference in structure means that the compound has different properties.

Organic compounds all contain carbon molecules, e.g. essential oils. They contain distinct parts known as a functional group. The functional group usually involves oxygen and nitrogen atoms. The rest of the compound involves carbon and hydrogen atoms. Differing combinations of atoms added to the functional group will give rise to different compounds, e.g.

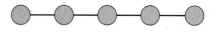

Aliphatic compounds

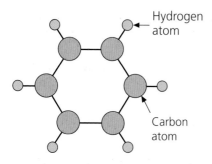

Hydrogen atom

Carbon atom

Aromatic compounds
Benzene ring

ester, alcohol, etc. When organic compounds react, only the functional group will undergo the chemical change.

Inorganic compounds do not contain any carbon molecules, e.g. water (H_2O).

Carbon compounds

Carbon is quite unique among the elements because of the very large group of compounds it can form. There are in excess of 10 million known carbon compounds.

(This will be important when we take a look at essential oils; see Chapter 11.)

Aliphatic compounds are a good example as these contain straight chains of carbon atoms:

$C - C - C - C - C$

Aromatic compounds contain carbon atoms joined together in a ring formation; a good example is benzene.

Polymers and macromolecules

Large molecular structures are known as macromolecules, e.g. polysaccharides and proteins. These are made of smaller molecules joined together in long chains and are known as polymers.

Chemical reactions and chemical bonds

The processes by which different combinations of elements are made or destroyed are known as chemical reactions. Many (but not all) involve the donation or receipt of electrons to form ions.

Atoms may be attracted to each other for a variety of reasons. This attraction may be strong and form groups of molecules, this is known as bonding. The atoms are held together because the electrons surrounding the nuclei mix together and become shared. This type of bonding is known as covalent bonding. It generates a 'holding power' or electro-negativity between the combined elements.

The number of bonds (combining power) an atom can make is called its valency, e.g. the oxygen in H_2O has a valency of 2, that is, it can make two double bonds by combining one oxygen atom with two hydrogen atoms.

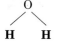

Covalent bond
H_2O

The outer shell of the oxygen atom has 6 electrons but has the potential to hold 2 more. It fills these spaces by sharing the electrons to form 2 hydrogen atoms.

The compound is described as stable as its electron capacity is full.

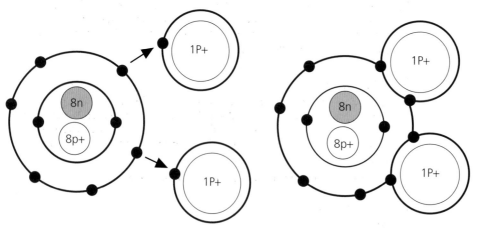

Covalent bonds

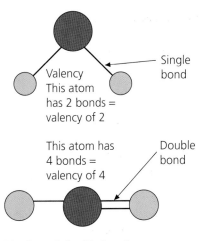

Valency
This atom
has 2 bonds =
valency of 2

Single
bond

This atom has
4 bonds =
valency of 4

Double
bond

Single and double bonds

The carbon in CO_2, carbon dioxide, has a valency of 4. The bond is shown as = because it bonds twice. i.e. it is a double bond:

O = C = O

Atoms can also make triple bonds.

When a compound is formed the total number of valencies of the different atoms in the compound will be the same. Bonds may be lost, shared or gained between atoms.

Where electrons are not shared equally, polar covalent bonds are formed and have a negative and a positive end.

Intermolecular forces

The electrons that form covalent bonds are constantly moving around. The change in the amount of electrons shared can create an electrical charge; the atom with more electrons will have a slight negative charge and the atom with fewer electrons a slight positive charge. This exchange will affect all the atoms within the molecule creating negative and positive areas. This separation of the charge is called a dipole.

If a molecule is next to another with an opposite charge they will be momentarily attracted. The electron will then move and the attraction will disappear. This is known as a London force.

Force

Some molecules possess an atom that is positively or negatively charged. A molecule with a negative end (i.e. one which is missing an electron) adjacent to another molecules with a positive atom (with an extra electron) at its end (and vice versa) will create an attractive force by donating or losing an electron. This is described as ionic bonding. The atoms are held by the oppositely charged atom to create a crystal lattice.

Hydrogen bonds are less able to attract shared electrons with an oxygen or nitrogen atom. This results in unequal shared electrons creating an attractive force. This creates a directional charge with the oxygen or nitrogen having a small negative charge and the hydrogen atom a small positive charge. An example would be hydrogen bonds, which are responsible for the large network of molecules that you will find in a glass of water.

Solids and liquids

Intermolecular forces are also the factor that determines whether a substance is liquid or solid. Solids have atoms or molecules that are closely held together. Intermolecular forces are responsible for many of the processes of the human body.

Changing states

Temperature determines the state of a substance. Some solids when heated change to liquids, and liquids to gases. This occurs because the molecules vibrate, weakening the bonds that hold their atomic structure together. When cooled the reverse happens as the atoms stop vibrating and the bonds strengthen.

Using water as an example, it has three defined stages:

1   ice when it is frozen

2   water

3   steam when it is heated.

Gases

In gases the forces holding the atoms or molecules are hardly noticeable and the atoms continually move about.

Why some compounds do not mix

Hydrogen bonds are also one reason why oil and water do not mix. The molecules of the oil cannot break the network of the hydrogen bonds holding the water molecules together so the two substances remain separate. Bonds between different molecules need to be compatible to mix. Some molecules mix naturally well together. A good example here is when essential oils are mixed together with carrier oil. They blend together to create a new aroma.

Emulsifiers are added to products in industry to stabilise substance that don't naturally mix, e.g. oil and water to create an emulsion. An emulsifier contains molecules that can be divided into two parts, one end has a positive charge and reacts well with water, and the other is non-polar and reacts well with oil.

Transfer of substances – how do molecules move?

Interesting fact

Kinetic theory states that 'particles of matter are constantly in motion'. The kinetic energy determines both the temperature and the way in which the matter behaves.

Substances move in a variety of ways, particularly within the body as cell membranes have selective permeability.

Osmosis is the movement of water molecules from a *weak or dilute solution to a more concentrated solution through a semi-permeable membrane*, to try to gain equilibrium or balance.

Diffusion is the random movement of molecules in a solute *from an area of high concentration to an area of low concentration* to create a more dilute solution.

Facilitated diffusion uses a specific carrier protein which temporarily binds to large molecules, e.g. glucose, outside the cell membrane and then changes shape, to facilitate its move into the cell interior where the substance is deposited.

Active transport occurs when substances required by a cell that are at a higher concentrate inside the cell than outside have to be moved (uphill). Carrier proteins carry out active transport and the molecules are pumped into channels using metabolic energy (ATP).

If the cell is surrounded by a weaker solution it will absorb water; if the surrounding solution is stronger it will dehydrate and distort. It is vital that the fluid surrounding cells does not become appreciably weaker or stronger so that the cell structure is maintained (*homeostasis*).

The pH scale – potential of hydrogen

Interesting fact

Acid is derived from the Latin word for sour.

The pH scale measures acidity and alkalinity – the 'pH' stands for potential of hydrogen. A standard scale has been devised to measure the hydrogen ion concentration. A pH solution below 7 indicates an acid solution; one above 7 indicates that the solution is alkaline. All body fluids have a pH value and this varies between different secretions, e.g. blood is slightly alkaline at 7.35–7.45 where as gastric juices are acidic at 1.5–3.5. Water is neutral and has a pH value of 7.

Interesting fact

Bases are compounds that neutralize acidity. *Alkalis* are bases that are soluble in water.

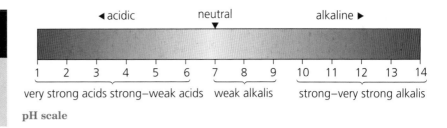

◄ acidic   neutral ▼   alkaline ►

| 1 | 2 | 3 | 4 | 5 | 6 | 7 | 8 | 9 | 10 | 11 | 12 | 13 | 14 |

very strong acids   strong–weak acids   weak alkalis   strong–very strong alkalis

pH scale

Knowledge review

1 Draw and label a simple diagram of an atom.

2 Define the following:
   (a) an element
   (b) a compound
   (c) an ion.

3 State three types of bonding.

4 Describe how molecules move.

5 What does a pH scale measure?

3 Understanding energy

Learning objectives

This chapter covers the following:

- **yin and yang**
- **meridians**
- **chakras**
- **Ayurvedic influences**

We often hear words and phrases such as 'imbalance', 'out of balance', 'balancing the chakras', 'running the meridians', 'too yin or too yang', but what do these words and phrases actually mean? They usually refer to an imbalance of 'life force energy' known as *Qi*. This life force energy flows along yin and yang meridians that run throughout the body. Any disruption to the flow disturbs the balance of yin and yang and leads to illness. Holistic therapy treatments improve the flow of this life force energy by applying different methods of treatment. For example, acupuncturists improve the flow of Qi by inserting needles into specific acupoints on the skin; reflexologists improve the flow by using specialized massage techniques on the feet; crystal and or colour therapists improve the flow through meditation and visualisation techniques using crystals, colours and the chakra energy system of the body. The theories and principles of yin and yang, the meridians, the chakras and Ayurveda to name but a few, all incorporate balancing the 'life force energy' in their teachings. When the circulation of this 'life force energy' is improved around the body, achieved by clearing blockages, both body and mind will function at an optimum level, increasing vitality and encouraging self-healing mechanisms. This chapter will give you a basic introduction and understanding into these techniques, and bring to your attention the complexity and importance of the subject, which may in turn inspire you to want to learn more.

Yin and yang

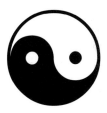

Ying and yang

Yin and yang

Yin	Yang
☯ cold	☯ hot
☯ empty	☯ full
☯ deep	☯ surface
☯ female	☯ male
☯ white	☯ black
☯ dark	☯ light
☯ passive	☯ active
☯ receptive	☯ creative
☯ negative	☯ positive

Whereas Western doctors start with a symptom, then look for a specific cause, Traditional Chinese Medicine (TCM) regards the symptoms as part of a 'pattern of disharmony'. Yin/yang is part of a theory that is used both to classify the pattern and to determine an effective remedy. The movement of energy is based on or is due to a relationship that sets up two opposing fields – a 'polarity'. In Chinese philosophy this polarity relationship is called 'yin and yang'.

Look at the yin and yang symbol and notice that within the yin is a little yang and within the yang is a little yin. The constant flow of yin into yang and vice versa is represented by the curved line. This well-known symbol is sometimes called the Tai Chi symbol. The Tai Chi is from the *I Ching* (Book of Changes) which records the foundations of Chinese philosophy. Nothing is ever *just* yin or yang – the symbol epitomizes the complementary nature of two opposing elements.

Yin and yang are opposite but complementary energy forces whose perfect balance within the body is essential for well-being. When yin and yang are balanced in your life, you will experience health. When there are imbalances, disease, disharmony and ill health can arise.

Yin signifies cold, damp, darkness, passivity and contradiction; yang signifies heat, dryness, light, action and expansion. The interaction of yin and yang gives rise to Qi (pronounced 'chee') which is an invisible 'life energy' that flows through meridians or channels, around the body. The ancient Chinese proposed that a balance of these two opposing forces of energy sustain every living thing. When yin and yang are out of balance in the body, this causes a blockage of energy (Qi) and subsequent illness. Yin and yang imbalances are caused by today's lifestyles which often result in excesses or deficiencies of work, stress, pollution, food, exercise, nicotine, alcohol, and physical and emotional issues when too much or too little of any can result in disharmony in our bodies, which eventually may result in disease.

Everyone is made up of both yin and yang elements. Yin exists within yang. Yang exists within yin. The solid organs of the body are considered to be yang and the hollow organs of the body are considered to be yin. The terms yin and yang are *relative* rather than *absolute* states. Just as there is a North Pole and a South Pole on a magnet, there are yin and yang polarities within the body and the life systems are energized by this flow of energy. Oriental thought recognizes an essence within in the body: Qi, the 'universal energy' or the 'life force energy', which is the origin of all things and of life itself. The channels along which this Qi energy flows in the body are called meridians.

Meridians

Meridians have a long history. The Chinese discovered the meridian system approximately 3000 years ago and it has been going from strength to strength. It is a logical progression to incorporate meridians into the realm of holistic therapies and an understanding of meridians can help holistic therapists to understand the disease pathway more comprehensively. A basic knowledge of how they work can be of enormous benefit in pinpointing problems.

Meridians are an energy force that can be felt but not seen. They can be described as channels of energy, or pathways through which energy moves through the body. They have been described as containing a free-flowing, colourless, non-cellular liquid that may be partly actuated by the heart.

Interesting fact

Pulses
Both Eastern and Western medical traditions assess health using the pulse in the radial artery of the wrist. Traditional Chinese and Ayurvedic practitioners distinguish up to nine pulses on each wrist, which are said to reflect the condition of internal organs and the flow of 'life energy' throughout the body. Western practitioners use only one pulse point on the wrist to check the rate at which blood pumps from the heart. From this they may diagnose heart disorders and circulatory problems.

Tip

When trying to remember the direction in which the meridians run, remember that the meridians which run along the 'inside' of the legs and arms are yin meridians. So – remember *'Inside for yin side'*.

These meridians have been measured and mapped using modern technological methods, electronically, thematically and radioactively. With practice, they can also be felt. There are specific acupuncture points along the meridians, upon which the practices of acupuncture, acupressure and reflexology are founded. In all these techniques, pressure is applied to specific points to clear blockages from the energy channels. These points are electromagnetic in character and consist of small, oval cells called Bonham corpuscles, which surround the capillaries in the skin, the blood vessels, and the organs throughout the body. There are some 500 points that are most frequently used by acupuncturists and therapists practising acupressure and reflexology; each point is worked upon in a definite sequence depending on the action desired.

Meridians are named by the life function with which they are associated. In most cases this name is similar to the name of a body organ with which we are familiar, for example, the liver meridian and the stomach meridian. Chinese physicians can detect imbalances in meridians by feeling the pulses, but this is a sensitive touch and it may take 10 to 20 years to develop proficiency with it.

Meridians are classified yin or yang on the basis of the direction in which they flow on the surface of the body. Meridians interconnect deep within the torso, but we work with the part that is on the surface and is accessible to touch techniques. Yang energy flows from the sun, and yang meridians run from the fingers to the face or from the face to the feet. Yin energy from the earth flows from the feet to the torso, and from the torso along the inside of the arms to the fingertips.

Since the meridian flow is actually one continuous unbroken flow, the energy flows in one definite direction, and from one meridian to another in a well-determined order. Since there is no beginning or end to this flow, the order of the meridians can be represented as a wheel. A blockage in any of the meridians will have a knock-on effect on all the other meridians.

When this energy flow in unrestricted, the body harmonizes the flow to optimize body functioning. Sometimes, however, the life we lead and the abuses we heap upon our bodies cause stress, and sometimes the stress is so intense or so constant that, in effect, it overloads the circuit, and a blockage occurs – this has an affect on all the other meridians.

There are 12 main meridians:

- lungs
- large intestine
- stomach
- spleen/pancreas
- heart
- small intestine
- bladder
- kidney
- pericardium
- 'triple warmer'
- gall bladder
- liver.

These 12 meridians can be subdivided into six main meridians that actually penetrate the major body organs and six other meridians that are situated in the arms and do not actually penetrate specific organs.

Closer study of the meridians reveals that the six main meridians are found in the feet, specifically the toes. Thus, massaging the feet is, in actual fact, stimulating and clearing congestion in the meridians. When congestion is cleared, energy is able to flow freely and the body is able to achieve a state

Major and minor meridians

The six main meridians are those that actually penetrate the major body organs	The other six meridians are situated in the arms and do not actually penetrate specific organs
Liver Spleen/pancreas Stomach Gall bladder Bladder Kidney	Lung Large intestine Pericardium/circulation Triple warmer/endocrine Small intestine Heart

 Interesting fact

Tongue diagnosis
According to TCM the tongue is linked to all the organs in the body via meridians, which act as channels for Qi, or 'life energy'. Disharmony in the body, based on a patient's pattern of symptoms, is believed to be reflected in the tongue before manifesting as disease.

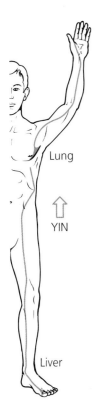

Lung meridian

of balance. With the six main meridians being represented in the feet, it is no wonder that reflexology treatments often report such dramatic positive results after treatment.

The Chinese maintain that the Qi circulates in the meridians 24 times a day and 24 times a night. In a sense there is only one single meridian that goes right around the entire body (the wheel effect), but many different meridians are described according to their positions and functions. There are the 12 main meridians, which are bilateral (paired) resulting in 24 separate pathways. Each meridian is connected and related to a specific organ from which it takes its name. It is also connected to a partner meridian and an organ with which it has a specific mutual relationship.

Within our bodies the yin organs are those that are hollow and involved in absorption and discharge such as the stomach and the bladder; the yang organs are the dense, blood-filled organs such as the heart, which regulate the body. There is constant interaction between yin and yang forces, and if the yin/yang balance between the organs is interrupted, the flow of Qi throughout the body will be affected and the person will be unwell.

The meridians in detail

The lung meridian

Partner meridian: large intestine
The lung meridian (yin energy from the earth) starts at the clavicle, passes over the shoulder and down the front of the arm, running along the biceps muscle, down the arm to the wrist and ends at the back of the thumb.

The lungs and large intestine control elimination: the former of carbon dioxide (CO_2), the latter solid faeces, unabsorbed waste products from the foods we eat. Since these meridians are partnered they can directly affect each other – for example, chest problems can be accompanied by constipation, and constipation can be accompanied by chest problems.

Physical symptoms

- Asthma
- Coughs
- Various forms of chest congestion
- Respiratory problems
- Wrist disorders, carpal tunnel syndrome
- Arthritis or stiffness in the thumb
- Shoulder pain

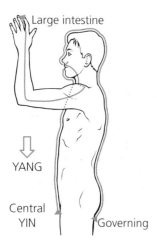

Large intestine meridian

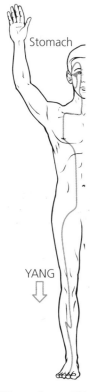

Stomach meridian

The large intestine meridian

Partner meridian: lung

The large intestine meridian (yang energy from the sun) starts from the top of the index finger, passes up the inside of the arm to the edge of the shoulder, before crossing to the back of the shoulder. It continues up the neck to the cheek, touches the upper lip and ends at the side of the nostril.

The large intestine forms the lower part of the digestive tract and is in charge of transporting, transforming and eliminating surplus matter. If these wastes are not eliminated regularly, it can have a toxic effect on the entire system.

Physical symptoms

- Constipation
- Diarrhoea
- Headache
- Shoulder pain (frozen shoulder)
- Nasal congestion
- Toothache
- Herpes/cold sores on lips
- Nosebleeds
- Tennis elbow
- Arthritis in index fingers

Stomach meridian

Partner meridian: spleen/pancreas

The stomach meridian (yang energy from the sun) starts under the eye and curves up to the temple and then continues down the body and ends at the toes. Below the kneecap, the meridian divides into branches, one that ends at the second toe and one that ends at the third toe.

The functions and activities of the stomach and spleen are closely related. The stomach controls digestion – it receives nourishment, chemically changes it and passes on the energy from food to be distributed around the body (via the small intestine). The spleen transforms some of this energy from food into Qi and blood. If the stomach does not hold and digest food, the spleen cannot transform it and transmit its essence. The stomach and spleen are interdependent meridians.

Physical symptoms

- Breast tenderness (sore nipples, lumps and inverted nipples)
- Diaphragm disorders (hiatus hernia, liver/gall bladder disorders)
- Distension of the upper abdomen
- Kidney/adrenal disorders, allergies
- Digestive problems (constipation, diverticulitis, colic)
- Appendix (right side) or ovarian problems, blocked fallopian tubes, infertility
- Thigh pain
- Knee pain
- Corns – problems with toes

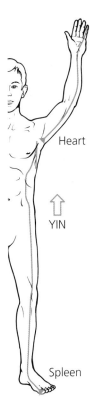

Spleen meridian

Spleen/pancreas meridian

Partner meridian: stomach

The spleen meridian (yin energy from the earth) starts at the inside of the big toe, runs along the inside of the foot up the leg before bending into the pelvis, then runs up the side of the abdomen ending at the shoulder.

The spleen is said to 'rule transformation and transportation'. It is the crucial link in the process by which food is transformed into Qi energy and blood. If this process of food transformation is not activated, nourishment and Qi energy are not available for the muscles so they become weak and the lips and mouth become pale and dry. If the spleen is imbalanced the whole body or some part of it may develop deficient Qi or deficient blood.

Physical symptoms

- Problems with outer breast (sore, lumps)
- Underarm complaints (eczema, boils, and lymph swellings)
- Abdominal pain
- Pelvic complaints
- Menstrual problems
- Groin pain, hernias
- Knee, thigh and shinbone problems
- Fungus, stiffness or ingrown toenails
- Hypoglycaemia or diabetes
- Heavy aching body

Small intestine meridian

Partner meridian: heart

The small intestine meridian (yang energy from sun) starts on the outside of the top of the little finger and passes upwards along the posterior side of the forearm, circling behind the shoulder along the side of the neck to the cheek and outer corner of the eye before entering the ear.

The small intestine meridian is in charge of assimilation as it continues the process of separation and absorption of food begun in the stomach. Because the meridian is in charge of this assimilation it has considerable influence over body nourishment and body–mind vitality.

Physical symptoms

- Ear problems – tinnitus, deafness
- Neuralgia in the face
- Swollen lymph glands in the throat region
- Fibrositis in the shoulder blade
- Shoulder complaints
- Tennis elbow
- Arthritis and stiffness in the little finger
- Difficulty in turning the head to one side
- Disorders relating to the small intestine

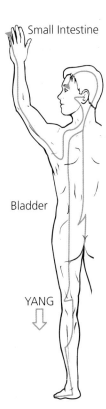

Small intestine meridian

Heart meridian

Partner meridian: small intestine

The heart meridian (yin energy from the earth) starts in the armpit, runs down the inside of the arm and ends at the back of the little finger toward the ring finger. (See spleen meridian figure.)

The heart and small intestine meridians are coupled. TCM explains this by saying that the heart controls the blood and unites with the small intestine. If the heart becomes heated, the heat will converge in the small intestine, producing blood in the urine. If the heart is strong, the body will be healthy and the emotions orderly; if it is weak, all the other meridians will be disturbed in consequence.

Physical symptoms

- Inner arm pain and weakness, numbness, angina
- Weak wrists
- Stiffness or pain in the little finger
- Irritability
- Nervousness
- Cardiovascular disorders
- Spontaneous sweating

Bladder meridian

Partner meridian: kidney
The bladder meridian (yang energy from the sun) begins at the inside corner of the eye, passes over the forehead and the top of the head, then continues down the back in four lines, two either side of the spine. The four lines continue over the buttocks and down the legs, where two meet behind each knee. A single line then passes down each leg along the centre line of the calf behind the outer ankle, and ends at the outer tip of the little toe. (See small intestine meridian figure on p.25.)

The partnership of the kidney and bladder meridians is one of the most obvious, and means that the bladder meridian has a role in stimulating and regulating the kidneys. The function of the bladder is to receive and excrete urine produced in the kidneys, and the meridian is therefore in charge of maintaining normal fluid levels in the body. The bladder is essential to life because if it is not functioning the rest of the system becomes poisoned. The bladder meridian strongly affects the spinal cord and nerves and is the most effective in releasing tensions along its route.

Physical symptoms

- Hair loss
- Neck tension
- Pain and stiffness in the spine
- Weak or lower back problems
- Bladder infections
- Incontinence
- Hip or sacrum problems
- Rounded shoulders
- Aching feet after standing
- Haemorrhoids
- Sciatica, varicose veins
- Cramps in calves

Kidney meridian

Partner meridian: bladder
The kidney meridian (yin energy from the earth) starts on the sole of the foot and ascends up the back of the leg. It emerges around the front of the lower thigh and ascends straight up the body to the sternum.

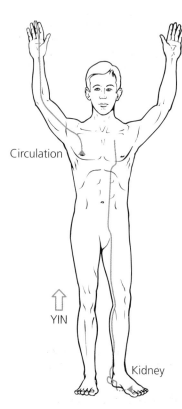

Kidney meridian

The kidneys have a special relationship with the other organs because the yin and yang of each organ ultimately depends on the yin and yang of the kidneys. The kidneys regulate the amount of water in the body. As fluid is essential to life, the flow of the fluid enables waste material to be collected and excreted in the form of urine. Enormous amounts of blood flow through the kidneys to be purified. If the blood does not flow as it should, symptoms such as high blood pressure or hypertension may result and there may be a build up of toxic substances that the body is unable to deal with.

Physical symptoms

- Foot problems
- Lung congestion
- Breast lumps (on the inner side of the nipple)
- Heart problems
- Reproductive problems
- Urinary incontinence
- Hair loss
- Darkness under the eyes
- Swollen inner ankles
- Phlebitis on inner calves

The pericardium/circulation meridian

Partner meridian: triple warmer
The circulation meridian (yin energy from the earth) starts internally at the surface of the heart and emerges just outside each nipple. It follows around the axilla and travels down the inside of the arm to the wrist, ending at the thumb-side corner of the middle fingernail. (See kidney meridian figure on p.26.)

The circulation meridian is known as a protective meridian as one of its main functions is to protect the heart, physically as well as energetically. The pericardium is a fibrous sac enclosing a slippery lubricated membrane that prevents friction as the heart beats. Stresses and shocks first affect the pericardium and do not penetrate the heart unless the pericardium is weakened.

Physical symptoms

- Swollen painful armpits
- Stiff elbows – tennis elbow
- Eczema or skin problems in the elbow crease
- Hot palms
- Red face
- Tension in upper chest
- Painful, stiff head and neck
- Arthritis to middle finger
- Carpal tunnel syndrome

Triple warmer meridian

Partner meridian: circulation
The triple warmer meridian (yang energy from the sun) starts on the back of the ring ringer, ascends up the arm and ends at the top of the outer corner of the eye.

The triple warmer meridian is the partner of the circulation meridian. Although there is no anatomical organ that correlates with the triple

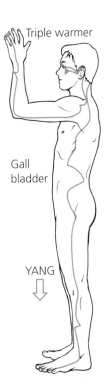

Triple warmer

Gall
bladder

YANG

Triple warmer meridian

warmer, the Chinese believe that all the organs in the body are guarded by it and that heat in the body is controlled by this function. The three 'heaters' or 'burners' correspond to divisions of the torso: the upper burner to the thoracic cavity; the middle burner to the abdominal cavity; the lower burner to the pelvic cavity. Their functions include control of the pituitary gland, regulation of body temperature, appetite and thirst, regulation of the autonomic nervous system and control of emotions and moods. Because of these functions, this meridian is also known as the endocrine meridian.

Physical symptoms

- Shoulder pains
- Pain behind and in the outer corner of eye
- Ear problems, eczema, deafness, pain behind the ear
- Elbow problems
- Slow metabolism – overweight
- Fast metabolism – hyperactive
- Stiffness and pain along the arm and wrist

Gall bladder meridian

Partner meridian: liver meridian
The gall bladder meridian (yin energy from earth) starts at the outer corner of the eye, crosses the temple and descends to the shoulder. It continues laterally down the body, in a zigzag pattern down the sides of the body, along the outside of each leg, over the front of the ankles and ends on the back of the fourth toe. The gall bladder meridian is also one of the longest meridians and one of the most well travelled, traversing almost the entire body except the arms. (See triple warmer meridian figure on p.27.)

TCM says that the gall bladder rules decision making, thus anger and rash decisions may be due to an excess of gall bladder Qi energy, while indecision may be a sign of gall bladder disharmony and weakness.

Physical symptoms

- Headaches – all types
- Eye and ear pain
- Joint stiffness and pain
- Neck tension
- Shoulder pains
- Gall stones
- Arthritic pain in hip
- Yellow colour in eyes

Liver meridian

Partner meridian: gall bladder
The liver meridian (yin energy from the earth) starts at the back of the big toe and ascends immediately up the leg. It runs past the inside of the knee and along the inner thigh to the genital region and continues upward to just below the nipple on the lower part of the sternum.

The liver is the primary centre of metabolism. Not only does it secrete bile, synthesize proteins, neutralize toxins and regulate blood sugar levels, it is also a store for fat-soluble vitamins and glycogen which it changes back to glucose when needed. Since the brain does not store any glucose, the liver's steady supply is crucial to life, and this is why the Chinese believed the

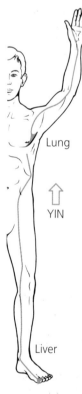

Lung

⇧ YIN

Liver

Liver meridian

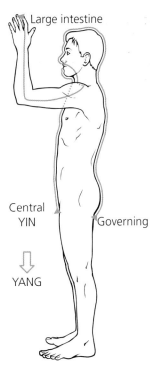

Large intestine

Central
YIN

YANG

Governing

Central and governing meridians

liver was vital to conscious and unconscious thought processes. The liver meridian helps control the functions of the nervous system and is important for psychological problems such as depression and anger.

Physical symptoms

- Liver problems (right side)
- Stomach/spleen problems (left side)
- Genital problems – herpes, low sperm count, impotence, low sexual libido, candida
- Problems with big toe – gout, ingrowing toenail, fungus, corns
- Knee and thigh pains
- Muscle spasms, seizures, convulsions
- Digestive problems

Central and governing meridians

In addition to the 12 main meridians there are two additional ones, often referred to as storage meridians. These storage meridians – called the central and governing meridians – run directly up the back and front of the body to the upper and lower lip. They help to create balance among the other 12 meridians by dispersing excess Qi energy to deficient meridians.

Central meridian

The central meridian starts in the pelvic cavity, drops down and emerges in the perineum, just between the anus and the genitals. It then crosses through the genital area to the top of the public bone, runs up the mid-line of the abdomen, chest and neck and ends just below the lower lip.

In TCM the central meridian is seen as the regulator of the peripheral nervous system and, along with the governing meridian, it controls the other 12 meridians. It creates balance by uniting the organ meridians, allowing energy flow to adjust when there is a blockage. In addition to providing energy to all of the peripheral nerves, the central vessel also governs menstruation and the development of the foetus in women.

Physical symptoms

- Asthma
- Coughing
- Epilepsy
- Laryngitis
- Lung problems
- Mouth sores
- Pneumonia
- Genital disorders

The governing meridian

The governing meridian begins in the pelvic cavity then drops down and emerges below the genital area. It passes to the tip of the coccyx from where it moves upwards across the sacrum and along the spine, up over the head and down the centre of the face, stopping at the centre of the upper lip.

In TCM the governing meridian is the regulator of the nervous system and, along with the central meridian, it allows excess energy to pass through it to other meridians that may be deficient in energy.

Interesting fact

Effleurage and the governing meridian
When you are performing effleurage during a back massage, you are actually working on the governing meridian, which runs directly up the back. Start at the coccyx (over the towel is fine) and end at the base of the neck. Do not worry about missing out the start and end of the meridian line – your work will still be of benefit to this meridian line.

Physical symptoms

- Headaches and pain in the eyes
- Stiffness in the spine
- Eye problems
- Haemorrhoids
- Insomnia
- Spinal problems

Chakras

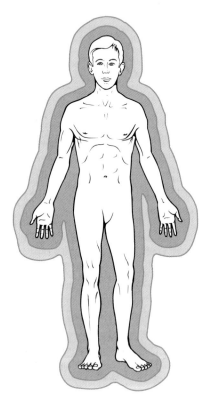

The subtle (non-physical) body

There is an energy field around every human being, which is described as the aura. This may be seen in colour or as a vague light. Much of the colour and energy of the auric field is supplied by the chakras. The aura usually stretches about four to six inches (10–15 cm) out from the physical body. All the time we are alive, this subtle energy field exists whether we can physically see it or not. However, once a person is truly dead there is no vitality in or around the physical body. The subtle energy field is no longer functioning; a vital essence has been withdrawn.

There are seven major chakras. They are located at the base of the spine, at the reproductive centre, at the solar plexus, the heart, the throat, the brow and at the crown of the head. These sites in turn represent the body's major systems: excretion, reproduction, digestion, circulation, respiration and the complex functions of cognition. The crown chakra is sometimes regarded as a unique centre of consciousness and not counted with the first six chakras. It is important to remember that there are other minor centres also in the hands, feet and behind the knees.

Chakra is a Sanskrit word meaning 'wheel' and denotes a point of intersection where mind and body meet. Chakras can also be called lotus flowers, symbolizing the unfolding of flower petals, which metaphorically describe the opening of a chakra. Lotus flowers are sacred in India. Growing from mud, they symbolize a path of development from a primitive being to a fully blossoming consciousness, mirroring the base chakra rooted in Earth, which evolves into a lotus flower with a thousand petals at the crown of the head. Like lotuses, chakras have 'petals' which vary in number from chakra to chakra. Beginning at the bottom with the first chakra, the petals number four, six, ten, twelve, sixteen, two, and a thousand petals. Like flowers, chakras can be open or closed, dying or budding, depending on the state of consciousness within.

The chakras are traditionally represented through symbols. Their functions and nature are described not through words but through symbolic images. This is the traditional approach of all *esoteric* traditions, for the symbol is richer in meaning than the word.

The chakras carry the colours of the rainbow spectrum, and a shape also represents each. The first five chakras also have animal symbols that express the nature of the chakra, and an elemental symbol. There are also common associations between the chakras and the glands of the endocrine system, so when we are 'balancing the chakras' we are, at a physical level, balancing the glands of the endocrine system. This is of course a very simplistic explanation of the chakra system of energy.

Base or root chakra – chakra 1

- **Location**: Perineum (the area mid-way between the anus and the genitals). The petals face downwards, between the legs, the stem faces upwards into the central.

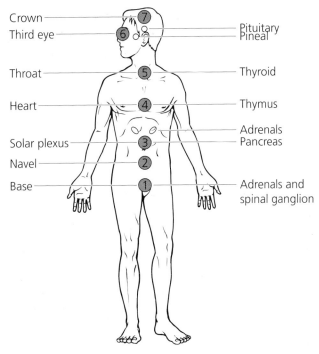

Crown — ⑦
Third eye — ⑥
Throat — ⑤
Heart — ④
Solar plexus — ③
Navel — ②
Base — ①

Pituitary
Pineal
Thyroid
Thymus
Adrenals
Pancreas
Adrenals and spinal ganglion

The chakras and their relevant glands

- **Key word:** Survival
- **Colour:** Red
- **Petals:** 4
- **Shape:** Square
- **Element:** Earth
- **Sense:** Smell
- **Endocrine gland:** Adrenals
- **Imbalance:** An imbalance in the base chakra can make a person feel as if they are ungrounded and unfocused; they may feel weak, lack confidence and be unable to achieve their goals.

Sacral chakra – chakra 2

- **Location:** The petals are approximately two fingers below the navel. The stem corresponds to the sacrum area of the spine.
- **Key word:** Reproduction
- **Colour:** Orange
- **Petals:** 6
- **Shape:** Circle
- **Element:** Water
- **Sense:** Taste
- **Endocrine gland:** Ovaries and testes – its energies also affect the urino-genital organs, the uterus, the kidneys, the lower digestive organs and the lower back.
- **Imbalance:** A person with an imbalance in this chakra may bury their emotions and be overly sensitive; an imbalance may also lead to sexual difficulties, infertility problems and blocks in creativity.

Solar plexus chakra – chakra 3

- **Location:** Just below the sternum, extending down the navel. The stem is in a corresponding position at the back.
- **Key words:** Personal power, will, self-esteem
- **Colour:** Yellow
- **Element:** Fire
- **Sense:** Sight
- **Endocrine gland:** Pancreas
- **Imbalance:** People who are under a lot of stress will show imbalances in this chakra. It is in this chakra that negative energies relating to thoughts and feelings are processed. Imbalances may result in depression, insecurity, lack of confidence and worries about what others think.

Heart chakra – chakra 4

- **Location:** On the same level as the physical heart but in the centre of the body. Stem is at the back.
- **Key word:** Love (unconditional)
- **Colour:** Green
- **Element:** Air
- **Sense:** Touch
- **Endocrine gland:** Thymus
- **Imbalance:** If the energy does not flow freely between the solar plexus and the heart, or between the heart and the throat, it can lead to energy withdrawal into the body; a person with an imbalance in this chakra may feel unloved, be afraid of loving, feel unworthy of love or be afraid of rejection. This chakra represents 'unconditional' love.

Interesting fact

The heart chakra is often referred to as the Rainbow Bridge. This is because it is a 'bridge' between the three lower, more physical, chakras, and the three higher, more spiritual, chakras.

Throat chakra – chakra 5

- **Location:** The neck, with petals at the front and stem at the back.
- **Key word:** Communication
- **Colour:** Blue
- **Element:** Ether
- **Sense:** Hearing
- **Endocrine gland:** Thyroid and parathyroid
- **Imbalance:** Imbalances in this chakra will have an impact on speaking one's mind. It also deals with issues of truth and expression of the soul. As well as speech, an imbalance in this chakra may affect one's willingness to hear.

Brow chakra – chakra 6

- **Location:** Above and between the eyes. The stem is at the back of the head.
- **Key words:** Inspiration, insight, completeness
- **Colour:** Indigo
- **Element:** Light

- **Sense:** There is no sense for this chakra
- **Endocrine gland:** Pineal
- **Imbalance:** Commonly known as the 'third eye', the brow chakra is central to 'seeing' past, present and future events. It is the storehouse of memories and imagination and is associated with intellect, understanding and intuition. Imbalances in this chakra may indicate someone afraid to look into the future, afraid of success, unassertive and undisciplined.

Crown chakra – chakra 7

- **Location:** At the top of the head with petals facing upwards and the stem going down into the central column.
- **Key words:** Knowledge, understanding, release
- **Colour:** Diamond, white, gold or violet
- **Element:** Thought
- **Sense:** There is no sense for this chakra
- **Endocrine gland:** Pituitary
- **Imbalance:** An imbalance in this chakra may be reflected in an unwillingness to open up to our spiritual potential.

Minor chakras

In addition to the major chakras described above, there are a number of additional chakras called minor chakras. These can be found:

- in the palms of hands (which are activated when you perform massage)
- in the soles of the feet
- at the front of each ear
- behind each knee
- behind each eye
- over the ovaries and testicles
- above each breast.

There is also a chakra positioned between the heart chakra and the throat chakra, called the *thymus chakra*. The thymus chakra is coloured turquoise and the key word for it is self-love (different from the unconditional love of the heart chakra). Until we can love ourselves, we are unable to love anyone or anything else – so having this chakra balanced is very important.

Website

Visit the companion website at www.thomsonlearning.co.uk/hairandbeauty/beckmann where you will find a chakra questionnaire that you can use to establish in which areas you or your client would most benefit from therapy.

Exercise – find your energy field

With practice you can become attuned to your own energy field. The following exercise may give you your first insight to your own energy.

Stage I

Quickly clench and unclench your fists several times. Sit with your palms facing, but not touching one another – about 1 inch apart. Slowly move the palms away from each other. Bring the palms back close together. Establish a gentle rhythm, moving together and apart in a bouncing motion. You may feel nothing at all. However, many will feel a tingling in the hands and some will experience what may be described as a magnetic force. The

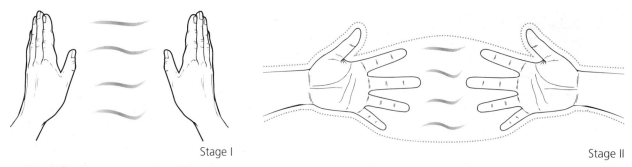

Stage I   Stage II

Feel the energy

sensation you are feeling cannot be confused with general body heat or warmth. It is a specific sensation – of your own energy field. Close your eyes. Become aware of your breathing and continue the exercise. When the feeling ceases, when the hands get too far apart, start again.

As with all things, practice makes perfect. The more often you do this exercise, the more success you will have.

Stage II

After practising Stage I above; develop the exercise by closing your eyes from the start. Become aware of your breathing and on the out breath visualize white light pouring out from the centre of your palms in a steady stream. You will be amazed and elated when you 'lock into' the energy. If you don't, just keep practising – empty your mind of everything and concentrate on what you are actually 'feeling'.

With experience you may begin to pull the hands further apart. Eventually the contact will break and you may start again. Palm-to-palm contact is easiest to work with at first. When you are comfortable with this you can make fingertip–fingertip contact, or use the fingertips of one hand against the palm of the other. The process of sensitizing the hands to the energy field will prepare you for making contact with your own chakra energy.

Ayurvedic influences

The major traditional holistic healing system of India is Ayurveda, which covers all aspects of health, encouraging physical, mental, emotional and spiritual well being. Practitioners believe well-being is affected by three *doshas*, or 'vital energies', which constantly fluctuate. Treatment aims to restore health, or doshic balance, through purifying techniques, diet, yoga postures, breathing exercises, massage and herbal remedies. Ayurveda is currently undergoing a government-sponsored revival in India and is attracting much interest in the West.

Main uses

Ayurveda can be used to combat the following:

- digestive problems, such as stomach ulcers
- heart disease
- rheumatoid arthritis
- allergies, asthma
- eczema, psoriasis and other skin conditions

- anxiety, insomnia
- wound healing
- viral infections, especially hepatitis.

Ayurveda is the Sanskrit word for 'science of life', and has been used in Indian since about 2500 BC. Derived from the *Vedas,* ancient Hindu texts, by *rishis,* or holy men, it is a sophisticated, comprehensive health system, and has similarities with TCM. Ayurveda teaches that there are five great elements – ether, air, fire, water and earth – which underlie all living systems and are constantly changing and interacting. They can be simplified into three doshas, or vital energies, existing in ever-changing proportions throughout nature. In the human body, the levels of the doshas are believed to rise and fall daily, affected by factors such as different foods, time of day, season, levels of stress and repressed emotions. Imbalances in the doshas are thought to disrupt the flow of *prana*, the life energy that enters the body through food and breath.

The doshas are three constantly fluctuating energy qualities that define all things on earth. Each is made up of a combination of two of the five great elements of Ayurveda:

- *vata* is formed from air and ether
- *pitta* from fire and water and
- *kapha* from water and earth.

Although the doshas cannot physically be measured or experienced, each has distinctive attributes that can be recognized in human beings and in the environment. Ayurvedic practitioners believe that good health depends on 'pacifying' excesses in the doshas and keeping fluctuations to a minimum. Each dosha has a 'seat' in the body that is able to absorb and eliminate small excess, but disease can result if the seat cannot cope with larger imbalances.

Constitutional types

Within the Ayurvedic principles, every individual has a unique combination of doshas – known as *prakriti* – determined by the doshas of his or her parents at the time of conception. Physiological strengths and weaknesses, intellectual capacity and personality are governed by one, or in some people two, doshas.

Vata types are either tall or short and of slight build; they are creative, with quick, nervous movements, but tend to waste energy. Their best seasons are autumn and early winter and the 'seat' of vata is the colon. Vata types should avoid raw foods.

Pitta types are evenly proportioned and of average height; confident and ambitious they can be aggressively competitive. Their best season is the summer and the 'seat' of pitta is the stomach. Pitta types should avoid red meat.

Kapha types are heavily built, slow moving and physically strong; they are stable and patient, but inclined to possessiveness. Their best season is the middle of winter and the 'seat' of kapha is the lungs. Kapha types should avoid dairy produce.

To be fully trained in the Ayurvedic holistic healing system takes many years. The training includes Ayurvedic nutrition, yoga, massage and preparing herbal remedies to name but a few of the subjects covered.

Many Western doctors accept that they cannot discount the medical systems of other cultures. Ayurvedic herbal remedies have been tried and tested by centuries of use, but their quality and efficacy cannot be guaranteed, since very few scientific tests have been carried out.

Marma therapy

All over the body are points through which the vital energy flows. They are positioned on the body where veins, arteries, tendons and bone meet. They are also junctions where vata, pitta and kapha gather (physical and astral; these points can be used to heal or harm!).

Marma points are grouped according to regions of the body and there are 107 in total. These points are similar to acupressure point; indeed their origins and positions are linked, but marma points are larger and easier to find than acupressure points. Like acupressure points they are sensitive to pressure. Major marma points correspond to the major chakras. Minor marma points are on the torso, limbs and head. There are 37 marma points located in the Indian head massage treatment area. Pressure and massage are applied on the marma point to ease the symptoms of ill health. Poor posture, injury, emotional blocks and trauma can cause the life energy to become blocked and stagnated.

Knowledge review

1 What does the curved line represent in the yin/yang symbol?

2 What is Qi?

3 What are meridians?

4 What exactly are acupuncture points?

5 There are 12 individual meridian channels in the body – why are they described as a wheel?

6 Name the six main meridians that actually penetrate the major body organs.

7 Where does the yin and yang energy come from?

8 Why do you think tinnitus may be a symptom of an unbalanced small intestine meridian?

9 What is the purpose of the central and governing meridians?

10 What is the aura?

11 What symptoms may someone with an unbalanced base chakra have?

12 What is the location, colour and keyword for the sacral chakra?

13 What is often referred to as the Rainbow Bridge?

14 If someone had problems with their thyroid, what chakra may be out of balance?

15 Give an example of the minor chakras.

16 What does the word Ayurveda actually mean?

17 What types of foods should vata types avoid?

18 How would you describe a kapha type of person?

19 What are the five great elements that are taught in Ayurveda?

20 State five uses for Ayurveda.

Anatomy and physiology

4

Learning objectives

This chapter covers the following:

- **terminology**
- **organization of the body**
- **integumentary system**
- **circulatory system**
- **lymphatic/immune system**
- **skeletal system**
- **muscular system**
- **respiratory system**
- **digestive system**
- **nervous system**
- **special senses**
- **endocrine system**
- **genito-urinary system**

It is essential if any treatment is to be performed safely and effectively that the therapist has at least a basic understanding of anatomy and physiology. An understanding of the systems of the body will also enable you to understand the implications of why certain conditions are contra indicated.

At the end of each section on a body system is a list of the more common conditions, disorders and diseases that relate to that particular system. In addition, and where relevant, there is some treatment guidance including essential oils to use, treatment and massage adaptations and reflexology points to work.

Terminology

Anatomical positions

- **Prone**: lying face down
- **Supine**: lying on the back (supine – spine side), face up
- **Anterior**: front of the body
- **Posterior**: back of the body
- **Lateral**: away from the mid-line of the body
- **Medial**: towards or closest to the mid-line of the body
- **Proximal**: nearest to the point of attachment of a limb
- **Distal**: furthest from the point of attachment of a limb
- **Superior**: above
- **Inferior**: below
- **Dorsal**: upper surface
- **Plantar**: sole of the foot

Movement

- **Abduction**: a movement away from the mid-line
- **Adduction**: movement towards the mid-line (*add*ing)
- **Extension**: straightening, or movement backwards from the mid-line
- **Flexion**: bending, a move forwards from the mid-line
- **Lateral flexion**: side bending
- **Rotation**: movement of a bone around an axis (180°)
- **Circumduction**: circular movement of a joint (360°)

Movements of the foot

- **Dorsiflexion**: top of the foot moved up
- **Plantar flexion**: sole of the foot moved down (toe pointed)
- **Inversion**: sole of the foot turned inwards
- **Eversion**: sole of the foot turned outwards

Movements of the hand

- **Palmar**: relating to the hand
- **Supination**: palm of the hand turned up
- **Pronation**: palm of the hand turned down

Organization of the body

There are 11 systems of the body, each of which is constructed from a basic cellular building block.

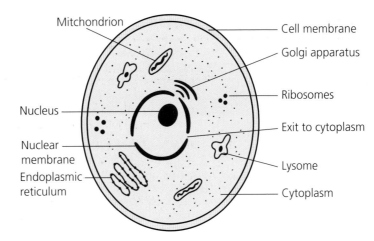

Structure of a cell

Cells

A cell is the smallest structure of the body capable of performing all the processes that define life. These include respiration and digestion. Cells are not all the same shape and they perform different functions, but all cells do have certain characteristics in common:

- growth
- reproduction
- excretion
- movement
- respiration
- metabolism
- sensitivity.

Typical structure of a cell

All cells are enclosed in a plasma (cell) membrane which behaves like a fluid to allow easy movement. It provides channels for the passage of molecules. The movement of substances passing in and out of the cell is semi-permeable, i.e. selectively controlled.

The **nucleus** is the control centre. It contains the cell's instructions or chromosome DNA (deoxyribonucleic acid). The nucleus contains the nucleolus, which enables cell division to take place.

Cytoplasm refers to all the cell contents outside the cell nucleus and is 75–90 per cent water.

Mitochondria are sausage-shaped structures in the cytoplasm. They comprise two membrane layers, one smooth, the other folded. It is the site of cell respiration providing chemical energy or ATP (adenosine triphosphate). It is often referred to as the powerhouse of the cell.

The **golgi body (golgi apparatus)** is a stack of flattened membranous sacks in which proteins are manufactured.

Endoplasmic reticulum are a series of membranous canals in the cytoplasm. There are two types: smooth and rough.

Tissues

Groups of cells can be classified according to their structure and function. A group of cells together performing the same function is called tissue. There are four main types of tissue: epithelial, connective, muscular and nervous. Tissues can have more than one function and therefore can be classified into more than one group.

Epithelial tissue

Epithelial tissue is always found in sheets. It is bound together by tight junctions formed between cells. It may be 'simple' (single layer) or 'stratified' (layered). There are four types of simple epithelial tissue: squamous, cuboidal, ciliated and columnar. Each has a slightly different structure to suit the purpose for which it is designed.

Epithelial tissue is found:

- covering the body
- lining cavities and tubes
- in glands.

Its function is:

- to protect underlying structures
- secretion
- absorption.

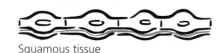

Squamous tissue

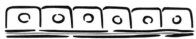

Cuboidal cells

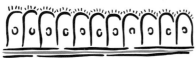

Cilated cells

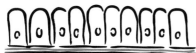

Columnar cells

Epithelial tissue

Connective tissue

Connective tissue comprises a diverse, widespread group of tissues. They include the blood cells, lymph, cartilage, bone and adipose tissue. The functions of connective tissue include:

- support
- binding and joining tissues together
- protection
- transport
- insulation.

There is a large quantity of inter cellular substance by which connective tissue cells are separated. There are several different types of cells found in connective tissue including fibroblasts, macrophages, plasma cells, mast cells, and fat cells.

Fibroblasts (fibre cells): fibroblast cells are particularly active in tissue repair. They bind together the cut surface of a wound or form scar tissue. Fibroblasts produce collagen, elastin and extra cellular material.

Macrophages: these are actively phagocytic, i.e. they engulf and digest cell debris, bacteria and any other foreign bodies.

Plasma cells: synthesize and secrete specific antibodies into the blood as part of the immune response.

Mast cells: found in loose connective tissue and in the lining of some organs. Mast cells produce histamine, which is involved in local and general inflammatory reactions. These are released when the cells are damaged by injury or disease.

Fat cells: the size and shape of fat cells varies according to their fat content. They are especially abundant in adipose tissue. Adipose tissue consists of fat cells containing large fat globules.

Areolar tissue: connects and supports other tissues. It is found under the skin, between muscles, supporting blood vessels, in the alimentary canal and in the glands.

Fibrous tissue: composed of a dense network of closely packed collagen fibres. Can be found:

- forming the ligaments which hold bones together
- as an outer protective covering for bone
- outer protective covering for some organs, e.g. kidney, brain
- forming muscle sheaths (muscle fascia) which extend beyond a muscle to become the tendon.

Elastic tissue: this tissue is capable of extension and recoil. Found in organs which need to alter their shape, e.g. in blood vessels.

Muscle tissue

Muscle tissue is highly specialized tissue which has the ability to contract and relax. There are three types: skeletal, voluntary or striated muscle; cardiac muscle; and smooth or involuntary muscle.

Nervous tissue

Two types of tissue can be found in the nervous system. *Excitable cells* are called neurones; they initiate, receive, conduct and transmit information. They include *motor* neurones, *sensory* neurones and *interneurones*. *Non-excitable cells* support neurones.

Organs

An organ is a group of tissues that perform a specific function. Organs can be grouped into systems which are a combination of tissues and organs.

Homeostasis

To remain healthy the body must be automatically regulated to maintain a relatively constant internal environment, or a constant state of internal equilibrium. To achieve this balance the following must be kept in check:

- removal of metabolites
- removal of urea
- balance of ions
- water content
- availability of oxygen and glucose
- temperature.

Communication within the body is essential for homeostasis and this is primarily accomplished by the nervous and endocrine systems.

Metabolism

Metabolism refers to all chemical reactions in the body. It uses absorbed nutrients to:

- provide energy by chemical oxidation of nutrients
- renew and repair body substances.

Interesting fact

Metabolites
A metabolite is a product of or substance taking part in metabolism e.g. carbon dioxide.

Types of processes

The *metabolic rate* is the rate at which energy is released from nutrients inside cells. As most processes require oxygen (O_2) and produce carbon dioxide (CO_2), the rate can be estimated by the measurement of O_2 uptake or CO_2 output.

The basal metabolic rate (BMR) is an individual's metabolic rate when at rest in a warm environment after having been without food for 12 hours.

Catabolism breaks down large molecules into smaller ones releasing chemical energy.

Anabolism builds up or synthesizes large molecules from small molecules and uses ATP.

Catabolism and anabolism usually involve a series of chemical reactions known as metabolic pathways.

Disorders and diseases of the tissues and cells

Cancer

Cancer is a generic word covering a variety of diseases. It is an abnormal unrestrained cellular growth in one of the body organs or tissues. Cancer cells spread and infiltrate the surrounding tissue. It has the ability to destroy nerves, bones and block passageways. Cancer cells (metastases) may spread via the lymphatic or blood vessels to other parts of the body to form secondary tumours.

Although we tend to view cancer as a single disease, symptoms are vast and vary according the site of the cancer, as does prognosis and suitable treatment. Cancer is more likely to occur in the main organs but can occur virtually anywhere in the body.

Treatment guidance: Refer to GP for advice before any treatment.

Specialized clinics are becoming increasingly common, offering holistic and alternative treatment under medical supervision.

There are several arguments for and against treating clients with cancer. Theoretically, if cancer cells spread through the circulatory and lymphatic system any treatment that stimulates these systems could be said to increase the risk of metastases. However, there have been no documented cases of this and in fact it has been shown in some recent studies that massage can actually be of benefit (see McNamara, P., *Massage for People with Cancer*): the body can achieve powerful things when in a deep state of relaxation.

The other debate concerns those who are terminally ill. At this late stage of the disease holistic treatment can do nothing more than make a patient feel cared for and relaxed, helping to relieve some of the troublesome symptoms.

Lupus erythematosus

Lupus erythematosus is an auto-immune disorder where the body's immune system attacks its own connective tissue causing inflammation. There is a heredity association and some link with hormonal triggers. There is no cure.

Symptoms vary both in severity and frequency, typically coming and going. Discoid lupus starts with a red circular rash on the face and scalp that changes to form thickened scar tissue. Systemic lupus is more serious and potentially fatal as it affects many systems of the body.

Treatment guidance: Refer to GP for advice before treatment.
Treat to boost the immune system and to alleviate the general symptoms.

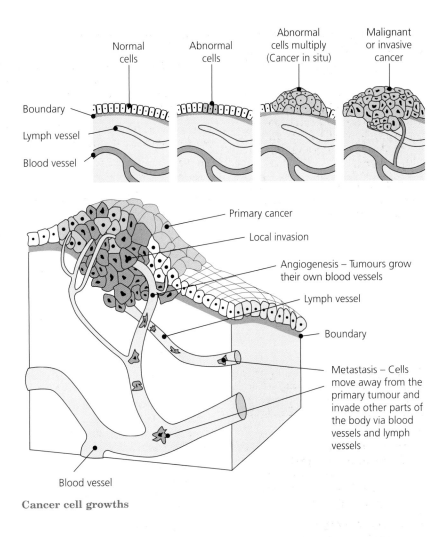

Cancer cell growths

The integumentary system

This comprises the skin and all its structures – nails, hair, sweat and sebaceous glands.

The skin

Functions of the skin

The skin is the largest of the vital organs and has the following functions:

 Interesting fact

The skin
The skin is the largest organ of the body covering approximately 1.7 → 1.9 square metres. It weighs approximately 2.3 → 3.2 kg. It comprises of 20% water. The skin is thinnest on the eyelids at around 0.04 mm and thickest on the sole of the feet at 6 mm, on average it is around 0.1 mm.

Tip

PASTES
Use the acronym *PASTES* to help you remember the functions of the skin.

Interesting fact

Acid mantle
The acid mantle is a protective layer on the surface of the epidermis. It comprises of a mixture of sebum, dead skin cells and sweat.

Interesting fact

Desquamation
The name given to the process of shedding dead skin cells, naturally or assisted.

Interesting fact

Keratinocytes
Keratinocytes cells are found in numerous quantities in the epidermis. These cells synthesis keratin. Keratin is a tough, fibrous insoluble protein. It imparts both strength and waterproofing to the epidermis.

Keratinisation the process by which cells change from living with a nucleus, to dead flat granular cells.

Protection: protects the moist, warm, internal environment from the dangers of the external environment in which we live.

- The acid mantle on the surface keeps the skin supple and provides a waterproof barrier to prevent the entry of pathogens and dehydration.
- Melanin cells absorb UV rays.
- Connective tissues cushion and protect the underlying organs.

Absorption: there is limited permeability through the skin but it can absorb certain substances, e.g. some drugs.

Sensory organ: nerve endings in the dermis relay sensations of pain, pressure, heat, cold and touch. These inform the central nervous system of changes in the external environment.

Temperature regulation: assists to keep the skin at a temperature of 37°C/98.6°F through vasodilation and vasoconstriction.

Excretion: sweat removes limited amounts of waste, e.g. urea, uric acid and ammonia.

Synthesis of vitamin D: certain fatty substances in the skin are converted into vitamin D by ultra violet (UV).

The skin has three layers:

- epidermis
- dermis
- hypodermis or subcutaneous layer.

Epidermis

The epidermis is the outer layer of the skin. It contains no blood vessels; all nutrients must pass from the blood vessels in the dermis and be transported from there to the epidermis.

Layers of the epidermis

Stratum corneum

- many layers of dead, flat, keratinized cells
- desquamation takes place
- first line of defence against entry of pathogens
- acid mantle provides a waterproof protective layer.

Stratum lucidum

- melanin disappears
- cells become flat and transparent
- light rays are able to penetrate.

Stratum granulosum

- keratinisation begins, cells begin to die and flatten, and granules appear in them.

Stratum spinosum

- four cells deep
- cells irregular in shape and connected by fibres
- cellular division still takes place (mitosis)

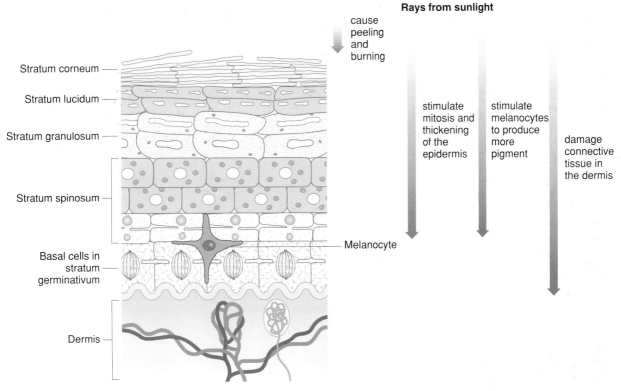

Rays from sunlight

cause peeling and burning

stimulate mitosis and thickening of the epidermis

stimulate melanocytes to produce more pigment

damage connective tissue in the dermis

Stratum corneum

Stratum lucidum

Stratum granulosum

Stratum spinosum

Basal cells in stratum germinativum

Melanocyte

Dermis

Section through the skin

Interesting fact

Mitosis

Mitosis is simple cell division and is responsible of the maintenance and replacement of cells as a result of growth and repair. The new cell created is an exact replica of the original cell.

Interesting fact

Melanin

Melanin provides protection against ultra violet (UV).

In Caucasian skins melanin tends to disintegrate as the cells move up the epidermis. In darker skin the melanocytes are more active and produce larger melanin granules.

- keratin production begins
- oxygen and nutrients diffuse between cells from the dermis.

Stratum germinatum (basal layer or malphigian layer)

- single layer of cells
- production of new epidermal cells (mitosis)
- melanocytes produce and inject melanin into keratinocytes.

Dermis

The dermis has two layers.

A superficial papillary layer consisting of loose connective tissue (collagen and elastin). Small finger-like projections extend into the epidermis to feed and nourish the tissues through an extensive capillary network.

The deep reticular layer consists of dense connective tissue.

- *Collagen* – a major constituent of the dermis and an important structural protein in the body. These wavy white fibres are arranged in an intricate network giving strength. It also resists stretching. It is collagen that makes meat tough.
- *Elastin* – also a protein. Consists of yellow fibres, which provide flexibility. Once stretched these fibres have the ability to snap back to their normal shape.

Other structures in the dermis are as follows:

- Blood vessels.
- Lymphatic vessels.

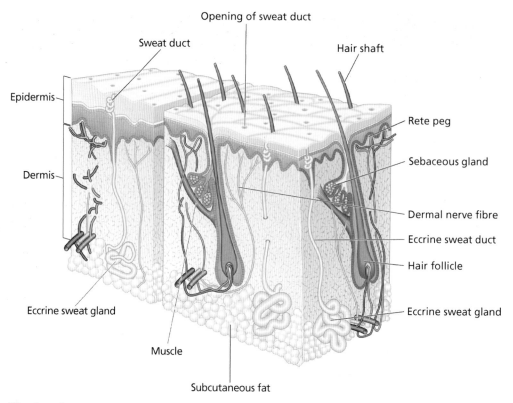

The dermis

- Nerves:
  - sensory for tactile sensation
  - motor for muscular tissue.
- Sweat glands: these help to regulate body temperature by excreting excess water. This evaporates, releasing heat off the surface of the body. There are two types.
  - Eccrine glands: these tiny coiled tubes extend up through the skin and open onto the surface. They are found all over the body. Their function is to regulate body temperature and eliminate waste materials.
  - Apocrine glands: these glands secrete into hair follicles and are found in the greatest numbers under the arms and groin. They develop and become active at puberty. The glands produce a thick sticky secretion. The odour only becomes unpleasant when bacteria multiply and decompose the sweat.
- Sebaceous glands: found all over the skin. Most open into hair follicles via little ducts. They are found in their greatest numbers on the scalp, face and back. The glands secrete an oily substance called sebum which contains waxes, fatty acids, cholesterol and dead cells. Sebum keeps the hair soft and the skin moist. It also provides an oily film that retards water loss from the surface of the skin and inhibits the growth of certain bacteria.

Interesting fact

Sweat
Sweat is formed by the active secretion of sodium at the base of the sweat glands under the influence of the sympathetic nervous system. (We all know how salty sweat tastes.)
The sodium attracts water to the gland. In addition to the potassium; chloride and urea are also secreted in the sweat.

Sweat accounts for about 14% of the heat loss from the body at room temperature.

Superficial skin healing

Once the skin has been damaged blood is released into the wounded area and the blood clotting mechanism is triggered. A protein in the blood plasma called fibrinogen is released. Fibrinogen forms a dense mesh, trapping blood cells and preventing further leakage. As this mesh dries out it forms a scab. Histamine is also released, making the blood vessels dilate and become leaky. This allows more blood to flow into the area to assist in the healing process.

First aid

All salons must have a first aid box. This should be located in an easily accessible and visible place. Modern first aid boxes are *green with a white cross*. The box should be kept tightly closed to keep the contents free from dust and moisture.

We have provided a 'First aid box' at the end of this book (Appendix 1, p.449), please refer to this for common areas of concern and the actions that need to be taken.

Fibroblasts are stimulated into action and produce collagen and actin. Actin gives the cells the ability to contract, slowly pulling the wound together. It takes 48 hours for a new surface of epithelial cells to form, growing over the next week into the normal layers of the skin. The scar may remain vascular (red) for 2–4 weeks.

Damage to the deeper layers of the dermis may take several weeks to heal depending on the size of the wound.

Different skins

Very dark pigmented skins are genetically different. Sudiferous and sebaceous glands are more abundant. The surface of the skin feels quite different as a result; it is shiny, soft and has a velvet texture. The additional melanin in the skin makes the skin thicker and firmer than Caucasian skin. Dark pigmented skin is still prone to all the same blemishes but the pigmentation masks skin variations to an untrained eye.

The function of the dermis is to provide nourishment to the epidermis. The cells of the dermis are separated by a complex mesh of dense extra cellular material (unlike the epidermis where the numerous cells are closely linked). The dermis consists of the following connective tissue.

Hypodermis or subcutaneous layer

The hypodermis is structurally unique. The fat cells are organized into chambers that are surrounded by strands of connective tissue. Its main purpose is to insulate and protect the internal organs. The subcutaneous layer is composed of adipose tissue, areolar tissue, blood, lymph and nerve endings.

Below the subcutaneous is the sub-dermal layer. This layer allows the skin to move freely over the muscular tissue beneath it.

Conditions, disorders and diseases affecting the skin

Common skin lesions

Listed below are terms commonly used to describe changes in the skin tissue.

Breaks in the skin's surface

- *Abrasion/scratch:* superficial removal of the epidermis by friction.
- *Fissures:* cracks in the epidermis, exposing the dermis underneath.
- *Ulcer:* an ulcer is an open inflamed sore on the skin or mucous membranes; it may be deep or shallow and there is a marked depression in the skin.
- *Weeping:* a continuous watery discharge (plasma) from an area of broken skin.
- *Crust:* dried, honey-coloured serum which has oozed from the body.
- *Scab:* a crust of dried blood that forms on the skin or on a mucous membrane where the skin is healing or infected.

Changes in texture

- *Flake:* dry loose cells on the surface of the skin.
- *Scales:* excess flakes of dry skin accumulated on the skin's surface; can be easily removed.

Fluid-filled lesions

- *Vesicle:* small raised blister containing serum and formed at the site of skin damage.
- *Blister:* larger than a vesicle, this is a raised area of skin filled with plasma.
- *Weal:* white raised area of skin containing fluid, the surrounding area of which is red; accompanied with itching; weals can vary in size, with larger ones blending together to form irregular patches of raised tissue; may appear and disappear very quickly.
- *Pustule:* a raised, infected area of skin containing pus.

Changes in shape

- *Papule:* small, firm area of unbroken skin up to 4mm in size; papules may be raised or flat; often becomes a pustule.
- *Nodule* or *cyst:* an abnormal, small, round swelling, larger than a papule at approximately 4mm to 2cm in size; may be fluid-filled and soft or filled with a semi-solid material; most are harmless but may affect the function of the tissues in which they grow.

Scar tissue

Scar tissue is a replacement of original connective tissue as the result of a wound leaving a marked changed in the skin's appearance.

- *Hypertrophic scars:* large unsightly scar tissue; some people are prone to this type of scarring regardless of the type and depth of the wound.
- *Keloid scar:* overgrown scar caused by excessive development of collagen; more common with darker skins.

Treatment guidance: The common practice is to avoid treating scar tissue for six months. However, where there are healing issues it may be possible to work over scar tissue once the initial inflammation has gone down (approximately 10 days). Always check with a GP before doing so. Friction movements over the area and the use of cicatrisant oils are very beneficial for hypertrophic scars and mobilization of the scar tissue keeps it supple and helps prevents tightness in the new collagen fibres.

Common skin blemishes

Moles or naevus

Moles are skin blemishes that can be flat, raised, pigmented or unpigmented. They may grow with or without hair growth and can vary in size. Pigmented moles can be brown to dark brown, blue, blue-black or red in colour and vary in size. In rare cases moles may become cancerous (melanoma).

Cause: An abnormality in the production of melanin.

Treatment guidance: Be aware of any changes.

Milia

Firm, pearly white spots commonly occurring around the eye and across the cheekbones. Caused by keratinization of the skin blocking a pore. There are many theories as to the contents of milia, ranging from sebum, uric acid or a build up of sweat deposits. The condition is associated with dehydrated skin or the use of mineral oils.

!

Health & Safety

Moles

Looking for moles should be part of your observation check. Draw the client's attention to moles, particularly those in difficult to see places such as the back. You may find it useful to a make a note of any prominent or suspicious moles on the client's record card.

Check for:

A = *Asymmetry*. Is the mole symmetrical in shape if you draw a cross through it?
B = *Border*. Moles usually have a smooth regular edge, check for ragged outlines.
C = *Colour*. Uneven distribution of pigmentation. Inflammation or redness around the edge.
D = *Diameter*. Is it bigger than the blunt end of a pencil or smaller than 6mm?

Also check for bleeding, weeping, irritation or itching.

Comedones/blackheads

A firm plug in the duct of the sebaceous gland preventing the sebum underneath from escaping. Sebum in comedones is grey/black due to oxidisation and melanin content rather than because of dirt.

Closed blackheads or congested pores

Blackheads are pores blocked with sebum that is still completely enclosed within the pore. Visible on close inspection of the skin as small raised areas.

Changes in pigmentation

(Either the increase or loss of pigmentation)

Macule

A macule is a small area of skin that may be lighter or darker than the surrounding skin. The blemish can be seen but not felt as there is no change in the texture of the skin, e.g. a freckle.

Ephilide

Ephilides or freckles are tiny oval patches of concentrated pigmentation activated by UV light.

Lentigo

Plural: lentigines. Often referred to as age spots. Flat discoloured area of skin, larger than a freckle. Some have a slight texture. They can occur on any area of the body and do not fade when exposure to the sun is avoided. A common condition with mature skins.

Chloasma or melasma

Also referred to as liver spots. Chloasma is an area of pigmentation noticeably darker than the surrounding skin (hyperpigmentation). There are several causes:

- friction – e.g. shoes, bra straps rubbing and stimulating the melanin
- excessive sunbathing causing irregular pigmentation
- pregnancy (mask of pregnancy) forming a temporary butterfly patch over the face
- contraceptive pill
- menopause
- Addison's disease.

Vitiligo

An area of skin lacking in pigmentation (hypopigmentation). The skin may appear to have a darker pigmentation ring around the edge. De-pigmentation commonly occurs around the creases at the joints, e.g. knees, elbows, neck, armpits, etc. Vitiligo is believed to be an auto-immune disorder that affects the production of melanocytes.

Treatment guidance: Care must be taken, as the skin may be ultra sensitive.

Albinism

Albinism is a genetic disorder causing a total absence of melanin. It includes the skin, hair (pure white in colour) and the iris (very pale blue eyes). Both

Tip

Reflexology for skin problems

Work the following points:

- lymphatic to stimulate immunity
- circulatory to increase nutrients and remove waste products
- endocrine system – particularly adrenals
- solar plexus and lungs to encourage deep breathing and calmness.

Interesting fact

Bruises

A bruise becomes blue as the oxygen is used up by the tissues, the oxygen cannot be re-supplied due to the tissue damage. The bruise changes to a yellowish colour as a result of the process of haemoglobin being broken down and removed by the white blood cells.

the skin and eyes are sensitive to light. With age, freckling occurs in areas exposed to the sun. Sufferers are prone to skin cancers.

Treatment guidance: Patch test skin for sensitivity. Work on the immune system to boost immunity.

Common disorders seen on the skin caused by a change in the circulation

Telangiectasia

An increase in the size or prominence of the small blood vessels beneath the surface of the skin giving the skin a diffused redness. Telangiectasia is often referred to as broken capillaries but this is not in fact strictly true. Common on the cheeks and thighs.

Spider naevus

Capillaries visible in the shape of spider, i.e. has a central red spot with lines travelling from in it. There are many causes of spider naevus, including damage to the surface of the skin and overexposure to the sun.

Angioma

Raised red area which may be as tiny as a pinhead or larger. Angiomas are caused by a benign tumour made up of a cluster of capillaries.

Vascular naevus

- *strawberry birthmarks:* bright red spongy growth
- *port-wine stains:* purple patches with a slight deviation in skin texture.

Both of the above are caused by malformations in the blood vessels.

Treatment guidance: Avoid excessive stimulation of the tissues.

Bruises

A discoloured area, usually blue under the surface of the skin. Bruises are caused by leakage of blood from damaged blood vessels. Swelling and pain are usually present.

Treatment guidance: Avoid area to prevent further tissue damage. Apply cool compresses, lavender, fennel, rosemary or witch hazel to draw the bruise out.

Common skin disorders

Bromhidrosis

Also known as body odour. Bromhidrosis is an unpleasant odour caused by bacteria decomposing the sweat from the apocrine glands in the armpits and pubic regions.

Treatment guidance: The client should shower before body treatments. Use essential oils with a deodorant and astringent effect.

Target the urinary system.

Cellulite

For many in the medical profession cellulite is not recognized and is purely an aesthetic term. However, the condition affects between 84–90 per cent of

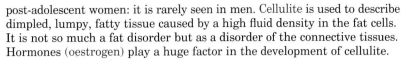

post-adolescent women: it is rarely seen in men. Cellulite is used to describe dimpled, lumpy, fatty tissue caused by a high fluid density in the fat cells. It is not so much a fat disorder but as a disorder of the connective tissues. Hormones (oestrogen) play a huge factor in the development of cellulite.

Cellulite occurs when the fat cells swell as lipid (fat) deposition increases. The chambers holding the fat cells apply pressure, restricting tissue drainage in the area. Capillary walls become excessively permeable allowing further fluid to accumulate. The tissues become impregnated with excess fluid and impurities.

The structure of the skin begins to change as collagen fibres become entwined around the fat cells, restricting circulation further. The fat chambers bulge causing the strands supporting the connective tissue to stiffen and become distorted, pulling down the skin at their point of anchor. The result is a dimpled appearance on the surface of the skin. Cellulite has a hard, grainy, nodular texture that can be felt when the skin is rolled between the fingers.

Cellulite is commonly found on the lower body, especially around the buttocks and thighs, and the condition becomes more exaggerated the heavier the weight gain. Cellulite can also occur on thin individuals.

There are several factors which contribute to the condition including:

- poor circulation
- inactivity and lack of exercise
- a poor diet high in refined foods and caffeine
- sluggish digestion.

Treatment guidance: A difficult condition to reverse. A change of lifestyle, diet and an increase in the level of exercise is important. Frequent regular massage with lots of deep percussion movements. Lymphatic massage is very beneficial as is skin brushing.

Target lymphatic, digestive and urinary systems.

Tip

Detecting cellulite
The dimpled appearance may be obvious; alternatively, clenching the muscles or gently squeezing the skin will determine the presence of cellulite (remember though that if you squeeze most tissues they will appear lumpy due to their structure).

Eczema/dermatitis

Dry, flaky, irritated and inflamed skin, which can be thickened with scaling. Wet eczema is characterized by vesicles and crusts. The condition is not contagious but may be very uncomfortable and poses a risk for easy cross infection as the skin is open. There are two categories of eczema:

- *exogenous eczema* caused by external agents, e.g. an allergy to chemicals (dermatitis)
- *endenous eczema* caused by an internal source via the bloodstream, e.g. an allergy to dairy produce.

Treatment guidance: Wet eczema is contra indicated.

Essential oils: For dry eczema use geranium, lavender, juniper, chamomile (patch test); calendula is an excellent carrier to use.

Reflexology: Solar plexus, digestive areas (including liver), adrenal and pituitary points.

Use hypoallergenic, perfume-free or products designed for very dry skin.

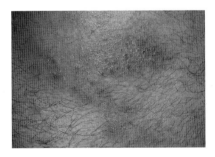

Eczema

Hyperhydrosis

Symptoms of hyperhidrosis include excessive sweating, which may be localized, i.e. affecting hands, feet, underarms, face, or generalized, i.e. affecting all the body's sweat glands. It has several possible causes including anxiety, exercise and hot weather. In some cases it is due to a nerve imbalance.

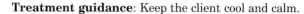

Treatment guidance: Keep the client cool and calm.

Target the nervous, urinary and endocrine systems.

Psoriasis

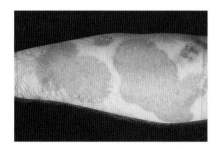

Psoriasis

An abnormal thickening of the skin producing red, often inflamed, patches with silvery scales. Skin is produced ten times faster than normal skin production. The skin may crack and bleed where there is excessive scaling. There may be intense itching. Sufferers may also experience swelling, stiffness and pain in the joints (arthritis).

Overproduction of skin cells will cause lifting of the nail plate or pit marks in the nail plate where the nails are affected.

In many cases this is a hereditary condition and it is believed that we all possess the potential to develop psoriasis. It is certainly linked to stress, illness and skin damage.

Treatment guidance: Be cautious and avoid direct contact where the skin is open.

Oil will calm some of the irritation, promote skin healing and keep the scales supple.

Target the nervous, endocrine and immune systems.

Seborrhoea (excessively oily skin/scalp)

Seborrhoea is caused by an overproduction of sebum. Androgen hormones are known to play a part but the exact cause is uncertain.

Symptoms: Sallow, shiny skin with excessive blackheads. If the scalp is affected the hair 'clogs' together with sebum, making it lank with a distinct odour.

Treatment guidance: Avoid excessive stimulation of the skin.

Target the adrenals and endocrine systems.

Sebaceous cyst (wen)

These are nodules under the skin on the face or scalp containing a smooth, yellow, cheesy material. The cysts can become very large and small capillaries can be seen running through the surface. May become infected.

Treatment guidance: Avoid area if tender or sensitive.

Sunburn

Burning caused by UV radiation.

There are four degrees of sunburn:

1. slight reddening which fades within 24 hours without soreness
2. marked reddening which fades in 2–3 days; slight irritation
3. red inflamed skin which is painful to the touch and lasts a week
4. as for 3 but with blisters.

Treatment guidance: Treatment of the affected area is contra indicated.

Recommend strict controlled exposure to the sun. Protect with sun block with a minimum SPF of 15+.

Urticaria/hives

Urticaria is caused by an allergic reaction to certain foods (e.g. strawberries), insect bites, pollens, drugs and plants. Also known as nettle rash.

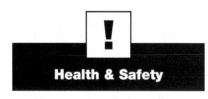

Health & Safety

Some medication can cause increased sensitivity to ultra violet rays.

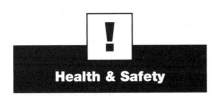

Symptoms: Eruption of weals (see p.48) and severe itching.

Treatment guidance: Do not treat.

Callus skin

An area of thickened skin caused by prolonged periods of pressure or friction. A callus can occur on the feet as a result of ill-fitting shoes, or on the hands due to hard labour (side of the middle finger = writer's callus).

Treatment advice: Refer the client to a chiropodist for treatment if the feet are affected and the callus is uncomfortable or painful.

Corns

A **corn** is a callus on a toe. They are caused by localized pressure, usually from ill-fitting shoes.

Treatment advice: Refer the client to a chiropodist if the corn is problematic.

Skin infections

There are four categories of micro-organisms which cause disease.

1. Bacteria

A single-celled micro-organism. Bacteria are abundant everywhere. Disease-causing bacteria are called Pathogens. There are several different types of bacteria and they are classified according to their shape.

Bacteria need the correct conditions to multiply

- **F**ood
- **O**xygen
- **D**arkness
- **W**armth
- **A**lkalinity
- **M**oisture

When the correct conditions are not available, some bacteria produce spores. These can lie dormant for long periods of time until conditions change.

2. Virus

The smallest known type of infectious agent, it is minute in size compared to bacteria.

It can be debated as to whether viruses are actually living organisms or just a collection of molecules capable of replicating. Their sole purpose is to invade and take over cells of other organisms disrupting the cells activities. Outside a cell a virus is totally inactive.

The body can effectively deal with some viruses but others deal a devastating blow and attack with such speed that the immune system does not have a chance to respond. Other viruses can lie dormant in the system causing recurrent infections. Viruses are difficult to treat as killing the viruses may involve killing the host cell, however, highly effective vaccines are available to protect against some viruses.

3. Parasite

A parasite is an organism that lives in or on another living organism (or host), benefiting from the process, however, the host may be disadvantaged.

The parasite obtains its nutritional needs from the tissues, blood or nutritional intake of the host. Viruses, disease causing fungi and bacteria are all parasites.

4. Fungi

Fungi are simple parasites and include yeast and moulds. Most are harmless and some are of a positive benefit to humans. Some fungi divide to form chains creating a complex network of filaments called mycelium. Some fungi can be hazardous such as the spores found on peanuts, which are thought to contribute to peanut allergies.

Acne vulgaris

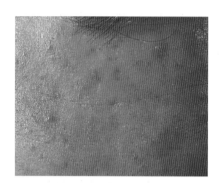

Acne vulgaris

Found where sebaceous glands are active on the face, chest, back and buttocks. Blackheads (comedones) are present, as are pustules and inflammation. Boils, nodules and cysts may also develop.

Cause: Bacterial infection (*staphylococci*) of overactive sebaceous glands which have been stimulated by an increase in the hormone androgen. Sebum oxidizes in the follicle, creating a blockage and allowing bacteria to breed. Condition can be aggravated by some medications such as steroids.

Treatment guidance: Direct contact with active acne is contra indicated as the infection can be spread. Aim to relax the client with massage and use essential oils which are suitable for acne and stress. These can be used over the adjoining areas and applied without massage to the affected areas.

Target the endocrine system.

Acne rosacea

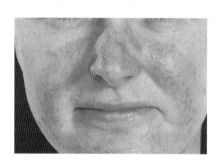

Acne rosacea

A chronic skin disorder affecting the superficial capillaries of the nose and cheeks. Contributory factors include overuse of corticosteroid creams, hormonal disturbances and intestinal disturbances.

Symptoms: Begins with chronic flushing of the face, developing into permanent dilation of the facial capillaries. The skin looks irritated and sensitive, with outbreaks of pustules. Unlike acne vulgaris, acne rosacea begins after the age of 30 and pustules generally affect the centre of the face in a butterfly pattern, i.e. across nose, cheeks and sometimes forehead.

Treatment guidance: Avoid any surface stimulation and where pustules are present avoid direct contact.

Target endocrine and digestive systems.

Boils (furuncles)

A deep bacterial infection (*Staphylococcus aureus*) in a hair follicle resulting in an abscess. Boils are attributed to poor hygiene, stress and an increase in androgens and bacteria can be carried naturally in the nose or groin and may be passed by direct and indirect contact, e.g. contact with towels.

Symptoms: Visible as an inflamed tender area, developing into a large painful pustule on the back of the neck, buttocks, groin or armpit. More common in young men.

Treatment guidance: Avoid area.

Carbuncles

A carbuncle is a number of boils (see above) clumped together, i.e. multi-headed, and often leaves a scar.

Treatment guidance: Avoid the area.

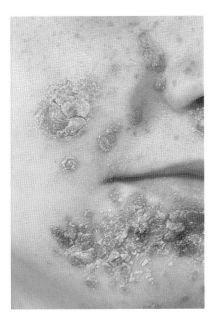

Impetigo

Impetigo

Bacterial infection by staphylococci and streptococci. Impetigo often occurs as a secondary infection after eczema, lice, scabies and herpes. Found commonly on the face around the nose and mouth but can occur on any area where the skin has been broken.

Symptoms: Red, raised areas of skin which quickly form small blisters. The blisters dry to become honey-coloured crusts. On removal of the crusts moist pink skin can be seen beneath.

Treatment guidance: Contra indicated; refer to GP.

Folliculitis

Folliculitis is a bacterial infection by staphylococci spread by indirect contact with contaminated equipment, poor hygiene, etc.

Symptoms: Inflammation of one or more hair follicles. May occur almost anywhere but commonly around the neck, thighs, buttocks and armpits. The hair may grow inwards causing further inflammation (pseudo-folliculitis).

Treatment guidance: Avoid area. Recommend application of tea tree oil to the infected area.

Herpes simplex

Commonly known as a cold sore. A recurrent viral infection that often develops when the sufferer is run down, under stress or after overexposure to the sun or wind. Once infected herpes simplex remains dormant in the skin.

Symptoms: Initially there is itching or irritation at the site of the cold sore. This develops into a red patch followed by blisters which progress into a moist, crusty patch. Common around the mouth but can occur anywhere.

Treatment guidance: Contra indicated as infectious when blisters are present. Spread by both direct and indirect contact. Recommend home treatment with neat tea tree oil.

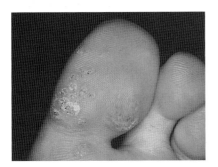

Wart

Herpes zoster (shingles)

After infection with the chicken pox virus, some of the viruses lie dormant in certain nerves that supply the skin. During periods of stress or weakened immunity herpes zoster re-emerges as shingles.

Symptoms: Painful rash with crusting blisters which appear four or so days after severe irritation along a nerve pathway. The pain may persist for months after the rash has disappeared. The rash follows a nerve pathway and may affect a strip on the side of the neck or part of the torso; occasionally part of the face is affected.

Treatment guidance: Contra indicated until all symptoms have cleared.

Warts/verrucae

Warts are caused by the 'human papilloma' virus of which there are thirty different types. The infection can be caught by direct and indirect contact. Warts affect the upper layers of the epidermis. They do not have roots, seeds or branches.

Symptoms:

- *Common:* firm, rough, raised area of skin occurring singularly or in clusters. Common on the hands.
- *Plantar* (verruca): occur on the soles of feet. The pressure from the weight of the body makes them grow inwards. Highly contagious.

Vurrucae

In both, black spots may be seen where capillaries have been caught in the rapid growth.

- *Filiform:* these are long slender filaments that commonly occur in clusters, often seen on the face, neck and under the bra line.

Treatment guidance: Direct contact is contra indicated as warts are contagious, especially when the wart has been damaged. Plantar warts are particularly contagious in damp, warm, moist conditions. Cover where appropriate with a non-porous dressing. Treat with neat lemon or tea tree essential oil.

Tinea

Tinea or ringworm is *not* caused by a parasite. It is a fungus, which produces a keratin-splitting enzyme. Different fungi affect different areas:

- *Corporis* is ringworm of the body; *capititus* of the head.
  Symptoms: Pink circular patch, sometimes scaly, with a defined outer red ring. Classically it heals from the centre as the infection spreads outwards in a ring, hence its name. It affects exposed parts of the body, i.e. face, arms and shoulders.
  Treatment consideration: Contra indicated; refer to GP.

- *Tinea pedis* (athlete's foot)
  Symptoms: Infection usually begins between the 4th and 5th toes. Skin appears sodden and white. Alternatively it may appear as tiny blisters which become red and peel away the skin becoming cracked or split. The area is often itchy and irritated. The infected skin may even rub off to reveal raw skin underneath. Often accompanied by a distinct odour.
  Treatment consideration: Contra indicated so avoid working on the feet.
  Essential oils: Apply neat tea tree.
  Reflexology: Mild cases only (between 4th and 5th toes only). Wipe feet with tea tree before and after treatment and avoid direct contact with affected areas.

Scabies

A parasitic mite called *Sarcoptes scabiei* which burrows into the skin where it lays its eggs. Scabies is a highly contagious disease.

Symptoms: The burrowing mites can be seen as tiny, grey, scaly swellings (ridges 3–10 mm long) usually between the fingers, wrists, armpits and genitals. Later, reddish lumps appear on the limbs and trunk. Infestation causes intense itching, hence its common name, 'itch mite'.

Treatment guidance: Contra indicated.

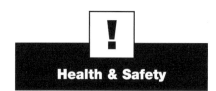

Health & Safety

Fungal infections

If you suspect that the client has a fungal infection on the skin advise them to consult their GP. There are so many skin blemishes, rashes and marks that the only way to be sure is to have a tissue scraping sent for skin analysis.

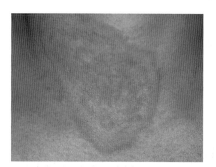

Tinea corporis

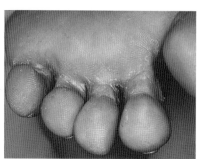

Tinea pedis

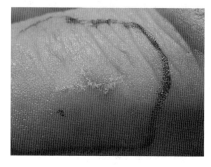

Scabies

The nail

The nail is an extension of the stratum lucidum layer of the epidermis and is composed of keratinized cells. Several chemicals are present in its composition and a small amount of fat. The nail is approximately 18 per cent water.

Functions of the nail

- Protection: forms a stiff backing to the soft, sensitive fingertips.
- Enhances finger sensitivity.
- Aids the fingers in picking up objects.
- Useful tool, e.g. for scratching.

Structure of the nail

The nail is divided into three parts:

- matrix
- nail plate
- free edge.

Matrix: The living part of the nail. Cells divide in the matrix and harden to form the nail. The matrix has an abundant supply of blood vessels and nerves. Injury to the matrix will result in the growth of the nail being affected, leading to temporary or permanent deformity. The nail may be lost completely if damage is severe.

Lunula: The visible part of the matrix, most prominent on the thumb. It is visible as a half-moon-shaped, pale pink, almost white area at the base of the nail plate. It forms a bridge between the living part of the nail and the dead cells after keratinization.

Nail plate: The visible portion of the nail. It is dead and has no blood supply or nerves. It is formed from three layers of hard keratinous cells tightly packed together and held in place by a cementing material.

Nail bed: As its name implies this is the area on which the nail plate lies. The dermis is arranged in a series of ridges, which fit into grooves in the prickle cell layer of the epidermis to form a firm adhesion.

Nail wall: The small fold of skin overlapping and framing the sides of the nail. It prevents the nail from becoming damaged and protects the matrix by making a tight waterproof seal. It also holds the nail plate in place.

Cuticle: Folds onto the base of the nail plate overlapping the lunula. Provides a barrier and seal against infection. It is divided into two parts:

- the *perionychium* covers a quarter of the developing nail and the outer portion surrounding the nail
- the *eponychium* lies beneath the perionychium.

Free edge: The nail which extends beyond the nail bed and is no longer attached.

The **hyponychium**: The epidermis under the free edge, seen as the white dividing line between the nail attached to the nail bed and the free edge.

Nail growth

The nail grows forward from its starting point in the matrix by cell division. Older cells are pushed forward as new cells are produced. They gradually harden as keratin is injected into the nail.

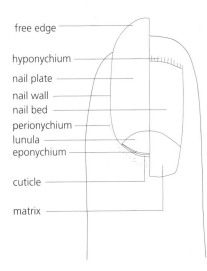

free edge

hyponychium

nail plate

nail wall

nail bed

perionychium

lunula

eponychium

cuticle

matrix

Structure of nail

Conditions, disorders and diseases of the nail

Adverse treatable nail conditions

Treatment guidance for the conditions below: Many treatable nail conditions will benefit from massage and stimulation of the circulation. In many cases you could recommend that the client has a manicure.

Blue nail: Nail bed is light or dark bluish in colour. Caused by poor circulation or heart problems.

Ridged nails:

- *Longitudinal ridges:* singular occurrence is generally associated with trauma or damage to the matrix; more generalized ridges are associated with illness, poor health or lifestyle, uneven nail growth and age.
- *Horizontal ridges:* these may be fine or deep corrugations; cause is as above.

Split nails (lamellar dystrophy): The nail layers have become separated so that the nail flakes away in sections. Common causes are poor health or diet and the use of strong alkaline products.

Leuconychia: White patches or spots on the nail. Occur as a result of injury to the nail causing the layers to separate, creating an opaque appearance.

Brittle nails (*fragitalitas ungium*): This condition may be congenital. It is usually caused by a low moisture content in the nail or poor circulation.

Eggshell nails: Ultra thin nail plates that are very flexible and transparent. They often curve at the free edge over the end of the fingertip. Associated with chronic illness.

Hangnails: Has nothing to do with the nail itself but concerns the skin around the nail. Threads of skin around the nail wall and cuticle become torn and untidy. Hangnails are usually a result of neglect or repeated cutting of the cuticle.

Common nail diseases

(These may be contra indicated.)

Atrophy of the nail
Atrophy occurs when the nail becomes wasted, loses it lustre and may actually come away from the nail bed. Caused by injury (e.g. deep bruising) or disease, including fungal infections.

Treatment guidance: Avoid area if in doubt of cause and refer client to GP.

Hypertrophy of the nail (onychauxis)
A thickened nail plate. Toenails tend to hypertrophy with age but this can be caused by internal disturbances and infections.

Stained nails
May be caused by several factors, from nicotine stains to fungal infections.

Treatment guidance: The first point you need to establish is the location of the staining within the nail plate – is it on the surface only or under the nail. This will help you to establish a cause.

Ingrowing nails (onychocryptosis)
Inflamed, swollen skin around the sides of the nail plate (usually one side) where the nail growth has extended into the tissues of the skin. Ingrowing toenails are common on the big toe. The condition is associated with incorrect cutting of the toenail and ill-fitting shoes.

Treatment guidance: Avoid area and refer client to a chiropodist or their GP.

Paronychia
Paronychia is caused by a bacterial infection.

Symptoms: Red, inflamed skin at the base or side of the nail plate.

Treatment guidance: Contra indicated; avoid area. Apply neat tea tree oil.

Tinea unguium (onychomycosis)
Fungal infection of the nail. Nails become thickened and yellow. As the fungus penetrates underneath the nail plate it may begin to lift. Often accompanied with scaling of the palms or soles of the feet.

Treatment guidance: Apply tea tree oil. Fungal infections of the nail are very difficult to treat and can take many months.

The hair

The hair is a fine thread-like structure of keratinized dead cells growing from the skin.

The hair itself can be divided into three layers: the *cuticle*, *cortex* and *medulla*.

Hair growth

The hair follicle undergoes periods of activity and rest. Hormones or drugs may influence these periods of growth. There are three stages:

1   **anagen** – active growth, approx. 80–90 per cent of hair
2   **catagen** – period of change, 1 per cent of hair
3   **telogen** – tired or resting stage, approx. 13 per cent of hair.

At certain times the anagen hair will come to the end of its growth cycle. It separates from the papilla at its base where the hair was produced. Over a period of several days the hair will rise up to the middle portion of the hair follicle. The bulb at the base of the hair begins to atrophy and forms a club shape. At this stage the hair is still attached to the follicle wall but the part of the follicle below the hair now begins to shrink upwards. It remains attached to the dermal papilla by a thread called the dermal cord. The hair is now in the catagen stage and lasts approximately two weeks. It continues to rise up to just beneath the sebaceous gland. The hair is now in the telogen stage; it can no longer be nourished and eventually disintegrates. The hair will loosen and either be brushed away or fall out.

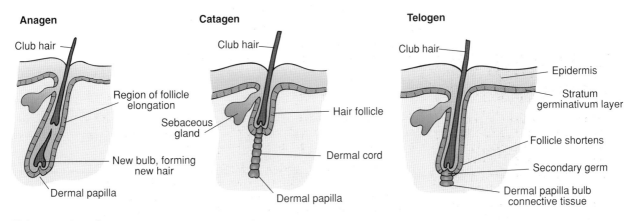

Hair growth cycle

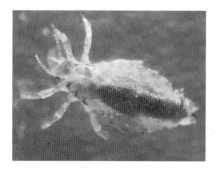

Head louse

Common scalp and hair disorders and diseases

Pediculosis capititis (head lice)

Lice are small, wingless, flat insects that feed on blood. Their eggs (nits) take 7–10 days to hatch. It takes 7–14 days for the lice to mature and mate. They survive for several weeks. Lice walk (they can't jump) from head to head so there must be direct contact.

Symptoms: Intense itching at the site of infestation. Nits are present on the scalp and appear as grey-coloured eggs attached to the hair shaft.

Treatment guidance: Contra indicated.

Treating head lice

To check for nits, lift sections of hair (best to start behind the ears) away from the scalp so that the light travels through the hair. This will help to make the nits, which can be seen as pearly spheres attached to the hair shaft, stand out. It is easy to mistake nits for loose bits of skin. If you are not sure, try to pull off one of the spheres; if it is firmly stuck it's a nit!

Home treatment must be ongoing for a minimum of 14 days. Special products can be bought but are not always effective. The hair must be meticulously combed through with a special comb to loosen and remove nits and lice on a daily basis for at least 7 days.

Try essential oils: tea tree, lavender, geranium and eucalyptus (avoid eucalyptus for young children). These can be mixed in with a conditioner and left on the hair for half an hour before rinsing out.

Vinegar is excellent for loosening the cement which holds the nits to the hair and has the added benefit of making the hair beautifully shiny.

Pediculosis pubis (pubic lice)

These are miniature insects that have crab-like claws (hence the common name of crabs). The females lay eggs which hatch after 8 days. Pubic lice are usually passed during sexual contact. They don't only live in the pubic hair, they also live under the arms, beards or eyelashes.

Symptoms: Intense itching at the site of infestation. Pubic lice look like miniature scabs as they partially bury themselves into the hair follicle causing further irritation.

Treatment guidance: Contra indicated.

Pityriasis simplex (dandruff)

Pityriasis simplex is an increased turnover of cells in germinative layer of the epidermis.

Symptoms: Small flakes of dead skin shed from the scalp. Can cause inflammation of the eyelid (blepharitis) or conjunctivitis.

Treatment guidance: Be careful not to overstimulate the scalp when working on this area.

Hirsutism

Hirsutism is abnormal excess hair growth in a male distribution, i.e. beard, chest, navel. The condition may be hereditary, as a result of some surgical procedures, certain medication, and hyper- or hypothyroidism.

Hypertrichosis

Symptoms: Hypertrichosis consists of an abnormal growth of excess hair.

Cause: Hormonal imbalance caused by disease (tumours, e.g. on pituitary) or injury.

Treatment guidance: Ensure client is consulting GP to investigate cause.

Talc or talc-free alternative may be appropriate for general massage.

Target reproductive and endocrine systems.

Alopecia (baldness)

Several different types of alopecia exist including androgenic alopecia (male baldness) and alopecia universalis (total loss of body hair). Possible causes include emotional stress, shock, underactivity of the thyroid gland or pituitary gland, iron deficiency and as a side effect of some medication and illnesses.

Symptoms: Loss of hair, thinning or receding hair growth.

Treatment guidance: Stimulate the blood supply to the scalp with massage to encourage healthy circulation and revive sluggish growth.

The circulatory system

The heart and circulation

Pulmonary circulation carries deoxygenated blood from the right side of the heart to the lungs and oxygenated blood back to the left side of the heart.

A second circulation, *systemic circulation*, carries oxygenated blood from the left side of the heart to the head and body. The right side of the heart receives deoxygenated blood from the body.

This keeps the oxygenated and deoxygenated blood separate. Blood alternates between the two circulations.

The heart

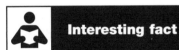

Interesting fact

A fit heart pumps more blood
A fit heart will pump 25% more blood per minute at rest and over 40% more blood during physical activity

The heart is a pear-shaped organ found in the thoracic cavity, lying slightly to the left. It is surrounded by a protective membrane which contains a fluid-filled cavity called the pericardium. This prevents friction between the heart and the surrounding tissues. The main blood vessels of the heart are as follows:

- vena cava: carries blood from the body into the right atrium
- pulmonary vein: carries blood from the lungs into the left atrium
- aorta: carries blood from the left ventricle to the body
- pulmonary artery: carries blood from the right ventricle to the lungs.

Blood vessels

Arteries are the blood vessels which transport oxygenated blood away from the heart (with the exception of the pulmonary artery). The blood is pure and bright red. Arteries vary considerably in size, but all have the same structure. They are thick walled and contain a layer of muscle. Their structure enables them to withstand the high pressure of the blood being pumped away from the heart.

Arteries becomes arterioles. Arterioles eventually break up into a number of minute vessels called capillaries.

The walls of a capillary are composed of a single layer that is very thin and permits the diffusion of small molecular substances such as oxygen,

Artery

Capillary

Vein

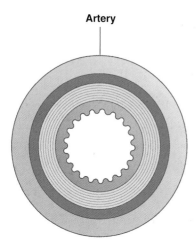
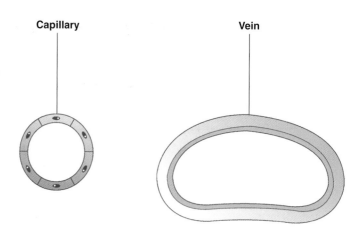

Blood vessels

vitamins, minerals, water and amino acids. These pass out from the capillaries into the interstitial fluid to nourish the cells. In return, substances such as carbon dioxide and water pass back. This simple process is known as *capillary exchange*. The capillaries form a vast network of tiny vessels that link the smallest arterioles to the smallest venules.

Veins transport deoxygenated blood to the heart from the body at low pressure (with the exception of the pulmonary vein). The blood is dark purplish red in colour. The walls of the veins are much thinner than those of arteries. Some veins have valves, which prevent the backflow of blood. Valves are abundant in the veins of the limbs but are usually absent from those in the thorax and abdomen. The smallest veins are called venules. Veins rely on muscular activity and breathing to push the blood along.

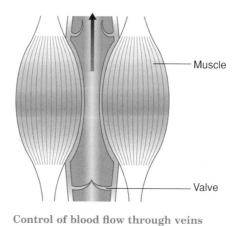

Muscle

Muscles squeeze the blood in the veins back towards the heart

Valve

Control of blood flow through veins

Interesting fact

Pulse rate
The normal resting pulse rate in an adult can vary between 60 and 80 beats per minute. It increases during stress; exercise, in some illnesses, while taking alcohol or as a result of injury. The pulse rate in very fit people is often slower.

Pulse

The pulse is the wave of pressure which passes along the arteries indicating the pumping action of the heart. It can be palpated where an artery is close to the surface (jugular, femoral, popliteal and radial).

Erythema

Erythema can be seen as a pink or red colour to the skin. The capillaries may become dilated and congested with blood as a result of external factors, e.g. heat or stimulation (massage). Superficial blood vessels dilate (vasodilation), bringing blood to the skin's surface so that heat can be lost to the atmosphere.

Blood supply to and from the head

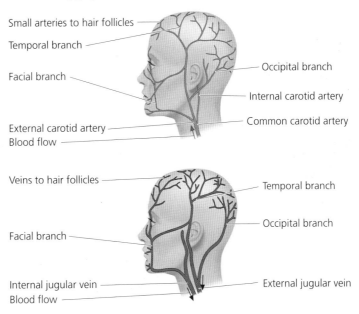

Small arteries to hair follicles

Temporal branch

Facial branch

Occipital branch

Internal carotid artery

Common carotid artery

External carotid artery
Blood flow

Veins to hair follicles

Temporal branch

Occipital branch

Facial branch

Internal jugular vein

External jugular vein

Blood flow

Blood supply to and from the body

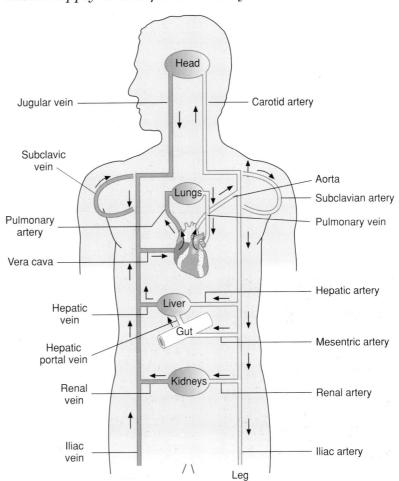

Head

Jugular vein

Carotid artery

Subclavic
vein

Aorta

Subclavian artery

Lungs

Pulmonary vein

Pulmonary
artery

Vera cava

Hepatic artery

Hepatic
vein

Liver

Gut

Mesentric artery

Hepatic
portal vein

Kidneys

Renal
vein

Renal artery

Iliac
vein

Iliac artery

Leg

Blood

Blood is a red, viscous, slightly alkaline fluid accounting for 7–9 per cent of the total body weight (approximately 4.6 litres). The volume and concentration of the constituents of blood are kept within narrow limits to maintain homeostasis.

Composition of blood

Plasma is a clear, slightly alkaline, yellow fluid. It is what is left of the blood when all the cells are removed and accounts for 44 per cent of the total volume of blood.

Erythrocytes or red blood cells account for 44 per cent of total blood volume. They are bi-concave circular cells which contain no nucleus. They contain the molecule haemoglobin; this combines with oxygen from the lungs to transport it around the body. Red blood cells are manufactured in the bone marrow of the short bones (e.g. ribs) and the proximal end of the long bones.

White corpuscles or **leukocytes** account for 1 per cent of blood volume and vary in size and shape. There are several different types, each with a specific function.

Granulocytes are formed in the bone marrow and play a major role in inflammation in response to injury. They include:

- *eosinophils* protect the body against foreign pathogens, they are phagocytic
- *basophils* contain heparin and histamine
- *neutrophils* are attracted to the site of an invasion by bacteria and fungal infections and are phagocytes.

Agranulocytes:

- *monocytes* originate in the red bone marrow and are phagocytic; some have an important function in inflammation and immunity
- *lymphocytes* are slow to reproduce; larger lymphocytes induce immunity and promote recovery. There are two functionally distinct types:
  - T-lymphocytes combat cells containing antigens
  - B-lymphocytes are involved in the production of antibodies that neutralize antigens.

Thrombocytes or **platelets** are small, non-nucleated discs/fragments in the blood and are involved in the clotting process.

The functions of blood

The functions of blood can be divided into two main areas: transport and protection.

Transportation

- Blood transports oxygen from the lungs to cells and removes carbon dioxide from the cells, returning it to the lungs for excretion.
- Transportation of nutrients to the cells.
- The blood removes waste products from the tissues and cells. These waste materials are transported to appropriate organs for excretion; these include urea and uric acid.
- Transports hormones and enzymes from their cells of origin to their target organs and tissues.

Composition of blood

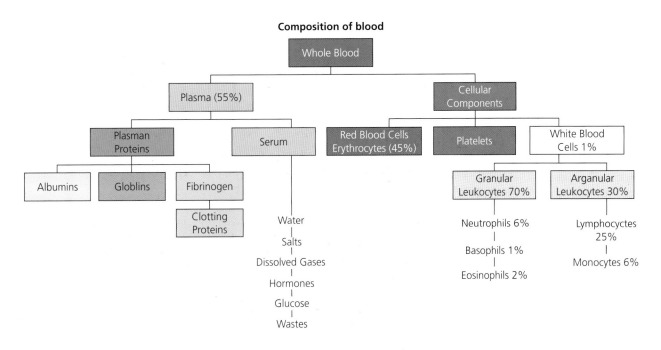

Protection

- Aids in the defence of the body against invasion of micro-organisms and their toxins due to the phagocytic action of neutrophils, monocytes and the presence of antibodies and anti-toxins.

- The clotting process prevents the loss of body fluid and blood cells.

- Plays a role in maintaining body temperature. Due to the chemical activity in the cells and tissues, heat is produced, warming the circulating blood. If too much heat is produced vasodilation occurs near the surface of the body, enabling heat to be lost. If the temperature of the outside atmosphere is low, vasoconstriction occurs and the superficial blood vessels constrict, preventing heat loss.

Blood flow through skin when hot   **and when cold**

Blood flows close to epidermis   Capillaries constricted

Epidermis

Shunt vessel constricted   Blood flows deep in dermis

Vasoconstriction/dilation

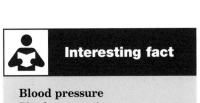

Interesting fact

Blood pressure
Blood pressure is measured by the use of a **sphygmomanometer** and is usually expressed in the following manner:

BP = 120/80 mm Hg or
BP = 16/11 kPa

Blood pressure varies according to the time of day, the posture, sex and age.

Blood pressure

Blood pressure may be defined as the force or pressure that the blood exerts on the walls of the blood vessels in which it is contained.

When the left ventricle contracts and pushes blood into the aorta, the pressure produced is known as the systolic blood pressure (systole = squeeze).

Diastole – heart fills with blood

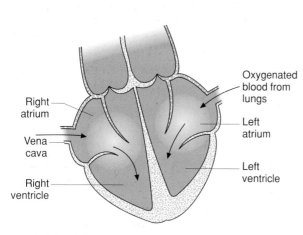

Right atrium

Vena cava

Right ventricle

Oxygenated blood from lungs

Left atrium

Left ventricle

Diastole/systole

Ventricular systole

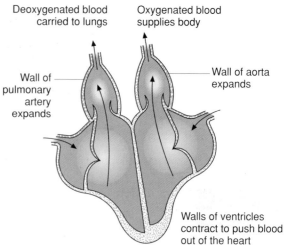

Deoxygenated blood carried to lungs

Oxygenated blood supplies body

Wall of pulmonary artery expands

Wall of aorta expands

Walls of ventricles contract to push blood out of the heart

When the heart is resting between contractions the pressure within the arteries is termed the diastolic blood pressure (diastole = dilate).

Conditions, disorders and diseases of the circulatory system

Haemorrhage

Haemorrhage is the medical term for bleeding or loss of blood. Blood loss may be internal and not obvious. The concern here for the therapist is contact with body fluids. The two conditions classified as haemorrhage that the therapist is likely to need to consider are:

- *nosebleeds*: these may start spontaneously and can be associated with high blood pressure and violent sneezing
- *heavy menstruation.*

Treatment guidance: Contra indicated. Avoid massage over the abdomen during the first couple of days of menstruation.

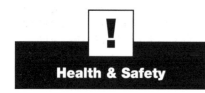

Health & Safety

- Always wear gloves when dealing with blood or any body fluids.
- Clean up blood spills using neat household bleach.
- Dispose of waste material in a sealed bag.

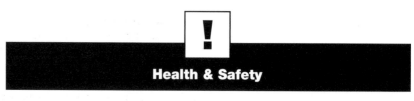

Health & Safety

Blood loss
If the blood loss is heavy the client may feel light-headed and dizzy. Avoid laying the client flat and/or letting him/her make any sudden movement.

Reflexology: Avoid heavy pressure over the uterus reflex the day prior to and the first couple of days into menstruation as this may stimulate bleeding.

Leukaemia

Leukaemia is a generic term for several types of cancer affecting the white blood cells. The condition is classified according to the white blood cells that are impaired and may be acute or chronic. The production of white blood cells and platelets is affected. The function of other organs may be disrupted by the infiltration of the leukaemic cells.

Symptoms: Fatigue, fever, night sweats, weight loss, anaemia, infections, bruising, tenderness, enlarged lymph nodes, liver and spleen.

Treatment guidance: Contra indicated; refer to GP.

Varicose veins

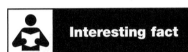

Interesting fact

Haemorrhoids
Haemorrhoids are a varicose vein sited in the rectum and anus.

The larger veins in the legs contain numerous cup-like non-return valves to keep the blood flowing back to the heart. When these valves deteriorate, the blood tends to pool and the veins become swollen and protrude. This condition is known as varicose veins. Because the leg veins are large and contain a large volume of blood, a sudden massive blood loss can occur when they are damaged or burst.

Treatment guidance: Do not massage over or below varicose veins as this puts further pressure on the valves. Drain the circulation by elevating the limb and massaging above the affected area. This will create a vacuum above the affected site, encouraging the stagnated blood to move.

Essential oils: Cypress, juniper, lavender, lemon, peppermint, rose, rosemary and sandalwood.

Reflexology: Circulatory system and leg reflexes.

Thrombosis

Thrombosis is a condition occurring when a blood clot (thrombus) interferes with the circulation by either partially or totally blocking a vessel. This may occur as the result of surgery or as a consequence of long haul flying but the client will usually be predisposed. The condition becomes a problem when individuals have a susceptibility to blood clots due to an ongoing systemic disorder (contraceptive pill, smoking, fractures, cardiovascular disease).

Treatment guidance: Contra indicated; refer to GP, particularly if the client is on medication for the condition. However, providing there is no history of incidence and there are no other systemic factors treatment can be given with care providing the thrombosis was not recent (i.e. not within a year).

Thrombophlebitis

An inflammation of part of a vein often accompanied by the formation of a blood clot (thrombus). Thrombophlebitis is associated with varicose veins but can also occur as a result of a minor injury to a vein after childbirth and certain blood vessel disorders.

Symptoms: Red, tender area over the affected vein. Usually there is obvious swelling and there may be a mild fever. There is a possibility of a more serious blood clot forming.

Treatment guidance: Contra indicated.

Embolism

An embolism is a blockage of an artery by a fragment of material travelling in the blood. This may be a thrombus, but could also be fat, a fragment of bone, air or other material.

Symptoms: Depends on the location and extent of the blockage.

Pulmonary embolism relates to the lungs and symptoms include breathlessness, feeling faint and chest pains. An embolism may also cause strokes and heart attacks.

Strokes

A stroke is caused by damage to the brain as a result of an interruption in the blood supply. Sensation, movement and function can all become impaired depending on the area damaged. There are three causes of strokes: *thrombosis*, *embolism* and *haemorrhage*.

Symptoms may develop over minutes or hours and may be mild/barely noticeable or, if extensive, fatal. There is usually weakness or paralysis. There are several factors which increase the risk of stroke including high blood pressure, smoking, heart disease, age, the contraceptive pill and HRT.

Treatment guidance: Refer to GP for advice before treatment. There have been some very positive results with reflexology for treating stroke victims who require a longer recovery period.

Atherosclerosis

A degenerative disorder generally associated with high blood pressure and age. Atherosclerosis is caused by a build-up of plaques of atheroma (cholesterol-rich fatty deposits). This eventually causes the arteries to thicken, restricting the blood flow. Thrombi form on the roughened plaque surfaces restricting blood flow further. If one of these thrombi should dislodge there is the risk of heart attack or a stroke. There are several related factors to atherosclerosis including smoking, excess weight, lack of activity and a genetic predisposition. It is also known that a diet high in cholesterol-rich foods is a contributing factor for those predisposed to the condition.

Symptoms: None in the early stages, but as the disease advances these may include angina or a heart attack.

Treatment guidance: Contra indicated; refer to GP.

Pacemaker

A device that is connected to the heart to supply an electrical impulse to maintain a regular heartbeat. The device may be internal or external (temporary). The pacemaker may be affected by electromagnetic pulses (powerful radio transmitters, diathermy machines, etc.).

Treatment guidance: Check with GP. What you need to be clear on is why the client has a need for a pacemaker and whether the condition that requires it is contra indicated rather than the pacemaker device itself.

Heart disease

Heart disease may be either congenital, i.e. a heart defect that has been present since birth, or ischaemic. Ischaemic heart disease is the most common type of heart disease and is caused by a reduction in the blood supply to the heart causing damage or the heart to malfunction. The reduced blood supply may be a result of a narrowing (atherosclerosis) or blockage of the coronary arteries. The two most common forms of heart disease are angina pectoris and heart attack.

Treatment guidance: Refer to GP before treatment. A more efficient venous return may assist the workload of the heart.

Angina

Angina is caused by an insufficient blood supply to the heart to meet the demands of exertion. There are several causes including heart disease, arterosclerosis, arrhythmia, narrowing of the aortic valve (aortic stenosis) and hyperthyroidism.

Symptoms include:

- a gripping central chest pain/pressure, spreading to the jaw and down the left arm
- shortness of breath and weakness.

Treatment guidance: Consult GP, as there may be other implications.

Essential oils: Black pepper.

Heart valve disorders

The valves in the heart prevent blood flowing backwards; any damage will make the heart work harder. Damaged valves generate distinctive heart sounds. Heart valve disorders may be hereditary or caused by a variety of illnesses. If severe enough the condition can lead to heart failure.

Treatment guidance: Refer to GP. Severe heart valve disorders are contra indicated.

Heart attack – myocardial infarction

A heart attack commonly occurs when the blood supply to the heart muscle is obstructed, e.g. by a blood clot in one of the coronary arteries. In myocardial infarction an area of heart tissue has died as a result of a lack of oxygen; this damage is permanent.

Symptoms: Like those described for angina.

Treatment guidance: Contra indicated until the client has recovered. Refer to GP before treatment.

Blood pressure disorders

Low blood pressure (hypotension)

If blood pressure is too low (hypotension), i.e. there is a loss of blood volume, the vital organs will be unable to function properly and the symptoms and signs of shock may develop.

- *Postural hypotension* is common and caused by a reduction in the blood pressure on sitting or standing up quickly.

Treatment guidance: Avoid lying client completely flat. Sit the client up after treatment slowly, possibly in stages.

Essential oils: Use hypertensive oils and keep massage fairly brisk.

Oils to avoid include sweet marjoram, ylang ylang and clary sage.

Oils to use should be more stimulating and include rosemary, black pepper and peppermint.

High blood pressure (hypertension)

If the blood pressure is continually too high hypertension occurs; this is common as age increases, and perhaps in association with hardening of the arteries. The blood vessels risk rupturing resulting in internal bleeding (e.g. cerebral haemorrhage, a form of stroke). There are many reasons for high blood pressure including obesity, smoking, lack of exercise and an inherited tendency. Hypertension also occurs as a result of other diseases including kidney and endocrine disorders.

Treatment guidance: Contra indicated; refer to GP for advice.

Generally, relaxing treatment will be beneficial in helping to bring blood pressure down. What needs to be considered more carefully is the cause of the condition and whether there are any other related contra indications.

Raynaud's disease

A disorder of the blood vessels, which on exposure to the cold causes the arterioles to contract suddenly. About 4 per cent of the population experience the condition.

Symptoms: On exposure to the cold the fingers or toes become white. The fingers may be numb and a tingling or burning sensation may be experienced. As circulation begins to return the fingers turn blue, becoming red once the circulation has returned.

Treatment guidance: Keep the hands and feet warm.

Chilblain

Interesting fact

Chilblains
Chilblains are more common in the young and elderly women.

An itchy, red swelling found on the finger or toe. It is caused by excessive vasoconstriction of the extremities during cold weather.

Treatment guidance: Treat carefully, working around affected areas; indirectly you will stimulate the circulation by working the surrounding tissue.

Advise the client to keep hands and feet warm during the cold weather. A little talc may help relieve the itching.

Disorders of the blood

Anaemia

Symptoms: Dizziness, tiredness, headaches, palpitations and pallor. Other symptoms will depend on the type of anaemia.

Cause: Insufficient haemoglobin due to a lack of iron in the blood means that there is not enough oxygen being carried from the lungs to supply the needs of the body. There are several different types of anaemia, the most common being 'iron deficiency' (common during pregnancy and heavy menstruation), faddish diets and unbalanced vegan or vegetarian diets (vitamin B12 and iron deficiency).

Treatment guidance: Check the cause and type of anaemia as this will depend on whether the condition is contra indicated or not. If you are unsure, refer to GP. Some types of anaemia make the body more susceptible to bruising and so caution should be taken.

Medical oedema

Although oedema is associated with the lymphatic circulation it is intricately linked with the venous circulation.

Symptoms: Abnormal accumulation of fluid in the body tissues. The condition may not always be noticeable. It can be localized, e.g. in the

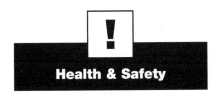

Health & Safety

Oedema
If the client is unsure or unaware they have oedema, refer the client to their GP to check underlying causes. *Do not treat*. There may be a more serious underlying medical problem.

---

ankles, or generalized. There are various causes of oedema, systemic (heart and kidneys), drug related and as a result of injury.

Excess fluid needs to increase by more than 14% before it becomes evident as swelling, prior to this it may only be evident as weight gain.

Pitting oedema can be detected by pressing a finger into the affected tissues. If an indentation remains only slowly regaining its natural shape oedema is present. This is a serious condition and is contra indicated.

Treatment guidance: Refer to GP before treatment. Medical oedema is contra indicated.

Massage may be beneficial but needs to be carried out carefully. The lower limbs should be elevated whilst working. Movements should be slow and drain from the top area first.

The lymphatic/immune system

The lymphatic system is a network of vessels and lymphatic organs supplying and draining excess fluid from the spaces between cells. The lymphatic system is made up of the following:

- lymph vessels and lymph
- lymph nodes or glands
- adenoids
- tonsils
- thymus
- spleen.

Functions of the lymph system

- Filtering lymph and preventing infection.
- Producing lymphocytes (T- and B-lymphocytes and antibodies in the nodes) which play a crucial role in immunity and protect against disease.
- Carrying digested fats away from the intestines.

Lymph/tissue fluid

Lymph is a pale, odourless, milky-coloured, slightly alkaline fluid. Its main component is water (94%) with a high concentration of lymphocytes. It contains no erythrocytes. Its composition is very similar to that of blood plasma but it contains less protein.

Lymph is formed by plasma seeping out of the capillaries where it bathes all the body tissues. It creates the environment that cells need in order to survive. It acts as a medium of exchange for transferring food, oxygen and water (nutritive materials) and receives urea and carbon dioxide (waste products) in return. The lymphatic system is one-way; it returns fluid to the bloodstream, but cannot collect it from there.

Lymph capillaries and lacteals

Lymph capillaries have a single layer of endothelial cells. Their walls are more permeable than blood capillaries, enabling them to soak up proteins and cell debris.

Interesting fact

Antigen
A general term used for any foreign material.

Antibodies
Antibodies or immunoglobulins are small proteins produced by the B lymphocytes in the lymph nodes and spleen. Antibodies bind themselves to antigens. This process enables other components of the immune system to precisely direct their attack. There are actually five classes of antibodies.

Interesting fact

Lymph drainage
Approx. 2–4 litres ($3^1/_2$–$7^1/_2$ pints) of lymph is filtered back into the venous bloodstream every day. Lymph is very slow, moving only a few millimetres per minute compared to blood which can pump round at 4–6 litres per minute.

Blood

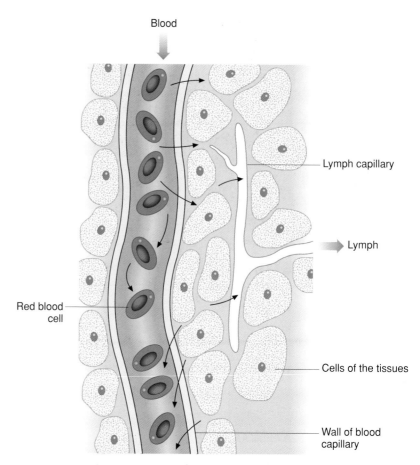

Lymph capillary

Lymph

Red blood cell

Cells of the tissues

Wall of blood capillary

Exchange of blood/tissue fluid

They are different from blood capillaries in that they have a blind end; blood capillaries have a venous and an arterial end, whereas lymph capillaries do not.

Inside the small intestine there are projections called villi. Villi contain a network of lymph capillaries called lacteals. Their function is to drain lymph from the small intestine. They also collect microscopic globules of fat from the small intestine; this gives lymph a milky appearance. Lymph returning back from the small intestine is called chyle. It travels through the lymphatic system before it is emptied into the bloodstream via the thoracic duct.

Lymph vessels

Large lymph vessels have numerous cup-shaped valves to keep the lymph flowing in the right direction. The lymphatic system, unlike the circulatory system, has no pump and mainly relies on muscular activity squeezing it back through the vessels towards the heart. The lymph vessels gradually get larger until finally the fluid is carried to the two largest vessels called lymph ducts. The thoracic duct drains lymph from both legs, the pelvic and abdominal cavities, the left half of the head, neck, thorax and left arm. The right lymphatic duct drains lymph from the right half of the head, neck, right arm and thorax.

Lymph is emptied into these two ducts after being filtered by the nodes and is then returned to the bloodstream via the subclavian veins.

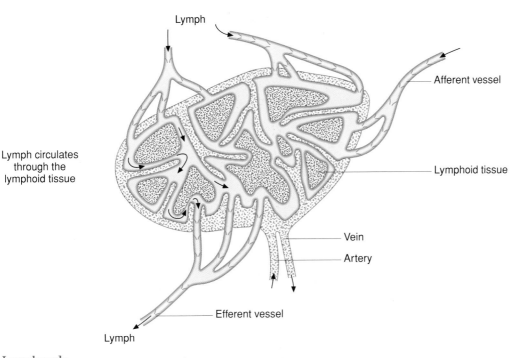

Lymph

Afferent vessel

Lymph circulates through the lymphoid tissue

Lymphoid tissue

Vein

Artery

Efferent vessel

Lymph

Lymph node

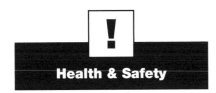

Lymph nodes

Lymph nodes vary considerably in size; some are as small as a pinhead and the largest about the size of an almond. They are situated in strategic positions throughout the body.

The main component of a node is reticular and lymphatic tissue which contains lymphocytes. These help to carry out the cleaning-up process. Lymph is filtered through several lymph nodes before it is returned to the venous bloodstream.

Major lymph nodes of the face

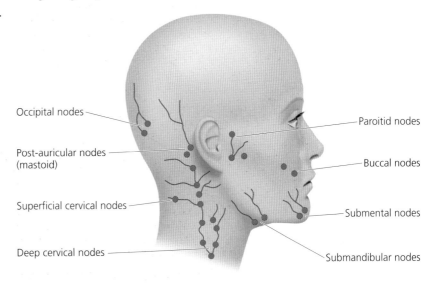

Occipital nodes

Paroitid nodes

Post-auricular nodes (mastoid)

Buccal nodes

Superficial cervical nodes

Submental nodes

Deep cervical nodes

Submandibular nodes

Lymph nodes face

Major lymph nodes in the body

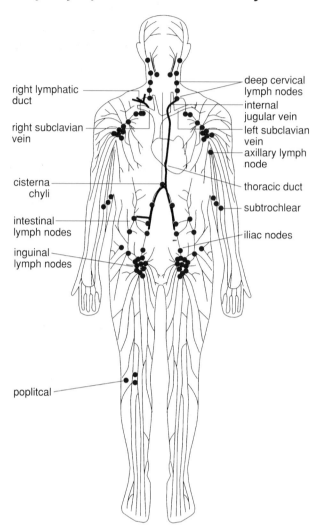

right lymphatic duct

right subclavian vein

cisterna chyli

intestinal lymph nodes

inguinal lymph nodes

poplitcal

deep cervical lymph nodes

internal jugular vein

left subclavian vein

axillary lymph node

thoracic duct

subtrochlear

iliac nodes

Lymph nodes body

Organs associated with the lymph system

Adenoids: A mass of lymphatic tissue at the rear of the nasal cavity. The two adenoids protect the upper part of the respiratory tract.

Tonsils: There are two tonsils at the back of the roof of the mouth, and a small pair (lingual tonsils) at the base of the tongue which are composed of lymphatic tissue. They help to protect the throat and airways from infection.

Thymus: A gland beneath the upper part of the sternum, lying close to the heart in the thoracic cavity. It is very large in young children but by adulthood it has become much smaller. The thymus gland produces T-lymphocyte cells. It is also involved with the endocrine system and produces several hormones important in early life to assist with growth and immunity.

Spleen: The largest of the lymph organs. It is found below the diaphragm, between the stomach and the duodenum. It contains lymph nodes, which produce lymphocytes and macrophages to fight infections. The spleen has several functions:

- erythrocytes are destroyed in the spleen and the by-products from the process passed on to the liver
- unwanted cellular materials are filtered and removed
- lymphocytes along with other blood cells are stored in the spleen and released when needed.

Disorders and diseases associated with the immune system

HIV (human immunodeficiency virus)

A person carrying HIV may not go on to develop AIDS (acquired immune deficiency syndrome). A carrier without symptoms is known as an asymtomatic carrier. An HIV carrier may experience the AIDS-related complex (ARC) which is a collection of symptoms and includes unexplained weight loss, fevers and swollen lymph glands but the individual does not yet have AIDS.

The virus is caught through direct contact with infected blood and semen, through sexual activities, sharing infected needles or, in the case of a foetus, from an HIV mother.

Cause: The HIV virus is a retro virus and infects the T-lymphocytes which are crucial for regulating the immune mechanism; this results in irreversible defects in immunity.

Treatment guidance: To treat or not? Unless there is a reason for testing, an individual may be a carrier and totally unaware. (A good reason for making sure you monitor your hygiene practices.) Because the treatments you are offering are not invasive you should not be at any risk, unless either of you have any open wounds.

Target nervous system, solar plexus, endocrine, lymph, circulatory reflexes.

AIDS (acquired immune deficiency syndrome)

With AIDS, the HIV virus has progressed and symptoms are established including fatigue and unexplained diarrhoea. HIV interferes with the immune system to make individuals susceptible to a variety of disease and cancers.

Treatment guidance: Refer to a GP who can refer the client to a specialized clinic which can cater for their treatment needs.

Hodgkin's disease

Progressive, painless swellings of the lymph nodes, which commonly starts in one of the nodes of the neck. Hodgkin's disease is a malignant disease and has no established cause.

Treatment guidance: Contra indicated; refer to GP.

Myalgic encephalitis (ME)

Also known as 'post viral syndrome' or 'chronic fatigue', some would dispute that ME is a separate disease. The condition commonly follows a viral infection of the upper respiratory tract, a gastrointestinal infection or glandular fever. There is believed to be a psychological link as tests rarely reveal any results. There has been some evidence however showing temporary changes in the brain tissue on MRI (magnetic resonance imaging) scans.

Symptoms: Chronic fatigue, malaise, depression, muscle pain, weakness, severe muscle fatigue, pins and needles, sleep disturbances, loss of concentration and nausea.

Treatment guidance: ME responds well to most holistic treatments, in particular reflexology, mainly because of the psychological boost. Symptoms typically tend to worsen before any improvement is felt.

Allergy

An allergy is an inappropriate response by the immune system to a substance (allergen) that is usually harmless to other people. An allergen may be ingested, inhaled or in contact with the skin and eyes. Allergens trigger the production of antibodies by the immune system, resulting in a variety of conditions. Not all allergic reactions are instant; some allergens cause sensitization that may take some time to build up in the body. Most allergies can be described as mild but others can be severe and even life threatening. On rare occasions a severe allergic reaction may result in anaphylactic shock where massive amounts of histamine are released into the body on exposure to the allergen. Symptoms include a sudden drop in blood pressure and constriction of the airways. Common causes are exposure to peanuts and insect stings. Emergency assistance should be sought immediately.

Treatment guidance: Hypersensitive individuals often know of their allergies and precautions can be taken in most cases. Patch test if necessary (see Chapter 10, p.224; also this chapter: hay fever, p.94, and urticaria, p.52).

Auto-immune disorders

Auto-immune disorders occur when the immune system produces antibodies against itself rather than to combat invading micro-organisms. The attack may be localized, e.g. vitiligo, or more general, e.g. multiple sclerosis, rheumatoid arthritis and lupus erythematosus. The exact reason why these changes occur is not yet fully understood.

Review also the individual disorders.

The skeletal system

Bone tissue

Bone is a rigid, non-elastic, connective tissue with cells called osteocytes. It is strengthened by the inorganic salts calcium and phosphate. Bone is the hardest tissue in the body.

Types of bone tissue

There are two types of bone tissue: cancellous or spongy, and compact (cortical) or hard bone. Hard bone forms the surface layer of all bones and the tubular shafts in long bones. Cancellous or spongy bone is found inside the hard bone. The spaces in spongy bone are usually filled with bone marrow where blood cells are formed.

Types of bone

- *Long bone:* these have a shaft (diaphysis) and are made of compact bone with a central canal. The ends (epiphyses) have an outer covering of compact bone with cancellous bone inside.
- *Short bone*, e.g. carpal.
- *Irregular*, e.g. vertebra.
- *Flat*, e.g. sternum, scapular, most skull bones.
- *Sesamoid,* e.g. patella.

Have a thin outer layer of compact bone with cancellous bone inside.

Haversian system

The Haversian system is a tubular arrangement of cells which gives bone its strength. Each structure consists of a central Haversian canal containing blood, lymph vessels and nerves surrounded by lamellae (lamellae are plates of bone tissue). There are further spaces between each structure, which contain lymph and osteocytes (bone cells).

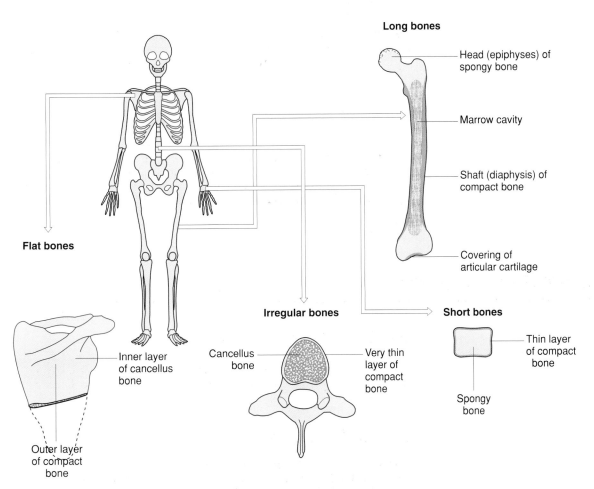

Long bones
— Head (epiphyses) of spongy bone
— Marrow cavity
— Shaft (diaphysis) of compact bone
— Covering of articular cartilage

Flat bones
Inner layer of cancellus bone
Outer layer of compact bone

Irregular bones
Cancellus bone
Very thin layer of compact bone

Short bones
Thin layer of compact bone
Spongy bone

Skeleton and types of bone

The skeleton

Functions of the skeleton

Support:

- maintains the shape of the body
- allows movement
- suspends the vital organs.

Attachment:

- bones have ridges to which muscles attach.

Protection:

- the skull protects the brain
- the spine protects the spinal cord
- the rib cage protects the heart and lungs.

Development of blood cells:

- all red blood cells and some of the white cells are made in the bone marrow.

Acts as a *calcium reservoir.*

The skeleton comprises 206 bones and is made up of two parts:

- the *axial skeleton* includes the skull, spine and thorax
- the *appendicular skeleton* includes the shoulder girdle, arms and hands, and the pelvic girdle, legs and feet.

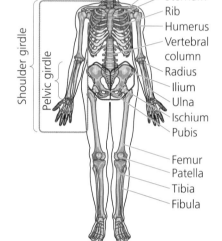

Cranium
Clavicle
Sternum
Rib
Humerus
Vertebral column
Radius
Ilium
Ulna
Ischium
Pubis
Femur
Patella
Tibia
Fibula

Shoulder girdle

Pelvic girdle

Skeleton

The axial skeleton

Skull

The skull consists of the cranium, which encloses and protects the brain. The cranium consists of 8 bones, which are fused together. There are also 14 facial bones.

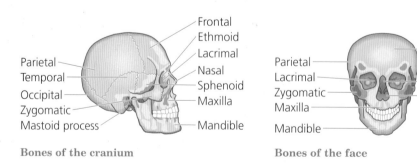

Parietal
Temporal
Occipital
Zygomatic
Mastoid process
Frontal
Ethmoid
Lacrimal
Nasal
Sphenoid
Maxilla
Mandible

Bones of the cranium

Parietal
Lacrimal
Zygomatic
Maxilla
Mandible
Frontal
Temporal
Nasal
Vomer

Bones of the face

The spine

The spine comprises 33 bones, 24 of which are moveable:

- cervical × 7
- thoracic × 12
- lumbar × 5

- sacrum × 5 (fused)
- coccyx × 4 (fused).

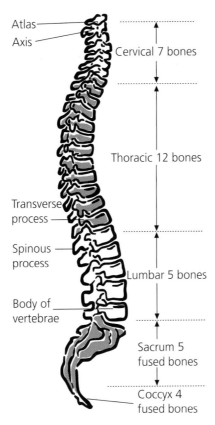

Atlas

Axis

Cervical 7 bones

Thoracic 12 bones

Transverse process

Spinous process

Lumbar 5 bones

Body of vertebrae

Sacrum 5 fused bones

Coccyx 4 fused bones

Vertebral column lateral view

Each vertebra has common features but each region of the spine has a specific shaped vertebrae.

The thorax

The thorax is the protective cavity for the chest and includes the ribs and sternum

The effects of spinal misalignment

The normal functioning of the body can be disturbed by misalignments of the vertebrae contributing or causing certain conditions. Such faults put pressure on both the nerves and blood supply to the surrounding tissues. Alternatively they may distend tissues to put pressure on the nerves, as with sciatica.

The appendicular skeleton

The shoulder girdle

Includes the scapulae, clavicle, humerus, ulna, radius and the bones of the hand.

The bones of the hand

- The fingers and thumbs are made up of 14 phalanges.
- The palm of the hand comprises 5 metacarpal bones.
- The wrist comprises 8 carpal bones.
- The forearm has two bones: the ulna, which runs in line with the little finger, and the radius, which is in line with the thumb.

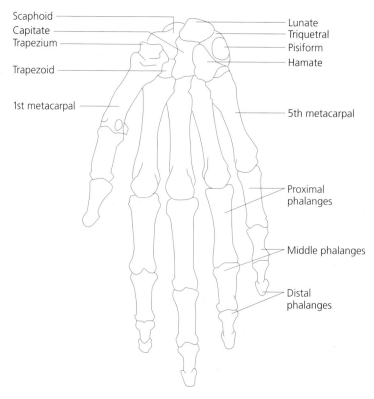

Scaphoid
Capitate
Trapezium

Trapezoid

1st metacarpal

Lunate
Triquetral
Pisiform
Hamate

5th metacarpal

Proximal
phalanges

Middle phalanges

Distal
phalanges

Bones of the hand

Interesting fact

The innominate bone
This is formed from three fused bones, the ilium, ischium and the pubis.

The pelvic girdle

Comprises the sacrum and the pelvis (formed from the two innominate bones).

The bones of the lower limb

These comprise the femur, patella, tibia, fibula and the bones of the foot.

The bones of the foot

- 14 phalanges make up the toes
- 5 metatarsals run from the ball of the foot to the
- 7 tarsals.

Cartilage

Cartilage is a special type of firm connective tissue. There are three types of cartilage: hyaline, fibrocartilage and elastic fibrocartilage.

Ligaments

Ligaments are made up of strings of connective tissue consisting of collagen. Their function is to hold together neighbouring bones where they meet to form a joint. Some ligaments hold bones together so tightly that they can hardly move; others are looser and allow the bones to change position. Ligaments are extremely strong, although they sometimes tear through injury, but it would take a very powerful pull to break them.

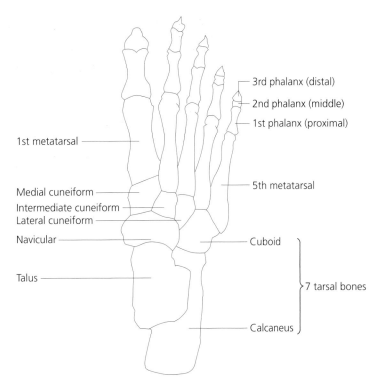

Bones of the foot

Joints

A joint is formed where two bones meet. Joints are classified by their structure or by the way they move.

- *Fibrous* or *fixed joints*, e.g. the skull. These joints, as their name suggests, are immovable.
- *Cartilaginous* or *slightly moveable joints*, e.g. joints between the vertebrae. They have a pad of fibrocartilage between the ends of the bones. This allows only a very slight movement.
- *Synovial* or *freely moveable joints*.

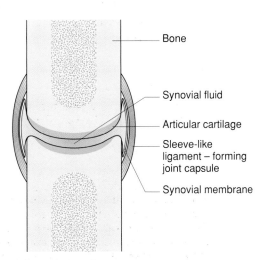

Typical synovial joint

Types of joints

Type of joint	Examples	Movement
Ball and socket joints	Hip and shoulder	Flexion, extension, adduction, abduction, rotation, circumduction
Condyloid/ellipsoidal joints	Wrist, ankle	Flexion, extension, adduction, abduction, circumduction
Gliding joints	Intercarpal and intertarsal joints	Movements limited to gliding or shifting
Hinge joints	Elbow, ankle, interphalangeal joints	Flexion and extension only
Pivot joints	Radio-ulna joint, atlas and axis	Rotation
Saddle joints	Carpo-metacarpal joint of thumb (base)	Flexion, extension, adduction, abduction, rotation (limited), circumduction

 Interesting fact

Bursa
These are little sacs of synovial fluid which are present in some joints e.g. the shoulder and act as a cushion between the bone and ligament.

Synovial joints are flexible and allow free movement between two bones. The bones that are in contact are covered with a special cartilage called hyaline cartilage. This provides a smooth articular surface. A sleeve of fibrous tissue called the capsular ligament surrounds the joint, holding the bones together. It allows movement and protects the joint from injury.

The synovial membrane lines the capsule and is composed of epithelial cells. These cells secrete synovial fluid into the capsule to act as a lubricant. The synovial fluid gives the joint stability and prevents it from being separated; it is also responsible for supplying nutrients to the surrounding tissues. Ligaments around the joints provide further stability and prevent the joint being dislocated. Supporting muscles and tendons stretch across the joint when movement takes place.

The six synovial joints are shown in the table above.

The arches of the foot

The bones of the foot are arranged to create a flexible bridge-like structure supported by 19 muscles and 107 ligaments. The arches of the foot distribute the weight of the body between the ball of the foot and the heel.

There are four arches in the foot:

- 1 medial longitudinal arch
- 1 lateral longitudinal arch
- 2 transverse arches (anterior and posterior).

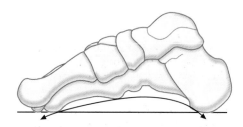

Arches of the foot

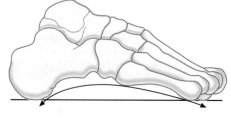 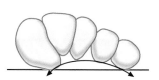

Arches of the foot (bones)

Conditions, disorders and diseases of the skeletal system

Fractures

A fracture is a crack or break in a bone.

Symptoms: Pain, swelling, tenderness and possible deformity in the bone shape.

Treatment guidance: The area is contra indicated until the fracture is healed. Massage is useful after the recovery period to ease stiffness and drain possible oedema if the area has been immobile. Remember that the older the client the slower the healing process.

Osteoporosis

With osteoporosis the amount of bone tissue is reduced causing it to become brittle and easily fractured. It is caused by an inability to replace bone during the normal process of bone replacement as it is naturally reabsorbed. The disease is associated with ageing, steroids, a high protein diet, poor exercise and hysterectomy. The condition may be progressive or temporary.

Symptoms: There may be no obvious symptoms. The first indication of any change in the bone mass may be after a fracture. Bone tissue which has been lost cannot be replaced easily and so the aim is to minimize any further loss. Regular sustained exercise is very beneficial as it helps to build and support the bones.

Treatment guidance: Avoid percussion and heavy movements. If you suspect osteoporosis, recommend that the client has a scan.

Osteomalacia

A demineralization of bone tissue due to a deficiency in vitamin D. It presents with similar symptoms to osteoporosis.

Arthritis

A disease of the joints of which there are several different types.

Rheumatoid arthritis

Rheumatoid arthritis (RA) is an auto-immune disorder where the body's immune system damages the synovial joints and its surrounding soft tissue. A chronic progressive inflammatory disease is the result.

Symptoms: Inflammation of the synovial joints of the hands and feet; in severe cases most of the synovial joints of the body are affected. The condition may flare up and then go into remission. The joints are damaged causing deformity, pain and loss of movement.

Osteoarthritis

Osteoarthritis is a common degenerative, non-inflammatory disease causing restricted movement and pain in the affected joints. The articular cartilage thins and eventually the articular surfaces degenerate through surface contact with each other. Usually associated with general wear and tear but other factors contribute.

Symptoms: Pain, swelling, stiffness and enlarged joints with possible loss of joint function. Commonly affects the hips, spine and knees. A reduction in the ability to use the joint causes further weakness.

Ankylosing spondylitis

Ankylosing spondylitis is an inflammatory disease which affects the joints between the vertebra of the spine and the pelvis.

Symptoms: Pain and stiffness in the lower back and hips, which is worse after inactivity and rest.

Treatment guidance (for all arthritic conditions): In milder cases, avoid the affected joints and massage above the affected area. In more severe cases refer to GP.

Target the immune system.

Gout

A metabolic disorder that causes attacks of arthritis, usually in a particular joint. Uric acid crystals are deposited in the joints and tendons. Only a single attack may be experienced or the condition can recur, resulting in progressively more joints being affected and damaged.

Gout is caused by high blood uric acid, either through overproduction or defective kidneys. The condition is more common in men than women.

Symptoms: Usually a single joint is affected (commonly the big toe); the joint becomes red, swollen and very tender. Pain may be intense so that no pressure can be tolerated on the joint.

Treatment guidance: Contra indicated during an attack. Ensure further checks have been given to the client. Diet is known to affect the condition so this should be monitored.

Spondylosis

Non-inflammatory wear and tear of the spine.

Symptoms: Normally none.

Treatment guidance: Caution when working over the affected area.

Skeletal terminology

The surface of all bones is very irregular and show a number of projections and depressions according to function.

Articular projections are smooth and form part of a joint. These include

- **head** when round like a sphere of disc
- **condyle** smooth oval projection of bone, which takes part in a joint.

Non-articular – are rough and give attachment to muscles and ligaments

- **process** rough projection for muscle attachment
- **spine** pointed rough projection, sharp ridge of bone
- **tuberosity** (large) ⎫
- **trochanter** (medium) ⎬ broad rough bony projection
- **tubercle** (small) ⎭
- **crest** long rough narrow projecting face/ridge

Non-articular depressions

- **fossa** a notch (hollow or depression) in a bone
- **groove** long narrow depression

Other terms

- **foramen** hole in structure
- **sinus** a hollow cavity in bone
- **border** a ridge of bone separating two surfaces

Bursitis

Inflammation of the bursa, a fluid-filled sac lying between bone and tendon the role of which is to prevent friction. Bursitis is usually as a result of friction or slight injury to the membrane surrounding the joint. It may also be caused by a bacterial infection.

Treatment guidance: Direct treatment is contra indicated. Allow joint to rest for a few days until the swelling has gone down. Home care advice is to apply ice.

Bunion (Halux vulgus)

Bunions occur when the base of the big toe bulges away from the foot causing the toe to displace and turn in. The skin over the joint becomes thickened, red and often painful. A bursa often forms due to pressure on the joint. There is some tendency towards bunions being hereditary. However, poor fitting shoes are the most likely contributor.

Treatment guidance: Avoid joint if painful; keep movements gentle.

The muscular system

Interesting fact

Muscles of the body
There are 640 named muscles in our body, 140 of these in the head and neck alone!

Tip

See Appendix 2 on page 453 for major muscle table.

Interesting fact

Skeletal muscle
Skeletal muscles account for between 40–50% of our body weight.

Functions of the muscular system

- Movement both internal and external occurs as a result of the shortening (contracting) and lengthening (extending) of muscles.
- Maintenance of posture.
- Heat production.
- Assists in venous return and lymph circulation.
- Some protection of abdominal organs.
- Defines our individual body shape.

Types of muscular tissue

There are three types of muscular tissue:

- *skeletal, striated* or *voluntary muscle*: under conscious control
- *cardiac muscle*: found exclusively in the heart
- *smooth* or *involuntary muscle*: not under conscious control.

Skeletal, striated or voluntary muscles

- Each muscle is made up of thousands of long cylindrical cells or fibres.
- A single muscle fibre is made up of large number of threads called myofibrils.
- Myofibrils consist of rows of minute protein filaments called actin and myosin; these lie side by side giving the muscle a striped appearance.
- These fibres are enclosed in a tough sheath of connective tissue. The sheath carries blood vessels and nerves to the muscles.

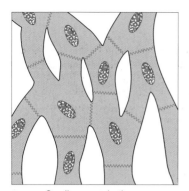

Cardiac muscle tissue

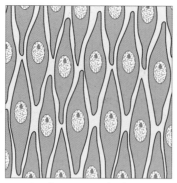

Involuntary muscle tissue

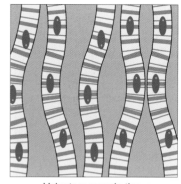

Voluntary muscle tissue

Types of muscular tissue

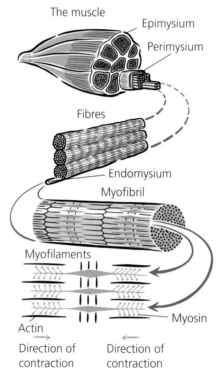

The muscle
Epimysium
Perimysium
Fibres
Endomysium
Myofibril
Myofilaments
Actin
Myosin
Direction of contraction
Direction of contraction

Skeletal muscle structure

- Each fibre is linked to the central nervous system (CNS) by a tiny nerve. Motor nerves carry messages from the CNS to the muscles to stimulate them into action.
- Fibres are grouped in bundles of 20–40, enclosed in a further connective sheath.
- The complete muscle is covered by a connective tissue layer called the fascia.

Cardiac muscle

Cardiac muscle is similar to skeletal muscle fibres but not identical. The fibres are striated. Each muscle cell has a close relationship with the next cell to ensure rapid and uniform spread of muscular contraction throughout the heart tissue. There is a small mass of specialized cardiac cells embedded in the wall of the right atrium that acts as the heart's pacemaker, regulating the heartbeat.

Smooth or involuntary muscle

Smooth muscle is found in the walls of hollow organs, i.e. blood and lymph vessels, the alimentary canal, respiratory tract, bladder, uterus and in the ducts of glands. Smooth muscle cells are small and structurally different from voluntary muscle cells. The fibres have the ability to contract spontaneously in a rhythmical fashion. They are constantly regulated by the autonomic nervous system and by hormones.

Tendons

A tendon attaches the ends of the muscle to bone or skin and is composed of fibrous connective tissue. When a tendon is pulled it moves the joint. Some tendons are broad and flat and are called aponeuroses (e.g. occipital joined to frontalis by the epicranial aponeurosis).

The fixed attachment of a muscle is known as the origin; the moveable point is known as the insertion.

How muscles work

When muscles require energy, a process called glycolysis (a series of metabolic pathways) takes place using glycogen and oxygen. Glucose is transported to the muscles by the circulation and stored as glycogen until it is needed. Adenosine triphosphate (ATP) is formed when these energy-providing molecules are broken down in the cells and is used to provide energy. If there is not enough oxygen to keep this process going, energy depletes and fatigue sets in. Carbon dioxide and water are produced as waste products from this process.

Muscle fatigue

Muscle fatigue occurs in the following instances.

- Fatigue is a result of overuse of a muscle. Muscle contractions become weaker and the muscle may begin to quiver.
- Lactic acid, carbon dioxide and waste products build up in the muscle.

Stretching exercises can help to encourage the natural process of waste removal. Massage also encourages removal by assisting lymphatic drainage and the circulation.

Muscle contraction

Muscles contract or shorten when stimulated to do so by the CNS, which carries a message via a motor nerve to a motor neurone in the muscle fibre. The more fibres that are stimulated, the shorter the muscle will become and the stronger the contraction will be.

Muscle tone

Some of the muscle fibres even when at rest remain in a contracted state. This is essential for maintaining posture. Muscle tone ensures an adequate blood supply to the muscles.

Poor muscle tone indicates undersized muscles that fatigue easily and are generally slow and weak on contraction. *Excessive tone* indicates overly tense muscles due to overdevelopment, which can lead to a shortening of the muscle tissue. The full range of muscle extension and joint movement may be limited as a result.

Muscles of the face and body

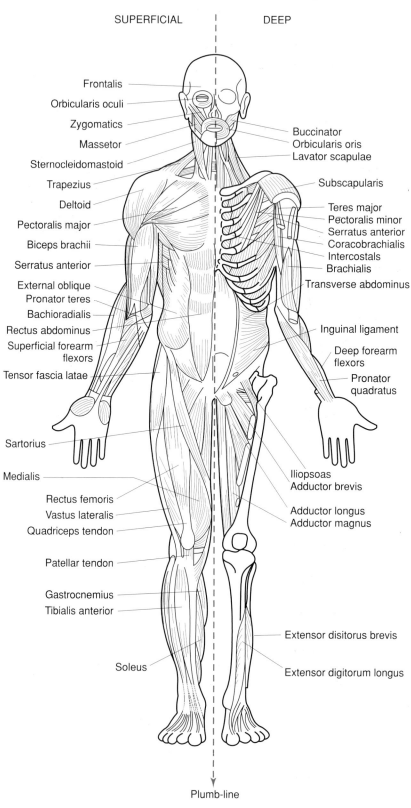

SUPERFICIAL   DEEP

Frontalis
Orbicularis oculi
Zygomatics
Massetor
Sternocleidomastoid
Trapezius
Deltoid
Pectoralis major
Biceps brachii
Serratus anterior
External oblique
Pronator teres
Bachioradialis
Rectus abdominus
Superficial forearm flexors
Tensor fascia latae
Sartorius
Medialis
Rectus femoris
Vastus lateralis
Quadriceps tendon
Patellar tendon
Gastrocnemius
Tibialis anterior
Soleus

Buccinator
Orbicularis oris
Lavator scapulae
Subscapularis
Teres major
Pectoralis minor
Serratus anterior
Coracobrachialis
Intercostals
Brachialis
Transverse abdominus
Inguinal ligament
Deep forearm flexors
Pronator quadratus
Iliopsoas
Adductor brevis
Adductor longus
Adductor magnus
Extensor disitorus brevis
Extensor digitorum longus

Plumb-line

Major muscles (anterior view)

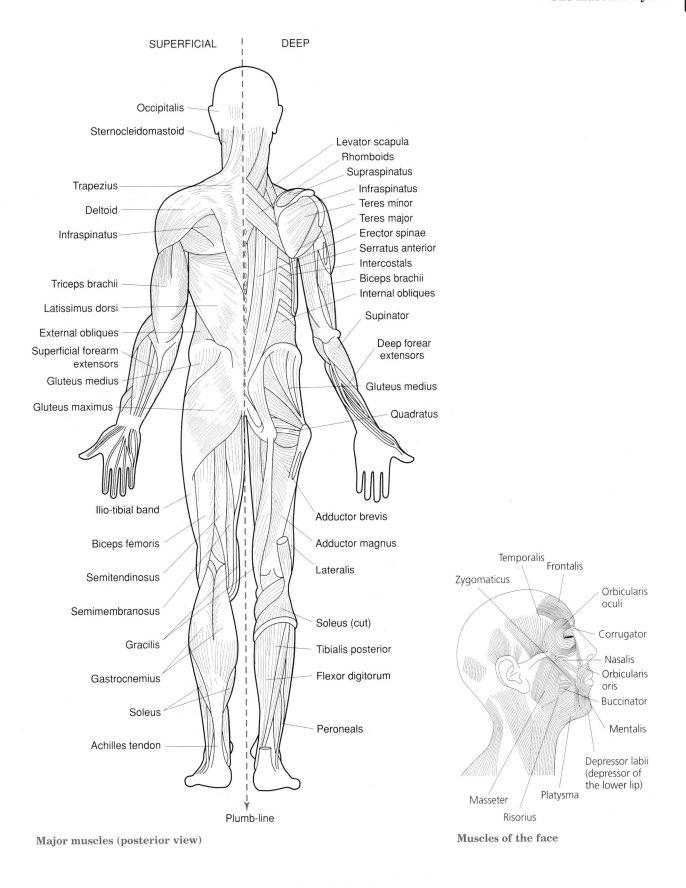

SUPERFICIAL   DEEP

Occipitalis

Sternocleidomastoid

Levator scapula
Rhomboids
Supraspinatus
Infraspinatus
Teres minor
Teres major
Erector spinae
Serratus anterior
Intercostals
Biceps brachii
Internal obliques

Trapezius

Deltoid

Infraspinatus

Triceps brachii

Latissimus dorsi

External obliques

Superficial forearm
extensors

Gluteus medius

Gluteus maximus

Supinator

Deep forear
extensors

Gluteus medius

Quadratus

Ilio-tibial band

Biceps femoris

Semitendinosus

Semimembranosus

Gracilis

Gastrocnemius

Soleus

Achilles tendon

Adductor brevis

Adductor magnus

Lateralis

Soleus (cut)

Tibialis posterior

Flexor digitorum

Peroneals

Plumb-line

Major muscles (posterior view)

Temporalis   Frontalis

Zygomaticus

Orbicularis
oculi

Corrugator

Nasalis

Orbicularis
oris

Buccinator

Mentalis

Depressor labii
(depressor of
the lower lip)

Masseter   Platysma

Risorius

Muscles of the face

Muscular disorders

Causes of muscular pain

Capsulitis

Capsulitis is a condition occurring when the capsule of a joint becomes inflamed. It is commonly found in the shoulder, where it may be called 'frozen shoulder'.

Treatment guidance: Allow joint to rest for a few days until the swelling has gone down before applying direct treatment.

Sprains

A sprain is caused when a sudden pull causes the ligament to tear or overstretch. The fibrous capsule may also be damaged. A partial tear takes 4–6 weeks to repair. If the ligament is ruptured it may need surgery.

Symptoms: Swelling and pain on movement.

Treatment guidance: Direct contra indication. You can work above the injury to improve drainage. Once the swelling has subsided gentle effleurage with pressure increasing as the injury improves.

Muscle soreness

Stiffness after doing unfamiliar or excessive exercise occurs 24 hours after the activity and usually peaks at 48 hours. This type of pain should be gone in 72 hours; if not, it may be the result of muscular strain or other injury.

Treatment guidance: Massage is beneficial for alleviating the symptoms; incorporate lots of drainage and effleurage.

Muscle strain

A strain is the result of a tear or overstretching of some of the muscle fibres:

- mild strain takes 2–14 days to heal
- severe strain takes 3–6 weeks to heal.

Treatment guidance: As for sprains, above.

Tendonitis

Inflammation of a tendon within its sheath. Usually due to repetitive stress or abnormal weight lifting.

Treatment guidance: As for sprains, above.

Disorders affecting both the muscular and nervous systems

Spasticity

A marked increase in the rigidity of a group of muscles, associated with damage to the motor neurones. The muscles become stiff and movement becomes restricted. Medical conditions where spasticity may be present include multiple sclerosis and Parkinson's disease. In spastic paralysis the muscles are ridged, and there is inability to move the muscles and the affected part of the body. Medical conditions where paralysis may be present include cerebral palsy and multiple sclerosis.

Treatment guidance: Dependent on the severity of the condition. You will need to consider the client's safety and how best to position them. It may only be possible to give a limited treatment.

Repetitive strain injury (RSI)

A term used to describe different types of soft tissue injury resulting from overuse. It includes carpal tunnel syndrome and tendonitis. Symptoms include pain and weakness in the wrist and fingers. The condition affects keyboard users, musicians and massage therapists.

Treatment guidance: Complete rest is recommended. Effleurage and deep tissue work of forearm muscles. Acupuncture may be useful.

Disorders affecting both the muscular and skeletal systems

Whiplash

Injury of the soft tissue, ligaments and spinal joints of the neck. Caused by the neck being forcibly or violently bent forwards then backwards (or vice versa). It is associated with car accidents but also occurs with head injuries. The damage is usually a minor sprain of the neck ligaments, however, in severe cases the vertebra may be fractured.

Symptoms: Neck pain and stiffness, which generally occurs 24 hours after the injury.

Treatment guidance: Refer to GP before soft tissue treatments.

After injury the neck is commonly immobilized. Osteopathy or physiotherapy is recommended. It may take several weeks to recover.

Rheumatism

See rheumatoid arthritis, p.83.

Hammer toes

Deformity of the first phalanx, which results in the toe to remaining bent up. It is caused by an abnormality of tendons in the toe. May be associated with ballet dancers.

Interesting fact

Pes
The term pes is used as a prefix and relates to the foot or any deformity of the foot e.g.

- Pes malleus valgus: hammer toe
- Pes planus: flat foot.

The respiratory system

The respiratory system consists of the following structures:

- nose
- pharynx
- larynx
- trachea
- bronchi
- alveoli
- lungs.

The nose

There are two nasal cavities. Each is lined with tiny hairs called cilia, which begin to filter the incoming air. The mucous membranes lining the cavity secrete a sticky fluid called mucus. Mucus helps to prevent dust and bacteria from entering the lungs. The nose has a role in the sense of smell.

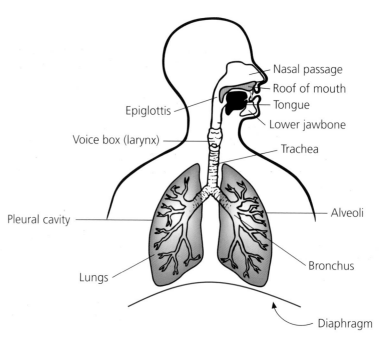

The respiratory system

The naso-pharynx is the upper part of the nasal cavity behind the nose. Air is moistened, warmed and filtered.

The pharynx

The pharynx is commonly known as the throat. It is a large cavity, 10 cm long, which lies behind the mouth and between the nasal cavity and the larynx. The pharynx continues to warm and moisten air as it passes through. The pharynx is both an air and food passage but cannot be used for both purposes at the same time or choking would result.

The larynx

The larynx is a short passage which connects the pharynx to the trachea. The vocal cords are located here. The larynx provides a passageway for air between the pharynx and the trachea.

The trachea

The trachea or windpipe is made up mainly of cartilage, which helps to keep the trachea permanently open. The trachea passes down into the chest and connects the larynx with the bronchi.

The bronchi

The bronchi are two short tubes that lead to and carry air into each lung. They are similar in structure to the trachea. The bronchi are also lined with mucous membranes and ciliated cells (cilia) which trap particles. Cilia move the particles upwards, preventing dirt from entering the delicate lung tissue. Like the trachea the bronchi contain cartilage to hold them open. The bronchi subdivide into bronchioles in the lungs. The bronchioles further divide yet again and finally end in alveoli.

Alveoli

Alveoli are minute air-filled sacs. They are only one cell thick and are the site of exchange of the gases oxygen and carbon dioxide.

The lungs

The lungs are cone-shaped, spongy organs situated in the thoracic cavity, one on either side of the heart. The function of the lungs is to facilitate the exchange of oxygen and carbon dioxide. The lungs are covered with an outer membrane called the pleura. This prevents any friction between the lungs and the chest wall.

The interchange of gases in the lungs

This process involves the absorption of oxygen from the air in exchange for carbon dioxide, which is released by the body as a waste product of cell metabolism.

- Oxygen is drawn in through the nose and mouth along the trachea and bronchial tubes to the alveoli of the lungs. The inspired air is rich with oxygen. Here it diffuses through a thin film of moisture lining the alveoli.

- The molecules come into close contact with the blood in the capillary network surrounding the alveoli.

- The oxygen then diffuses across a permeable membrane wall surrounding the alveoli to be taken up by red blood cells and carried to the heart.

- Carbon dioxide, collected from the respiring cells around the body, passes in the opposite direction by diffusing from the capillary walls into the alveoli, passes through to the bronchi, trachea and eventually is exhaled through the nose and mouth.

During inspiration, when we breathe in, the diaphragm (a large muscle) contracts, increasing the volume of the thoracic cavity and filling the lungs with air. The external intercostal muscles located between each of the ribs contract, pulling the ribs up and outwards.

During expiration, when we breathe out, air leaves the lungs due to relaxation of the diaphragm. If the body needs to force air out during physical exertion the internal intercostal muscles contract assisted by the abdominal muscles.

Interesting fact

Lung capacity
The lung when fully inflated can hold 4.4 litres of air, but only $\frac{1}{2}$ a litre of air is taken up during restful breathing. Even during strenuous exercise we will only use about 2 litres of the potential capacity.

Interesting fact

Rate of breathing
- Controlled by respiratory centre of brain and is regulated according to levels of CO_2 in blood

- On average we take 12 to 20 breaths per minute

- The level of activity increases both the rate and depth of breathing.

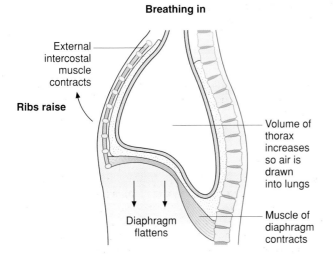

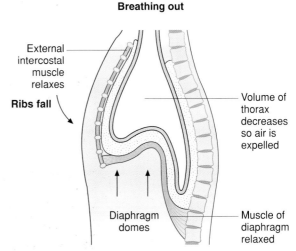

Inspiration and expiration

Conditions, disorders and diseases of the respiratory system

Asthma

Recurrent attacks of breathlessness and wheezing caused by inflammation of the bronchi. During an attack the lining of the bronchi become swollen and the airways become constricted, reducing the amount of airflow both in and out the lungs. There is an excessive secretion of mucus which further restricts airflow. The severity of attacks varies, as does duration. Asthma can start at any age but characteristically begins in childhood.

Other factors which are known to trigger an asthma attack in those who are susceptible are cold air, emotional stress, strenuous exercise and an infection of the upper respiratory tract.

Symptoms: Breathlessness, wheezing, dry cough and a tight feeling in the chest.

Types of asthma

There are two types of asthma:

- **extrinsic** develops in childhood and is caused by a hypersensitivity to an allergen. These include house dust, animal fur, pollen, tobacco smoke, air pollution or a food allergy
- **intrinsic** develops later in life and is associated with a chronic inflammation of the upper respiratory tract.

During an asthma attack inspiration is relatively normal but there is difficulty in expiration, causing the lungs to become hyper-inflated. In a more severe attack breathing becomes increasingly difficult, causing distress, anxiety, rapid heartbeat and sweating. There are occasions when the attack is so severe that the amount of oxygen in the blood becomes critically low and urgent medical assistance is required.

Treatment guidance: Stop treatment if an attack occurs.

Bronchitis

Bronchitis is an inflammation of the bronchi. An attack may be described as acute or chronic:

- *acute*: sudden onset and short in duration; caused by a viral or bacterial infection or air pollution
- *chronic*: persistent bronchitis; associated with lung disease or smoking.

Symptoms: Wheezing and shortness of breath, persistent, possibly painful chesty cough with yellow or green phlegm (acute).

Treatment guidance: With acute bronchitis rest is recommended.

Hay fever

Hay fever is a seasonal inflammation of the mucus membranes lining the nose due to an allergy to pollen.

Symptoms: Sneezing, runny nose, congested nasal cavities, itching sensation in the throat and eyes.

Treatment guidance: Target respiratory, adrenal and immune systems.

The digestive system

Food, whether liquid or solid, needs to be processed by the digestive organs. Before the body can absorb nutrients they have to be broken down by specialized proteins called enzymes.

Enzymes speed up the breakdown of a substance, and once this has happened the small molecules can be absorbed into the body. The nutrients are circulated to provide energy and raw materials required for growth and repair of body structures. Food that cannot be digested becomes waste material and is expelled from the body by defecation (urination).

The digestive system comprises two parts:

1 The *alimentary canal* or *gastrointestinal tract*. This is a long tube (approx. 9 metres in length). It commences at the mouth and ends at the anus. It includes the:

- mouth
- pharynx and oesophagus
- stomach
- small intestine: duodenum, jejunum, ileum
- large intestine: caecum, appendix, colon, rectum and anus.

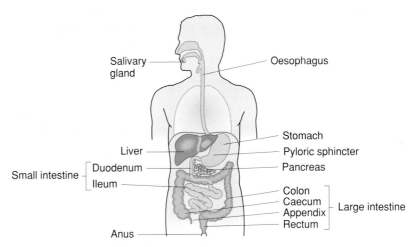

The digestive system

2 *Accessory organs*
- liver
- gall bladder
- pancreas.

The alimentary canal/ gastrointestinal tract

Mouth

In the mouth food is cut, chewed and ground down by the teeth as it is mixed with saliva.

Saliva is secreted from three pairs of salivary glands connected to the mouth. It is a slightly acidic solution of salts containing a number of components. It helps food move down the throat by forming it into a soft mass or bolus.

Pharynx

Also known as the throat. Approximately 12 to 14 cm long it lies behind the nose, mouth and larynx (voice box).

Oesophagus

The oesophagus is a thick-walled muscular tube about 24 cm long. It carries food from the mouth to the stomach by peristalsis. These are waves of contraction and relaxation in the muscles, which propel the food along.

Stomach

The main function of the stomach is to store food, to begin protein digestion and to control the entry of food into the duodenum. The stomach is a J-shaped muscular bag which lies beneath the diaphragm. It churns food and mixes it with gastric juices secreted by the gastric glands in the stomach lining to form chyme, a soup-like mixture of liquid and small particles. Food usually stays in the stomach for about four hours before the partly digested food leaves the stomach and passes into the duodenum, beginning with carbohydrates, followed by proteins and finally the fats.

Small intestine

The small intestine includes the duodenum, jejunum and ileum. It is about 3 m long and 4 cm in width. The main task of the small intestine is to continue digestion and absorption. Nutrients and water begin to be absorbed into the bloodstream.

There are a variety of digestive juices that are secreted into the small intestines including bile, pancreatic juice and intestinal juice. Absorption of digested food mainly takes place in the ileum. The surface area of the ileum is greatly increased by villi – tiny projections that contain a network of capillaries and lymph vessels called lacteals. This huge surface area absorbs nutrients into the blood and lymph vessels.

Large intestine

The large intestine is made up of the caecum (appendix), colon, rectum and anus.

It is approximately 1.4 m long and about 6.4 cm in width. The main function of the colon is to convert liquid from the small intestine into faeces. It does not carry out digestion but does absorb small amounts of digested food. Mucus is produced to help lubricate the passage of faeces, which it also stores.

The colon making up the main part of the large intestine is divided into four parts:

- ascending colon
- transverse colon
- descending colon
- sigmoid colon.

The main function of the colon is to absorb water (it absorbs 90%), turning the liquid entering the colon into a solid mass – faeces. The rectum is the last part of the large intestine. It is a short chamber about 4 inches long and its function is to hold the faeces. Muscles contract to remove faeces by expulsion through the anus.

Interesting fact

First foods to be absorbed
Alcohol, water and glucose are absorbed into the blood stream directly from the stomach.

Interesting fact

Villi
The combined surface of all the villi in the intestine creates an area the size of a tennis court.

Interesting fact

Gut bacteria/flora
Not all bacteria are bad! We have around 1.4 kg of bacteria in the gut. There are between 300–400 different bacteria inside us. These assist in the breakdown of some foods.

Accessory organs

Liver

The liver is located in the upper right-hand side of the abdomen under the diaphragm. It is a vital organ with several major functions.

- *Regulation of blood sugar levels:* absorbs excess glucose and stores it as glycogen, releasing it when blood sugar levels fall.
- *Regulation of fat metabolism:* converts fats into a form that can be stored or broken down to release energy.
- *Vitamin storage:* including A, D and B12.
- *Mineral storage.*
- *Protein metabolism:* amino acids are collected and either used to make proteins or broken down if not required.
- *Bile production:* bile is an alkaline consisting of water, mineral salts, mucus, bilirubin (bile pigments), bile salts and cholesterol, the main function of which is to emulsify (break up) fat droplets.
- *Regulation of toxic substances:* toxic substances such as drugs, poisons and waste products are removed from the blood, broken down and converted into safer substances.
- *Hormone breakdown:* removes hormones not required from the blood.
- *Excretory function:* breaks down old red blood cells.
- *Heat production:* a result of the cellular activity within the liver.

Gall bladder

The gall bladder is a small, muscular sac lying underneath the liver. Its functions are to store and excrete bile from the liver. Approximately 400–1000 ml of bile is produced daily.

Pancreas

The pancreas is a gland, about 12–14 cm in length. It lies adjacent to the duodenum and stretches upwards behind the stomach. Its functions are to:

- produce pancreatic juices rich in enzymes that break down carbohydrates, proteins, fats and nucleic acids in the duodenum
- produce the hormones insulin and glucagon which control the level of glucose in the blood.

Disorders and diseases of the digestive system

Coeliac disease

Coeliac disease is the result of an abnormal immune reaction to the protein gluten (found in wheat, rye, barley and other cereals). The body destroys the villi in the small intestine causing problems in absorption of nutrients. This disease has a hereditary tendency.

Symptoms: Severity of the disease varies, with some individuals never developing problematic symptoms while others develop symptoms over a number of years or suddenly. Symptoms include bulky, pale, greasy, smelly faeces, tiredness, weight loss, abdominal pain, diarrhoea, vomiting, anaemia and in some a distinctive skin rash.

Treatment guidance: If the hypersensitivity extends to the skin avoid using wheat- (or cereal-)based oils.

Inflammatory bowel disease (IBD)

Crohn's disease

A chronic inflammatory disease which can affect any part of the gastrointestinal tract. There is patchy inflammation causing thickening of the intestinal walls; pus-filled ulcers may also be present. The cause of Crohn's disease is uncertain but it is linked with an adverse immune response.

Symptoms: Spasmodic pain, sickness, diarrhoea, anaemia and weight loss.

Colitis

A chronic inflammatory disease of the colon and rectum that eventually results in ulceration and infection. Colitis may be caused by an infection and occasionally antibiotics.

Symptoms: Diarrhoea, often with blood and mucus; abdominal pain and fever.

Diverticular disease

Diverticular are pouches of intestine that protrude externally into the abdomen. When the pouches become ruptured and inflamed diverticulitis occurs, resulting in abscesses forming in the surrounding tissue. Faeces can become trapped and stagnate, causing inflammation.

Symptoms: Abdominal pain, vomiting and fever; there may be bleeding from the rectum.

Treatment guidance (IBD): Avoid abdominal massage if the client is experiencing discomfort.

Irritable bowel syndrome (IBS)

IBS is a distressing change in bowel habits which on investigation shows no known disease. The involuntary muscle of the large intestine becomes erratic in its function although there is no abnormality in its structure. Influencing factors include:

- *dietary*: food intolerance to milk, wheat, yeast or hydrogenated fats, a diet high in refined foods and sugar and too little fibre
- candida albicans and laxative abuse
- hormones and stress.

To establish a cause the client needs to be prepared totally to re-evaluate their diet and what they eat.

Symptoms: An intermittent cramping pain with abdominal bloating, flatulence, diarrhoea, constipation or a fluctuation between both. Additional symptoms may include back ache, agitation, tiredness, loss of appetite, weakness and fatigue.

Treatment guidance: If the client has not been to their GP, advise them to do so in order to rule out any other cause.

Interesting fact

IBS
Irritable bowel syndrome affects 10–20% of adults and is twice as common in women as in men.

Interesting fact

Candida
Around 1/3 of the population suffer with candida albican complications such as IBS and thrush.

Abdominal massage may be omitted depending on client preference. Remember that massage will stimulate the peristalsis action which may aggravate some symptoms.

Target digestive, adrenal and endocrine systems.

Candida albicans

(See Thrush, p.117.)

A naturally occurring yeast that lives on the skin, and in the digestive tract and mucus membranes. When candida is kept in check it does no harm but changes in the pH of its habitat can trigger an imbalance. A candida imbalance can be spread from one area of the body to another.

In its yeast form candida albicans can reproduce itself but remains in the intestinal tract. Contributing factors causing the yeast to multiply include:

- the use of antibiotics which kill too many good bacteria and lower resistance
- high sugar, refined diets
- contraceptive pill.

Symptoms: Linked to ME, IBS, thrush. Becomes a common complication with HIV and AIDS.

Treatment guidance: Boost the immune system: offer dietary advice (avoid sugar, yeast and refined foods); bio yoghurts are excellent for replacing good bacteria. Check for tinea (see p.56) as this is common due to weakened immunity. Skin infections are contra indicated.

Hepatitis

Hepatitis means inflammation of the liver. There are several causes but the main concern for therapists is viral hepatitis. A hepatitis carrier may not exhibit symptoms but can still infect others and the virus is very infectious even during incubation when no symptoms are apparent.

There are several hepatitis viruses including A, B, AB, non-AB, C, D, E.

Hepatitis A – infectious hepatitis

There may be no symptoms or typical acute hepatitis which includes yellowing of the skin and whites of eyes due to jaundice. Urine becomes darker, faeces paler; there is also a loss of appetite, nausea and fever (flu-like symptoms). It is caught by direct contact with infected faeces, faecal contaminated water and food or infected individuals. The incubation period is between 3–6 weeks after infection.

Hepatitis B – serum hepatitis

Often more severe than hepatitis A with a greater risk of the condition becoming chronic and progressing to additional liver disease such as cirrhosis of the liver or liver cancer. It is caught by direct contact with infected blood, including dried blood. Generally spread through the use of infected needles or through sexual intercourse. Incubation of the virus is from a few weeks to several months. The virus is very hardy and can survive for several years outside the body.

Hepatitis C

As for hepatitis B.

Treatment guidance: Contra indicated.

The nervous system

The nervous system is the main communication system for the body. It receives and interprets information from both inside and outside the body. The nervous system works intimately with the endocrine system to help regulate body processes and maintain homeostasis.

The nervous system has two main divisions:

- the *central nervous system (CNS)* comprising the brain and the spinal cord
- the *peripheral nervous system,* comprising all of the nervous system excepting the brain and spinal cord, which consists of 31 pairs of spinal nerves and 12 pairs of cranial nerves.

Nerve cell/neurone

A neurone is a specialized nerve cell designed to receive stimuli from the body and conduct impulses to the CNS. Each neurone comprises a cell body, a central nucleus and processes called axons and dendrites. Dendrites are long branches that receive messages from other nerve cells.

There are three main types of nerve impulses.

- *Sensory* or *afferent* neurones: receive stimuli from the sensory organs and sensory receptors (including heat, cold, pain, taste, smell, sight and sound) and transmit the impulse to the CNS.
- *Motor* or *efferent* neurones: conduct impulses away from the CNS to muscles and glands to stimulate them into carrying out their activities.
- *Associated* or *connecting* neurones: these connect sensory and motor neurones and are found in the brain and spinal cord.

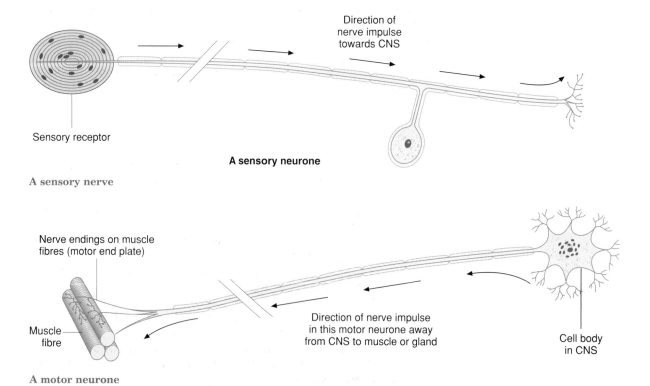

Sensory receptor

Direction of nerve impulse towards CNS

A sensory neurone

A sensory nerve

Nerve endings on muscle fibres (motor end plate)

Muscle fibre

Direction of nerve impulse in this motor neurone away from CNS to muscle or gland

Cell body in CNS

A motor neurone

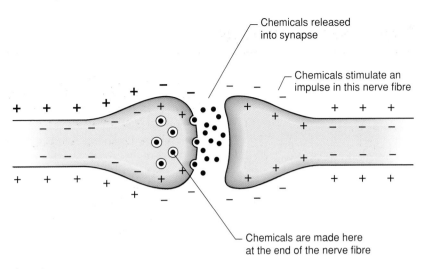

Chemicals released into synapse

Chemicals stimulate an impulse in this nerve fibre

Chemicals are made here at the end of the nerve fibre

A motor nerve

The transmission of nerve impulses

The function of a neurone is to transmit impulses from their origin to their destination. The nerve fibres of a neurone are not actually joined together but have a minute gap called a synapse. It is at this point that nerve impulses are transmitted from one neurone to another.

Impulses are a change of electrical charge that is carried down the axon fibre until it reaches a synapse. A chemical substance called a transmitter is released by the neurone to carry the impulses across the synapse to stimulate the next neurone. The synapse will only carry the impulse in one direction. If the level of the stimulus does not reach a certain intensity then the next nerve will not respond.

The motor point is the point at which the nerve supply enters the muscle. A special kind of synapse occurs at the junction between a nerve and a muscle and the area of contact is called a neuromuscular junction. Tiny neurones branch off from this to make contact with individual muscle cells.

Neurones

- Action potentials normally move in only one direction along the axon and can transmit at speeds of between 0.2 and 100 metres per second.

- Action potentials are 'all or none' i.e. they either occur in full or not at all.

- A neurotransmitter is a chemical synthesized in the cell. It is stored at the terminal of a neuron and released in response to the arrival of an action potential into the synaptic cleft. A neuron is characterised by the neurotransmitter that it synthesises, stores and releases at a synapse.

- The surface of the cell membrane is uniquely sensitive and influenced by a particular neurotransmitter.

- The effect of the neurotransmitter can be one of excitation or inhibition, depending upon the properties of the neurotransmitter and its receptor.

The central nervous system

The brain

The human brain is a complex mass of nervous tissue lying within the protection of the skull. The function of the brain is to co-ordinate stimuli received and initiate the correct response. It is also the site of consciousness and intellect. It can be described as the main communication centre of the nervous system.

The outer surface of the brain (cerebrum) consists of grey matter about 2–6 mm thick and this contains the cell bodies of the nerves. Below this is the white matter containing nerve fibres (axons).

Important structures in the brain

Cerebrum: Largest part of the brain; forms two distinct parts. Functions include mental activities, e.g. memory, thinking, intelligence, sensory perception and initiation of voluntary movement.

Cerebellum: Facilitates smooth, precise movement, balance and posture.

Medulla oblongata: Continuation of the spinal cord; controls the autonomic nervous system.

Hypothalamus: Located in the centre at the base of the brain. Controls automatic body processes, regulates appetite, water balance, body temperature and libido. It also plays an important role in motivation and emotion, influencing feelings of pleasure, fear and anger.

Thalamus: Located in the centre of the brain at the base of the cerebrum. Comprises a mass of nerve cells that act as a sensory relay station for nerve impulses coming up from the spinal cord and down from the higher brain centres (cerebrum). Interprets and directs sensory information.

Limbic system: Comprises a group of closely interconnected structures including areas of the hypothalamus, thalamus, hippocampus, amygdala, olfactory nerves, bulb and tract and other regions of the brain. It affects the emotional behaviour and plays a role in emotional response, autonomic reposes, subconscious motor and sensory drive, sexual behaviour, biological rhythms and motivation.

Brain stem: Contains centres that regulate many survival functions, e.g. heartbeat, respiration, blood pressure, digestion, swallowing.

Interesting fact

The brain
Although the brain makes up 2% of the body's weight it needs 20% of the body's blood.

Blood–brain barrier
This is a selective barrier that protects the brain from chemical variations in the blood.

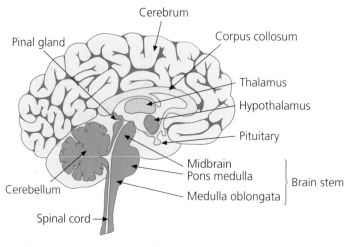

The brain

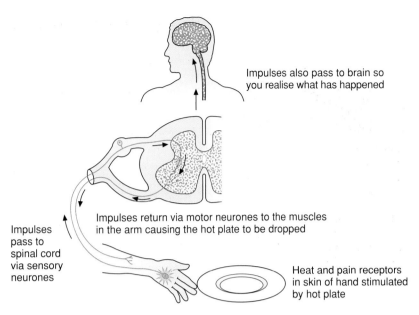

Impulses also pass to brain so you realise what has happened

Impulses return via motor neurones to the muscles in the arm causing the hot plate to be dropped

Impulses pass to spinal cord via sensory neurones

Heat and pain receptors in skin of hand stimulated by hot plate

Simple reflex action

Cerebrospinal fluid (CSF): A clear fluid produced in the brain protecting it from mechanical forces and infections. Contains lymphocytes, proteins and glucose.

Meninges: Membranes and connective tissues that cover, protect and supply nutrients to the brain and spinal cord.

Spinal cord: The spinal cord is an extension of the brain stem and extends from the base of the skull down to the second lumbar vertebra. Its function is to relay impulses to and from the brain.

The spinal cord is also the centre for reflex actions. Spinal reflex actions provide a fast automatic response to external or internal stimuli and do not require involvement of the brain: examples include a knee jerk, dropping a hot object, or the iris of the eye responding to light changes. On these occasions you will notice that the body has often responded before you are conscious of any sensation.

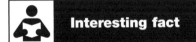

Interesting fact

The Spinal cord
The spinal cord on average is about 43 cm long.

The peripheral nervous system

The peripheral nervous system comprises the parts of the nervous system excepting the brain and the spinal cord. It includes the following:

- 12 pairs of cranial nerves, which connect directly to the brain. They provide a nerve supply to the sensory organs, muscles and skin of the head and the neck.
- 31 pairs of spinal nerves, which link it with the autonomic nervous system. Spinal nerves receive sensory impulses from the body and transmit motor signals to specific regions of the body. Each of the spinal nerves is numbered and named according to the level of the spinal column from which it emerges.
- The autonomic nervous system.

The somatic nervous system

The somatic nervous system is also referred to as the voluntary nervous system. It includes all muscular activity over which we exert voluntary

Interesting fact

Cranial nerves

- V/4th cranial nerve or trigeminal nerve has three branches and supplies the skin teeth nose and mouth.
- Vll/7th cranial or facial nerve has five braches and supplies the muscles of facial expression the ear, tongue and palate.
- Xl/11th cranial nerve supplies the muscles of the neck.

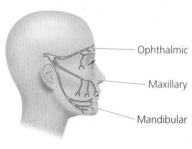

Ophthalmic

Maxillary

Mandibular

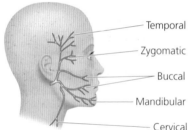

Temporal

Zygomatic

Buccal

Mandibular

Cervical

5th and 7th cranial nerve

control i.e. skeletal muscles movement. (Although reflex actions also use the same muscles.)

The autonomic nervous system

This is the involuntary part of the nervous system and controls the automatic body activities of smooth and cardiac muscle and the activities of the glands. It comprises two parts: the sympathetic and the parasympathetic nervous system. The two systems work together and there is a fine balance to provide for the optimum functioning of organs.

Sympathetic nervous system

The sympathetic nervous system is responsible for sympathetic stimulation, which produces a series of changes to prepare the body for vigorous activity, i.e. 'fight, flight and frolic'. Stimulation includes:

- increased cardiac output, increasing the rate and force of heart contraction
- bronchi in the lungs dilate, increasing breathing capacity
- vasodilation to allow increased blood flow
- secretions from the adrenal and sweat glands increase
- digestion slows down, the salivary and digestive glands secrete less
- more glucose is produced in the liver and released into the bloodstream to provide energy
- the pupils dilate to enhance perception.

The sympathetic stimulation of the autonomic system is increased by the release of the hormone adrenaline.

Parasympathetic nervous system

The parasympathetic nervous system system has an inhibitory effect, preparing the body for inactivity. It conserves and restores the body's energy, slowing down the body's processes (with the exception of digestion and the functions of the genito-urinary system).

Disorders and diseases associated with the nervous system

Migraine

Classified as a severe headache accompanied by visual disturbances, nausea or vomiting. The symptoms may last anything from two hours to a few days. A migraine may be a single occurrence or recurrent. There is no single cause of migraine but there is a tendency for them to run in families. Factors associated with the onset of a migraine are:

- stress
- food related, including chocolate, wine, cheese, citrus fruits to name a few
- sensory related and induced by bright lights and loud noises
- menstruation
- contraceptive pill, HRT.

There are two categories of migraine.

- *Common*: pain develops slowly and is made worse by movement or noise.
- *Classical*: headache is preceded by visual disturbance, with an area of expanding blindness surrounded by a crackling edge. This lasts for about 20 minutes and is usually followed by the symptoms of common migraine. Temporary weakness on one side of the body and a sensitivity to light is not uncommon.

Treatment guidance: Realistically it is unlikely a client would wish to be treated during an attack and it would be unadvisable anyway. There are occasions where clients susceptible to migraines may experience one as part of a healing crisis.

Parkinson's disease

Parkinson's disease is a neurological disorder caused by the degeneration of the nerve cells in a small part of the brain called the substantia nigra. The brain becomes deprived of a chemical called dopamine (a neurotransmitter). This is crucial for proper movement, a lack affecting muscle control and co-ordination.

Symptoms: In the early stages these present as a trembling of muscles in a hand or leg, stiffness, decreased movement and postural instability. The trembling becomes increasingly difficult to control. Secondary stages of the disease are characteristically diagnosed by rigid posture, difficulties with dexterity, co-ordination, speech and swallowing and problems within the gastrointestinal and urinary systems. There are changes to both skin and blood pressure. Dementia is experienced in the very late stages but otherwise intellect is unaffected.

Treatment guidance: Chances are that your contact with this disease will be through an existing client who is diagnosed rather than a new client. Refer to GP.

Reflexology: Has shown positive results with management of symptoms.

Multiple sclerosis (MS)

A progressive disease of the CNS whereby scattered patches of the protective covering of the nerve fibres (myelin) in the brain and spinal cord are destroyed. The exact cause of MS is unknown but it is thought to be an auto-immune disorder.

Symptoms: These may begin and then go into remission (i.e. resume later). Symptoms vary according the parts of the brain and spinal cord that have been damaged. General symptoms include tingling and numbness, fatigue, vertigo, clumsiness, weakness, slurred speech unsteadiness. Progressive symptoms may include incontinence and paralysis. Some individuals may have mild relapses and remission for long periods whilst others see a rapid onset of symptoms which soon leave them debilitated.

Treatment guidance: This will depend on the stage and severity of symptoms of the disease. Always refer to GP before treatment.

Anxiety

Anxiety is best described as an unpleasant emotional state ranging in severity from a feeling of unease to intense or irrational fear. A certain amount of anxiety is normal to us all, but it can become a problem if experienced when there is no obvious threat and when it starts to disrupt day-to-day activities. It may be caused by a variety of factors including

Interesting fact

Migraine
Migraines occur in over 10% of the population. It is three times more common in women than in men.

Interesting fact

Parkinson's disease
Approximately 1 in 200 people have Parkinson's disease. The disease is more common in men than women and mainly affects the elderly.

- a naturally raised level of arousal in the CNS
- repressed experiences
- loss of a loved object/person/animal
- learned response to an experience, particularly if the experience was unpleasant.

Symptoms: These are numerous, with some experiencing the whole spectrum of symptoms. They include palpitations, tight chest, light-headedness, breathlessness (either hyperventilating or hypoventilating), dizziness, headaches, restlessness, dry mouth, nausea, diarrhoea, a frequent need to go to the loo, burping, swallowing air, sweating, blushing or pale pallor, a feeling of impending doom, fatigue, insomnia and irritability.

Treatment guidance: Refer to GP who may suggest counselling. Be cautious: anxiety can lead to a dependency on others, a good therapist being one of them. All treatments will help to calm anxiety and boost self-esteem. Include breathing and relaxation techniques. Target pituitary, adrenal and nerve reflexes.

Depression

We all get depressed at times; events in life do not always go according to plan; a close relative or friend may pass away and naturally we will feel emotional. Depression becomes a problem when the depressed state is not just a temporary blip but persists, deepens and is accompanied by a range of psychiatric illnesses. True depression is not just a mood that someone can shake themselves out of. There is often no single cause but the condition may be triggered by a particular or series of events that cumulate in a depression. Alternatively, depression may be triggered by a systemic disorder or viral illness. It is also not uncommon after pregnancy (post-natal depression).

Symptoms: These depend on the severity of the illness. Mild symptoms include anxiety, variable moods and a need to weep for no apparent reason. More serious depression may result in a loss of appetite, insomnia, general lack of interest, fatigue, loss of concentration and general lethargy. The illness may become extreme, with delusions and an intense feeling of guilt and lack of self-worth; the sufferer becomes withdrawn and there may even be suicidal thoughts.

Treatment guidance: All treatments are of great benefit. As there are so many possible causes for depression it is recommended that the client is referred for counselling and to their GP. The client also needs to be aware that symptoms may worsen before they feel an improvement. As the client is already feeling low they need to understand that this may be part of the healing process.

Epilepsy

A temporary alteration in the functioning of the brain or recurrent seizures. A seizure is caused by brain dysfunction and is a result of abnormal electrical activity therein. There are several causes of epilepsy including head injury, brain infection, birth trauma, drug induced or a metabolic disorder. There may be no found reason (idiopathic epilepsy). The frequency of seizures varies, with many epileptics leading normal lives with no other symptoms between seizures.

There are two classifications of epileptic seizures.

Generalized seizure

This involves a loss of consciousness and affects the whole body. There are two types.

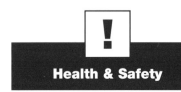

Interesting fact

Depression
No one should be made to feel ashamed or belittled. Depression is a very common illness and affects around 10–14% of the population at some time during their lives.

Health & Safety

If the client is on medication do not suggest that they change or stop taking it; refer them back to their GP for support.

- *Grand mal*: this seizure results in a loss of consciousness, collapse and the entire body alternates between stiffening and twitching. After the seizure, the body muscles relax. The person will be confused and disorientated and usually just want to sleep as the seizure is very exhausting. Some individuals experience an aura before the onset of a seizure and have some warning that one is imminent.

- *Petit mal* (absence): here there is a momentary loss of consciousness creating a blank period and the person is unresponsive. It looks like the individual is daydreaming.

Partial seizures

These are more limited and can be described as simple or complex. The effect on the brain may spread, leading to a generalized seizure. There are two types.

- *Simple*: the person remains conscious but there is an abnormal twitching movement, tingling or other sensory sensation (heightened sense of smell, taste) lasting several minutes.

- *Complex*: conscious awareness of the surroundings is lost and the sufferer becomes dazed and may exhibit strange behaviour.

Treatment guidance: In the case of recurrent epilepsy always refer to GP before considering treatment. Although this condition is a contra indication it can be argued that the calming effects of massage and aromatherapy may be beneficial. The question which is more important is how comfortable would you feel treating a client who *may* have a seizure? Seizures normally have set triggers such as flashing lights or electrical impulses.

The following oils should not be recommended for use on a client with epilepsy:

- fennel
- hyssop
- sage
- eucalyptus
- (possibly rosemary although there is conflicting opinion).

Ylang ylang is a particular beneficial oil to use, as are basil, juniper and lavender.

Sciatica

Pressure as a result of an inter-vertebral disc pressing on the nerve or local muscle spasm squeezing the nerve can cause sciatica.

Symptoms: Include pain radiating along the nerve; this can be in the buttock, thigh or travel along the entire length of the leg to the foot.

Treatment guidance: dependent on the cause. Providing there is no damage, and the sciatica is due more to muscular tension or postural faults, deep tissue work to the gluteals and lower back muscles will be beneficial.

Carpal tunnel syndrome

Carpal tunnel syndrome is a common occupational hazard primarily affecting those who frequently use a word processor or keyboard. The condition also occurs with some other medical diseases, is frequent during pregnancy and is not uncommon in massage therapists. It is caused by pressure on the median nerve in the lower arm where it passes from the wrist in to the hand (a gap called the carpal tunnel).

Interesting fact

Seizures
The correct term is a seizure not fit.

About 1 in every 200 people suffers with some form of epilepsy.

Interesting fact

Sciatic nerve
The sciatic nerve is the longest nerve in the body. It supplies the hip joint, thigh muscles, the skin behind the thigh, the lower knee, ankle joint, muscles of the lower leg and foot, skin below the knee.

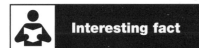
Symptoms: Pain, tingling and numbness in the thumb, index and middle fingers on one or both hands. The condition tends to be worse at night-time.

Treatment guidance: Effleurage, ice and elevation. Encourage rest.

Anaesthesia

A loss of sensation that may be local or generalized. There are several diseases with which anaesthesia may be experienced. Of particular importance to the therapist is diabetes.

The special senses

There are five senses:

- touch (see p.43, integumentary system)
- sight
- smell (see p.110, olfactory system)
- hearing (see Chapter 18, p.393)
- taste (the sense of taste is not covered here because it has no direct relationship to our treatments).

Each of the senses has its own specialized nerve endings. These link with the brain where they undergo complex processes of perception.

The eye

The eye is a sense organ and enables us to focus and receive light rays. Information is transmitted to the brain via the optic nerve. The *optic nerve* does not transmit a stream of pictures (like a TV) but transmits information about the light patterns reaching the eye for the brain to interpret.

Each eye has a separate structure but the eyes generally function together. The eye itself is almost spherical in shape and around 2.4 cm in diameter. It is protected by the bony walls of the orbital cavity and by fatty tissue.

The structure of, and passage of light into, the eye

The *sclera* and *cornea* are the outer layer or the white of the eye. The cornea is clear and acts to bend or refract the light rays to focus light on to the retina. The *conjunctiva* is a continuation of the epidermis and covers the front of the eye (with the exception of the cornea) and lines the inside of the eyelids. It is kept nourished by tears to prevent friction and keep the eye clear of dust and dirt.

The *iris* is the coloured, visible part of the eye. It consists of circular and radial muscles that regulate the amount of light entering the eye

- the circular muscles contract, reducing the amount of light entering the eye
- the radial muscle when contracted opens the iris.

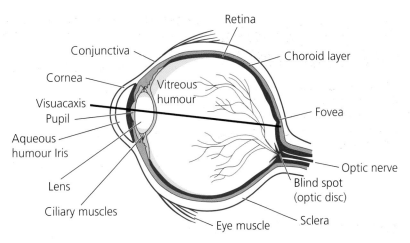

The eye

The *aqueous humour* is a watery fluid behind the cornea and in front of the lens: it protects the pupil and lens. The *pupil* is a small hole in the centre of the eye which allows light to pass through the *lens*. The lens is made up of a transparent jelly that focuses the light's rays on to the retina. The *ciliary muscles* continually change its shape to give focus.

Inside the eye itself is the *vitreous humour*, a jelly-like fluid that helps to maintain the shape of the eye. All light rays striking the eye from one point in space are brought to a focus at one point on the innermost layer of the eye called the *retina*. This comprises specialized tissue which contains two types of cells:

- *cones*: sensitive to light, these have a colour-sensitive pigment each for red, green and blue; there are 7 million cones in each eye
- *rods*: sensitive to light intensity.

A small depression called the *fovea* has concentrated amounts of cones (no rods) and is the area where vision is the sharpest. A second area called the *blind spot* or optic disc has no field of vision; this spot marks the area where the optic nerve leaves the eye.

Behind the retina lies the *choroid* layer. It is rich in blood vessels and absorbs the light passing through the retina, preventing it from reflecting within the eyeball.

Disorders of the eye

Conjunctivitis

Inflammation of the mucus membranes that line and cover the eye. Conjunctivitis is commonly caused by an allergy or bacterial (staphylococci) infection but may also be the result of a viral infection associated with a cold. It is spread by both direct and indirect contact.

Symptoms: Red, often swollen eyes with itching, discharge, and occasionally there is sensitivity to light. Eyes may feel gritty. With infective conjunctivitis the discharge may contain pus and may cause the eyelids to stick together in the morning.

Treatment guidance: Contra indicated; refer to GP.

The sense of smell
The sense of smell is 10,000 times more sensitive than the sense of taste.

Smell and taste work in unison, when you are unable to smell you lose about 80% of your ability to taste.

Primary odours
It is thought that man can detect between 4–10,000 odours. Some scientists suggest that there may be seven primary odours, others say odour is subjective. These seven are: floral, peppermint, ethereal, musky, camphouraceous, pungent and putrid.

The nostrils
The nostrils play no part in smell other than to act as filtering tubes.

The olfactory system

Smell and taste are two chemical senses stimulated by molecules of odour and flavour.

Before an odour can be smelt, it must be:

1. volatile, i.e. in the air
2. capable of dissolving in the water-based mucus
3. lipid soluble, to react with the receptor membrane.

The sense of smell

An odour comes from particles of gas or vapour. They are not smelled unless the smell-bearing molecules come in contact with the sensitive surface of the inner nose.

There are two receptor sites about the size of a postage stamp in an exposed cavity located behind the eye sockets at the roof of the nasal cavity. Each site has a membrane covered with yellowy-brown mucus called the olfactory epithelium. They are also covered with millions of hair-like projections which extend through the mucus and make contact with the air as it passes through to the throat and lungs. The odour molecules dissolve into the mucus. Fibres from these cells link up with olfactory areas in the brain.

Normal airflow only allows a small amount of air to make contact with the sensory mucus. To enhance odour perception breathe deeply through the nose. You can still smell even if you hold your nostrils together and breath. A small amount of air still comes in contact with the sensory mucus.

Different odour molecules are like keys, and for a smell to register with the brain it must fit into the right lock or receptor. Once the receptor is activated the signal is conducted to the brain via the olfactory bulb. From here the odour passes to the olfactory stalk, to the limbic system. As a result of stimulating the limbic system a response can be triggered resulting in a range of responses, e.g. the smell of bread baking may induce hunger and the smell of a certain aftershave or perfume may remind you of a particular person.

Structures of the olfactory system

1st cranial nerve: the olfactory nerve. Its fibres arise in the mucous membrane of the nose and join the olfactory bulb.

The *olfactory lobe* is situated on the under-surface of the frontal lobe of the brain. It comprises two areas: the anterior and posterior lobes.

The *olfactory bulb* rests on the ethmoid bone. The under-side of the bulb receives the olfactory nerves fibres which pass upward through the ethmoid bone from the olfactory region of the nose.

The *olfactory tract* is a band of triangular-shaped white matter. It lies under the surface of the frontal lobe of the brain. It divides into two parts which connect to the amygdala and hippocampus regions of the brain.

Amygdala
The primitive emotional centre of the brain where action is sensed. It is involved in fight, flight and frolic responses.

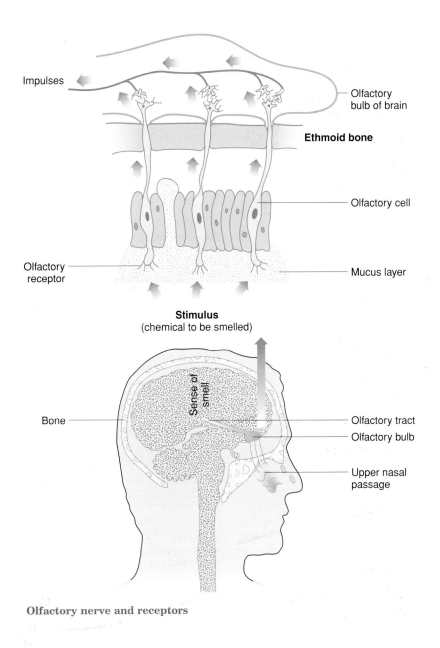

Olfactory nerve and receptors

The ear

It is important that you know about the anatomy of the ear when doing thermal auricular therapy. We have covered this in detail in Chapter 18.

The endocrine system

The endocrine system consists of 14 endocrine glands and the hormones that they secrete and/or store. The secretory cells of the endocrine gland cluster around blood capillaries inside the gland so that hormones can pass readily into the blood for transportation.

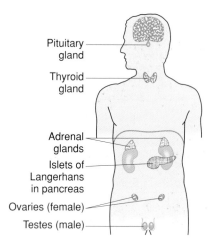

Pituitary gland
Thyroid gland
Adrenal glands
Islets of Langerhans in pancreas
Ovaries (female)
Testes (male)

Glands of the endocrine system

Hormones can be described as chemical messengers as they become attached to plasma proteins and are transported around the body to initiate a response in a target organ. They work like a chemical key in that the key must fit the target site to produce the desired response. Hormones may affect a number of target organs, which can be widely separated in the body.

The endocrine system works with the nervous system to control and co-ordinate the body's activities.

Feedback mechanisms

These control and regulate the production of hormones to maintain homeostasis. Homeostasis involves the pituitary gland and the target organ. Once a hormone has been released the feedback system may release another hormone (positive feedback). Alternatively it can inhibit the release of a hormone (negative feedback) once a response has been achieved.

The endocrine glands and their hormones

Interesting fact

Number of hormones
There are approximately 100 different hormones with about 40 circulating in the blood stream at any one time.

The endocrine glands, their hormones and associate disorders

The pituitary gland (master gland)

The pituitary gland is about the size of a pea and lies at the base of the skull. It is attached to the hypothalamus by a stalk. These two act as one unit regulating the activity of nearly all the other endocrine glands. The pituitary gland consists of two lobes: the anterior and posterior

Hormones of the anterior lobe

Growth hormone

Action	Hypersecretion	Hyposecretion
Controls the growth of the skeleton and muscles ensuring that chemical substances necessary for growth are available	Gigantism – in childhood, limb bones increase in length	Dwarfism
	Acromegaly – in adults, enlarged hands, feet, nose, jaw and ears	

Thyroid-stimulating hormone (TSH)

Action   TSH is released to stimulate the thyroid into activity when the levels of thyroxin circulating in the blood are low

Adrenocorticotrophic hormone (ACTH)

Action   ACTH regulates the activity of the cortex and adrenal glands controlling both growth and steroid hormone output

Hormones of the sex glands

These hormones are responsible for the onset of puberty. They stimulate and control the development and function of testes and ovaries. They regulate the menstrual cycle in women and the production of spermatozoa in men

In the female the following hormones are produced:

Prolactin	stimulates activity in the corpus luteum and causes milk to be secreted from the breasts
Gonadotrophic hormones	stimulate the ovaries or testes
Follicle stimulating hormones (FSH)	causes the rapid growth of the Graaffian follicle
Luteinising hormone (LH)	must be present in certain proportions with FSH for an ovum to be produced

In the male two hormones are produced:

Interstitial cell stimulating hormone	stimulates the cells of the testes to produce the hormone testosterone
Follicle stimulating hormone (FSH)	stimulates the production of spermatozoa

Posterior lobe of the pituitary gland

Anti-diuretic hormone	regulates the amount of water passed by the kidneys
Oxytocin	stimulates the contraction of the uterus
	initiates the release of milk during breast feeding

Pineal gland

Small gland situated under the brain. Connected to the brain and hypothalamus by a short stalk containing nerves

Melatonin	exact function is not fully understood
	stimulated by light entering the eye and fluctuates during each 24-hour cycle
	associated with co-ordination of body biorhythms (body clock)
	inhibits the onset of puberty (atrophies after the onset)

Thyroid gland

The thyroid gland is an H-shaped gland positioned at the front of the neck. The function of the thyroid gland is to secrete the hormone thyroxin and store iodine

Thyroxin

Action	Hypersecretion	Hyposecretion
Responsible for mental and physical development Controls the stability and functioning of the nerves and cardiovascular systems Controls the utilization of oxygen. Therefore the rate of the basal metabolic rate is controlled by thyroxin, which stimulates metabolism in the tissues and is essential for normal growth; carbohydrate, protein and lipid metabolism; healthy skin and hair	*Goitre* – thyroid gland increases in size forming a swelling in the neck. Eyes may bulge due to accumulation of fluid behind the eyeball *Hyperthyroidism* (thyrotoxicosis) – increase in mental and physical activity with extreme nervous excitability. The skin is moist and the sweat glands are overactive. The hair is lank and greasy in appearance. There is weight loss, yet appetite is increased. Body temperature is raised and the pulse is rapid	*Hypothyroidism* – in childhood, cretinism: mental, physical and sexual development is retarded *Myxoedema* – in adults the metabolic rate is slow and body weight increases. Mental activity is slow. Skin becomes coarse and dry. Hair becomes thin and brittle. Oedema is present *Goitre* – persistent iodine deficiency

Parathyroid glands

There are four of these glands positioned behind the thyroid gland

Parathormone (PTH)

Action   Controls the excretion of phosphate; indirectly controls the amount of calcium in the blood and bones

Adrenals

There are two adrenal glands one situated on either side of the vertebral column on the posterior abdomen wall, capping the upper end of each kidney. The adrenals are embedded in fat. Each adrenal consists of two parts: a *cortex* and *medulla*

Cortex

Glucocorticoids (cortisol)

Action	Hypersecretion	Hyposecretion
Regulates the metabolism of carbohydrates (availability of energy) Resists the effects of stress Plays a part in water balance	High blood pressure or high stress levels. High levels of glucose in blood and urine, nervousness and increased sweating. Could result in a tumour	*Cushing's Syndrome* – weight gain, body fat is redistributed, i.e. very thin legs, large moon face, and shoulder hump, enlarged abdomen. Blood pressure is raised and face appears flushed. Bruises easily. Increased hair growth in women (hirsutism). Bones become soft and fragile Also Addison's disease (see below)

Aldosterone

Action	Hypersecretion	Hyposecretion
Reacts on the kidneys to maintain the balance of water, sodium and potassium in the body	–	*Addison's disease* – muscular weakness, weight loss, mental lethargy. There is insufficient glucose in the blood for tissue cell respiration, particularly skeletal muscle. Increased potassium and decreased sodium in the blood leads to reduced blood pressure and dehydration. Bronzing of the skin occurs on pressure areas. Women lose axillary hair

Androgens

Action	Hypersecretion	Hyposecretion
Regulates the development and maintenance of the secondary sex characteristics	Virilism in women and development of male sexual characteristics, such as facial hair	–

Medulla

Adrenalin

Action	Hypersecretion	Hyposecretion
Prepares the body to withstand extenuating circumstances – the 'fight, flight or frolic' response Dilation of the arteries, increasing the blood supply Dilation of the bronchi allowing a greater amount of air to enter the lungs Constriction of the blood vessels to the skin causing an increase in blood pressure Increases the amount of available glycogen Slows digestion Increased activity of the sweat glands	Over long periods, results in anxiety and stress	–

Noradrenalin

Action   Balances the effects of adrenalin

Pancreas

Scattered throughout the pancreas are abundant, pinhead-sized groups of specialized cells called the 'islets of Langerhans'

Insulin

Action	Hypersecretion	Hyposecretion
Regulates the level of glucose in the blood	–	Insufficient insulin in the body leads to *diabetes mellitus*. Also where there is a high blood glucose level (hyperglycaemia). Some diabetics have to have commercial insulin preparations injected at regular intervals Symptoms include high blood pressure, thirst and a frequent need to pass urine because of the high concentration of glucose. Excessive amounts of water can be excreted leading to dehydration Further problems associated with diabetes include circulatory problems (particularly in extremities), altered skin sensation, eyesight problems, poor healing *Type I*: insulin-dependent, usually starts before age 35 *Type II*: usually has a gradual onset and typically develops age 40+; linked to obesity

Glucagon

Action   Raises the level of glucose in the blood

Thymus

Located in the chest behind the sternum

Thymosin

Action   Required for the development of T-lymphocytes

Sex glands

The ovaries are the female gonads or sex glands and the testes the male. The testes secrete the hormone testosterone and androgens after puberty

Ovaries

The ovaries are almond in shape and lie on either side of the pelvis. Each is attached to the upper part of the uterus and to the back by ligaments.

Oestrogen

Action	Hypersecretion	Hyposecretion
Controls the development and function of the female sex organs. Controls the development of secondary sexual characteristics	Reproductive problems	Hirsuitism Infertility

Progesterone

Action	Hypersecretion	Hyposecretion
Prepares for and maintains pregnancy	Premenstrual tension and reproductive problems	Infertility

Testosterone

Action	Hypersecretion	Hyposecretion
Results in male sexual characteristics	Virilism in females	–

Androgen

Action	Hypersecretion	Hyposecretion
Controls the development and function of the male sex organs Controls the development of secondary sexual characteristics	See adrenals above	–

The amount of hormone released by an endocrine gland is determined by the body's need for that hormone at any given time. The body is normally regulated so that there is no over- or underproduction of hormone. There are times when the regulating mechanism does not operate properly and hormonal levels are too high or too low. When this happens, endocrine disorders result.

 Interesting fact

Stress and hormones
During times of stress the hormones are released from the hypothalamus, pituitary, adrenals. Blood pressure and sugar levels increase ready for action. Problems occur when these levels are maintained but no body response is actually taken.

Disorders and diseases of the endocrine system

We have covered individual disorders of the endocrine system in the table on pp.112–115, but below is some general advice.

Treatment guidance: For endocrine disorders, refer to GP for advice.

Effects of massage: General massage, by alleviating the symptoms of stress, can support the endocrine system in maintaining homeostasis.

Essential oils: May affect either a particular system or gland through the action of phytohormone (plant hormones) on a corresponding human hormone. Use balancing oils such as geranium and rose.

Reflexology: It must be noted that it is possible to stimulate a gland to produce more of its hormone and the client must be made aware of this possibility, e.g. if they suffer with insulin dependence. The reflex point may be excluded if dysfunctional until medical advice has been given.

The genito-urinary system

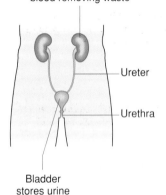

Kidney filters the blood removing waste

Ureter

Urethra

Bladder stores urine

Urinary system

This comprises two systems: the urinary and the reproductive. They are often referred to as a combined system as some organs are shared between the two.

Renal or urinary system

The main function of the renal system is to regulate the volume and composition of body fluids. Waste products such as urea and uric acid, in addition to excess water and mineral salts, must be removed from the body in order to provide a constant internal environment (homeostasis) and to prevent disease.

The urinary system consists of the following:

- kidneys
- ureters
- urinary bladder
- urethra.

The kidneys

The kidneys lie on the posterior wall of the abdomen, one on either side of the spine. The left kidney is situated slightly higher than the right.

The kidneys have the following functions:

- filtration of impurities and metabolic waste from blood
- regulation of water and salt balance in the body, maintaining blood pH
- formation of urine.

The role of the kidneys in fluid balance

The kidneys control the balance between water intake and water output. The amount of fluid taken into the body (mainly through digestion) must equal the amount of fluid excreted from it (faeces, urine, sweat, moisture in exhaled breath). This is necessary for the body to maintain a constant internal environment.

There are several factors that affect the fluid balance in the body:

- if the body temperature increases, water is lost from the body in sweat
- a high salt intake can result in increased water re-absorption, which reduces the volume of urine produced
- diuretics such as alcohol, tea and coffee can also increase the volume of urine
- nervousness can result in an increased production of urine (sympathetic nerves constricting the blood vessels)
- when the blood pressure inside the kidney tubules rises, less water is re-absorbed and the volume of urine will be increased; when the blood pressure inside the kidney tubules falls, more water is re-absorbed into the blood and the volume of urine will be reduced.

The ureters

The ureters are two very fine muscular tubes. They transport urine from the kidneys to the urinary bladder.

The urinary bladder

This is a pear-shaped sac that lies in the pelvic cavity. The size of the bladder varies according to the amount of urine it contains. The functions of the bladder are to store urine and expel it at intervals.

The urethra

This extends from the neck of the bladder to the outside of the body. A muscle usually prevents urine being release until it consciously relaxed.

Disorders and diseases of the urinary system

Cystitis/urethritis

Cystitis literally means bladder inflammation, but strictly speaking it affects the inner lining of the bladder. The term is often incorrectly used to include urethritis, which is an inflammation of the urethra. Cystitis is usually caused by a bacterial infection but there are other causes such as food irritants, chemicals and contraception. There is a risk if the condition is not treated that the infection may travel up to the kidneys so treatment should be sought.

Symptoms: Urgency or frequent need to urinate, but only passing small quantities (even drips). A burning, stinging sensation is experienced when passing water. Sometimes the pain is agonizing. The urine may be dark and have a strong odour. Occasionally there may be discomfort in the lower abdomen.

Candida albicans (moniliasis/thrush)

See Digestive system, p.99, for description.

Symptoms of candida on the mucus membranes, i.e. mouth, vagina (thrush) moist skin, include:

Interesting fact

Nephrons
There are approximately a million nephrons in each kidney. Each nephron is a functional unit that filters and processes urine.

Interesting fact

Length of urethra
The female urethra is shorter than the male being approximately 4 centimetres in length, compared to the male urethra at approximately 18 to 20 cm.

Interesting fact

Diuretics
A diuretic is a substance/ drug which helps to eliminate excess fluid from the body, by increasing urination.

Essential oils which help with fluid retention include bergamot, cedarwood, chamomile.

- intense itching, irritation
- rash with white creamy raised patches in the mouth
- cottage cheese-like discharge from the vagina and (possibly) some discomfort when urinating
- on infected skin appears as an itchy red rash with flaky white patches (nappy rash).

Some women however experience no symptoms. For men the infection is known as balanitis.

Treatment guidance: Contra indicated if the skin is infected.

The reproductive organs

The structure of the male and female reproductive organs

The main organs of the reproductive system are located within the pelvic girdle.

The *male* genitalia include the penis, prostrate gland, testes and vas deferens.

After the onset of puberty the testes continually produce sperm. During ejaculation sperm is released through the vas deferens.

The *female* reproductive organs include the uterus, ovaries, fallopian tubes, cervix and vagina.

Life changes

Puberty

Puberty usually begins between the ages of 10–14, stimulated by the gonadotrophic hormones. The following changes occur as the reproductive organs reach maturity:

- pubic and axillary hair begins to grow.

In men:

- marked increase in the growth of muscle and bone
- enlargement of the larynx and deepening of the voice
- growth of hair on the face, chest and abdomen
- enlargement of the penis, scrotum and prostate gland
- maturation of the testes and production of spermatozoa
- thickening of the skin and increase in sebum production.

In women:

- the uterus, uterine tubes and ovaries reach maturity
- the menstrual cycle and ovulation begin
- the breasts begin to develop and enlarge
- the width of the pelvis increases
- fat deposits in the subcutaneous tissue increase.

Menstrual cycle

Puberty (or menarche) marks the beginning of the reproductive years. The ovaries are stimulated by the gonadotrophin hormones released from

Interesting fact

The ovaries
The ovaries are composed of two parts:

The medulla: consists of fibrous tissue, blood vessels and nerves.

The cortex: surrounds the medulla. It has a framework of connective tissue covered by epithelium tissue containing the ovarian follicles.

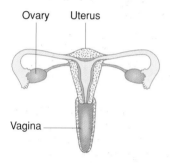

Female reproductive organs

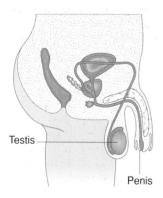

Male reproductive organs

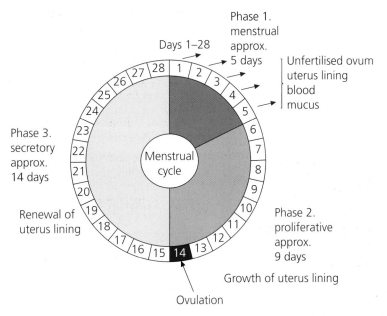

Menstrual cycle

The corpus luteum
This is a small mass of temporary endocrine tissue. It develops from the Graafian follicle on the surface of the ovary after ovulation has occurred. If pregnancy occurs it remains active secreting progesterone and oestrogen otherwise it degenerates after approximately 10 days.

Fertility
Ovulation occurs approximately 14 days prior to the next menstrual cycle (and not in the middle of the cycle unless cycle is 28 days long). The first day of the menstrual cycle is the first day of bleeding.

the anterior pituitary gland (the follicle stimulating hormone (FSH) and luteinising hormone (LH)).

The menstrual cycle is a series of events that occurs regularly in most females every 23–34 days. It consists of the following stages.

The *menstrual phase*, lasting approximately 4–5 days. High levels of progesterone in the blood inhibit the activity of the pituitary gland and LH is reduced. The withdrawal of this hormone causes the corpus luteum and progesterone to decrease. The uterus begins to degenerate and the menstrual flow begins.

The *proliferative phase*, lasting approximately 10 days. The ovarian follicle is stimulated by FSH, and begins to mature and produce oestrogen. Oestrogen stimulates reproduction of the cells of the uterine walls in preparation for implantation. It also inhibits FSH, preventing development of further follicles, and reduces oestrogen. This phase ends when ovulation occurs.

The *secretory phase*, lasting 14 days. LH brings about ovulation and causes the Graafian follicle to change into the corpus luteum. It also stimulates the corpus luteum to secrete the hormone progesterone. Progesterone causes the uterus to become thick, vascular and secretory, ready for implantation, and there is an increase in mucus secretions.

If fertilization does not occur the cycle begins again.

The unfertilized ovum may survive for only a short period of time (around 24 hours). The spermatozoa may only be capable of fertilizing the ovum during this time (although spermatozoa have the potential to survive for several days if conditions are right). If the ovum is fertilized there is no breakdown of the endometrium and no menstrual flow. The ovum travels through the uterine tube and becomes embedded in the wall of the uterus where it produces the hormone human chorionic gonadotrophin (HCG). This hormone keeps the corpus luteum intact so that pregnancy develops.

Contraceptive pill

The contraceptive pill uses synthetic hormones to increase the hormone levels of progesterone and oestrogen. These hormones interfere with the production of the pituitary hormones FSH and LH preventing ovulation.

HRT
Hormone replacement therapy (HRT) is the use of a synthetic or natural chemical to replace a hormone.

Symptoms of the menopause
The menopause can be easy sailing for some experiencing few symptoms, others may experience all of the following:

- changes in the menstrual cycle – abnormal bleeding, irregular periods
- fatigue
- headaches
- nervousness, lack of confidence
- insomnia
- dizziness
- palpitations
- depression
- hot flushes, night sweats
- crawling/creeping sensation under the skin
- numbness
- incontinence
- libido decreases, painful intercourse
- loss of bone mass (osteoporosis)
- superfluous hair yet axillary and pubic hair become sparse.

The mini pill contains progesterone only, its main action is to change the mucus lining the cervix to make it impenetrable to sperm.

Menopause

The menopause is the opposite of puberty. It marks the end of the fertile years and is part of natural progression. It usually begins between the ages of 45–55 and may occur over several years. This process is determined by several factors: hereditary, racial and physiological. It is also influenced by environmental conditions, diet and level of fitness.

Changes in the hormone levels occur and the ovaries gradually become less responsive to the FSH and LH. The ovaries become inactive, there is a decline in hormone production and the menstrual cycle ceases.

During the menopause several physical changes occur:

- the ovaries reduce in size
- the lining of the uterus atrophies
- vagina narrows and vaginal tissue thins
- skin becomes thin, dryer, scaly and inelastic
- there is a loss of subcutaneous fat
- breasts droop
- increase in susceptibility to osteoporosis
- increase in superfluous hair.

The breast

The breasts are positioned on the top of the pectoral muscles. The breast does not contain muscular tissue but consists of mainly glandular, fibrous and fatty tissue. The firm breast shape in youth is maintained by the support of powerful ligaments (Cooper's ligaments), acting against gravity and giving support. Lymph is drained mainly through the axillary lymph vessels and nodes. There are some internal mammary nodes where lymph can drain should the superficial route become obstructed.

Pregnancy and breast-feeding

The function of the breast is to produce milk for breast-feeding and the size of breast does not determination the ability to produce milk. The breast tissue increases at around the third month of pregnancy when the lactiferous sinuses become active in preparation for storing milk.

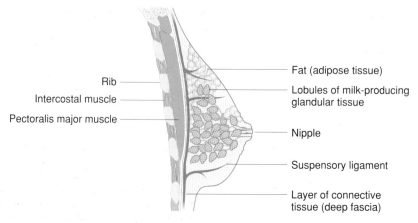

The breast

Conditions related to the reproductive system

Pre-menstrual syndrome (PMS)

PMS is a collection of emotional and physical symptoms that begin after ovulation and continue until menstruation starts. Hormonal influences have a clear effect on PMS and the two offending hormones are oestrogen and progesterone. There have been links with deficiencies in vitamin B, magnesium and pyridoxine.

Symptoms: Include some or all of the following: irritability, tension, depression and fatigue. Physical symptoms include tender breasts, fluid retention, headache, backache and lower abdominal pain.

Treatment guidance: PMS responds well to regular treatment with reflexology and aromatherapy to balance the body.

Essential oils: Chamomile, citrus, clary sage, geranium, frankincense, juniper, lavender, marjoram, neroli, rose, sandalwood, vetiver and ylang ylang.

Treatment guidance in pregnancy

It can be debated whether treatment should be given during pregnancy. There is an issue particularly here if the client has a history of miscarriage and is either trying to conceive or is in the early stages of pregnancy; if something were to go wrong it is only natural to look for a reason why, whether it is a legitimate reason or not.

There are many who would suggest that all body treatments and reflexology should be avoided, but this is a matter of personal opinion and confidence.

Massage and aromatherapy: Treatment directly over the abdomen is best avoided, although oil can be applied with superficial effleurage. Many women suffer with a variety of aches and discomfort which massage will help to alleviate. Circulation in the legs is notoriously sluggish for many, especially in the later stages. The weight of the foetus restricts the circulation to the legs. Quite early on it becomes uncomfortable to lie on the abdomen and so any massage will need to be adapted.

Essential oils: Any oil that is described as an emmenagogue should be avoided (lavender and chamomile may be used if diluted well). It is advisable to avoid aromatherapy treatment in the first trimester (12–16 weeks) of pregnancy.

After the fifth month some of the oils can be used in a 1 per cent dilution with some beneficial results but caution should always be observed.

There is no reason why a client cannot use oils for inhalation or in the bath provided they are carefully chosen (and the bath is not too hot). Always check the client's medical history, particularly if there is a history of miscarriage.

Reflexology: It may be advisable to avoid working the uterus point until the very late stages of pregnancy.

Endometriosis

A common uterine condition where fragments of endometrial tissue migrate and begin to grow outside the uterus (including the ovaries, uterine tubes and pelvic structures). There is inflammation of the uterine lining often caused by an infection. The tissue still reacts to the sex hormones causing menstrual bleeding where the tissue has formed (i.e. internally). Complications of endometriosis include adhesions and fertility problems.

Interesting fact

Premenstrual syndrome (tension)
Commonly referred to as PMT or PMS. 90% of fertile women endure the symptoms of PMS at some stage during their lives. Some have such severe symptoms that it seriously affects their life.

Tip

Oils to avoid during pregnancy
Following is a list of oils to be avoided when massaging during pregnancy or if you suspect a client is trying to conceive. It is important that you are familiar with oils that are safe before working on a pregnant client.

*basil

*cedarwood

*clary sage

*fennel

*hyssop

*jasmine

*juniper

*myrrh

~peppermint

~rose

~rosemary

*sweet marjoram

*sage

*thyme.

* Avoid completely.
~ Can be used after the fourth month.

Symptoms: In some cases there are no symptoms, but typically they include lower abdominal pain, back pain, heavy periods, occasionally digestive disorders and fertility problems

Treatment guidance: If there is great discomfort it may be wise to avoid abdominal massage, with the exception of soothing, gentle effleurage.

Knowledge review

1   Why is it important that a therapist has an understanding of the systems of the body?

2   Define the term *homeostasis*.

3   Name the four main types of tissue.

4   List the functions of the skin.

5   Make a list of common contagious and non-contagious skin diseases/disorders.

6   Make a table and compare and contrast the differences between veins and arteries.

7   List the cells found in blood.

8   Make a table and compare lymph and blood circulation.

9   List four functions of the skeleton.

10   List the functions of the muscular system.

11   What are the three types of muscular tissue?

12   Review the figures on pp.88–9. Make sure you can identify and describe the functions of the following muscles:

   (some should indicate individual muscles, other groups of muscles) – deltoid, biceps, triceps, brachialis, radialis, trapezius, latissimus dorsi, erector spinae, pectorals, intercostals, diaphragm, rectus abdominis, obliques, gluteals, hamstrings, quadriceps, abductors of the upper leg, gastrocnemius, soleus, tibialis anterior.

13   Briefly describe how oxygen and carbon dioxide are exchanged in the lungs.

14   List the functions of the liver.

15   Name the two main division of the nervous system and list their components.

16   Describe the sense of smell, from a molecule entering the nose to it reaching the limbic area of the brain.

17   List the eight main endocrine glands and name the hormone(s) secreted by each.

18   What is the function of the renal system?

19   What is meant by the term 'fluid balance'? List the main life changes that occur in a female.

20   What considerations would you take before treating a pregnant client?

Client care

5

Learning objectives

This chapter covers the following:

- **first impressions**
- **interpersonal skills**
- **counselling skills and the therapist**
- **protecting yourself**
- **preparing for treatment**
- **consultation techniques**
- **contra indications**
- **after care and advice**

This chapter will look at a variety of skills to ensure that you give your clients the service they deserve. Many therapists forget too quickly that the client has a choice. It is a privilege – not a right – that the client has chosen *you* to be their therapist. There is only one opportunity to make a good 'first impression'. Make sure it is the right one.

First impressions

Creating the right atmosphere

Colour

The colour you choose to decorate and accessorize your salon or clinic should reflect the general atmosphere you want to create. Your colour theme needs to appeal to the clients (male and female if treating both sexes). Colour themes should be carried through to include towels and bedding.

Lighting

Lighting in the treatment room should be subtle to induce relaxation. Avoid lights in places the eyes may rest upon. Lighting also helps to create a good environment and atmosphere. Inadequate lighting can lead to poor visibility, eyestrain and headaches. There are several different types of lamps which all produce different lighting effects. Dimmer switches are useful as these allow the amount of light to be varied depending on the desired effect.

Sound

Therapeutic music may be played to create the right mood. Choose music without vocals, as these may be distracting. Themed tapes can help set a scene for the client to relax into, e.g. during Indian head massage traditional Indian music could be used. It may even be preferable to work in a quiet atmosphere.

General salon sounds should be monitored to avoid unnecessary noise:

- move containers quietly and keep movement to a minimum during treatment
- open and close doors quietly
- move about slowly
- don't whisper as it attracts attention
- leave tidying up until the treatment has finished – you can do this as the client is coming to after treatment.

Temperature

Heat stress

The optimum working temperature is about 18.3°C with a working range between 15.5–22°C (or 70°F). The recommended temperature is 20°C. It is higher than for other businesses as the clients are usually semi-clothed. The temperature in a salon should be maintained and should not fluctuate unnecessarily causing discomfort.

Air conditioning

An effective air-conditioning system

- controls temperature – effective for both keeping temperature warm when cold as well as cool when hot
- maintains humidity – moistening or drying the air
- filters pollutants – dust and dirt.

Although very effective, air conditioning is also expensive to install. Both permanent and portable apparatus is available dependent on need.

Humidity

The amount of water vapour or 'dampness' in the air is called humidity; it can be increased through

- sweating
- breathing
- steamers/steam baths.

Comfortable humidity is 30–50 per cent. Humidity should be controlled and should not exceed 70 per cent as this leads to discomfort and heat stress; the body is unable to cool itself naturally as sweat is unable to evaporate. When the air can hold no more water it is described as saturated. The higher the temperature the more water vapour it can hold. When the water content cools it forms condensation.

Ventilation

Ventilation is the replacement of stale air with fresh air. Fresh air contains approximately 21 per cent of oxygen; in the salon this is normally about 16 per cent. Good ventilation is essential to ensure that stagnant air does not build up as this will lead to fatigue and an increased risk from cross-infection. The air in the salon should be changed 3–4 times every hour.

- *Natural convection* (ventilation without the assistance of fans): Generally stale air exits from a high point directed upwards and fresh air enters from a lower level (not floor level as this causes draughts), e.g. louvered windows.
- *Controlled or artificial ventilation:* Movement of air assisted by electric fans, e.g. extractor fans in walls or windows.

Inadequate ventilation will lead to:

- build up of micro-organisms
- increase in temperature – stuffy atmosphere
- a build up of CO_2
- condensation and damp.

Aroma

Aromatherapy creates its own distinct aroma. Masseuses may choose to create their own pleasing smell using a diffuser or a burner; this may even enhance the treatments effects. Burning incense sticks can also to help create a calming atmosphere.

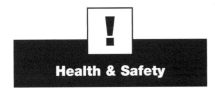

Health & Safety

Fire hazard
Be careful of burners which use night-lights. Essential oils are volatile and electric burners are a safer option.

Interpersonal skills

As with any industry demand is high for excellent customer service. It is the level of service provided that can make the difference between an average therapist and an excellent one. Sadly we are all too ready to criticize the poor service and complain (on average to at least 10 people!). It is far more cost effective to maintain the clients you have than to continually generate new business because the client base is unstable. If clients are not returning you need find out why and address the issues.

Interesting fact

During the first seven seconds of contact, people will make eleven decisions about you!

Personal presentation

Posture

Adopt good posture and non-verbal communication (NVC). These will not only portray confidence but make you feel confident too.

To ensure you are familiar with posture see Chapter 7.

Presentation

As a professional you should dress the part. Would you take a nurse seriously if they wore jeans and a scruffy T-shirt? Wear an appropriate uniform that is clean and pressed. If you have a sloppy appearance it may indicate to the client that this is the level of service they can expect from their treatment. Make sure your uniform gives you room to move and doesn't expose you (either end!), especially when you are leaning forward; this is particularly important for females working with male clients.

Review Chapter 1, p.12, for additional guidance on personal presentation.

Communication skills

What is communication?

Communication is a way of conveying, receiving and responding to thoughts, feelings and information. It is important that you develop good communication skills as poor communication leads to confusion, misunderstanding and mistakes.

We communicate in a variety of ways, both verbal and non-verbal, the latter including body language and written text.

How do we receive information?

In the clinic, for the majority of time we are face to face with a client. We receive and analyse information in the following ways. During conversation only 7 per cent of communication is from the words you use: 38 per cent is the tone you use, how you say it, 55 per cent is NVC or body language.

Tip

Never assume.

Break the word up:
Ass + U + Me.

Always be clear with information.

It's not what you say, but how you say it!

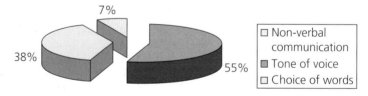

Non-verbal communication
Tone of voice
Choice of words

Non-verbal communication (NVC)

Paralanguage is a term given to NVC. It is defined as:

> That which is left after subtracting verbal content from speech.

Para – is how it is said.

Language – is what is said.

NVC includes:

- gestures
- limb movements
- facial expressions and head nods ('your face can speak a thousands words!')
- eye contact
- posture.

NVC can reinforce or contradict verbal communication. People see what you mean; true feelings can be given away.

By monitoring the client's responses you can ensure that their treatment is as effective as possible. The words may say something quite different from what the body language shouts. Is the client really relaxed and enjoying the treatment or simply being polite and just saying they are?

Gestures (NVC) are like words in a sentence – to make sense you need to look at gesture clusters, avoid interpreting a solitary gesture.

A smile

'A smile costs nothing.' The simplest way to impress, a smile will relax both you and the client. A smile says 'I am pleased to see you' and makes a client feel welcome. When handling an awkward situation it's amazing what you can get away with if you keep your body language open and smile! But don't overdo it.

Stressed body?

Many of the clients having treatments today do so to help them relax and combat the stresses of modern living. The following when clustered are good indicators of a stressed or anxious client:

- avoiding eye contact, frequent or prolonged blinking
- touching or pulling ear (symbolic of shutting out noise)
- touching, scratching nose
- touching or rubbing eyes (symbolic of don't like what they see)
- fidgeting, fiddling
- folding arms (a comfort gesture but can also be a sign of guarding or protecting the body).

Dishonesty! Retreat and negativity

Be aware of the defensive body. When carrying out a consultation it may be useful to be aware of the client who may not be being quite honest or who is evasive. Look for the opposite of effective NVC in the table on p.128.

If a client is being defensive, ask yourself why. Are you trying to give them the hard sell? Leaning away from you, crossed legs with the crossed leg pointing away from you, and crossed arms are all signs to look for that the client is ready to retreat!

Verbal communication

- Listening
- Questioning

Interpersonal skills

Top NVC turn offs	**Effective NVC**
Common NVCs indicating a lack of interest. Avoid them – they will make the client feel unwelcome, intimidated or as if they are being judged	*Use these to give a positive impression*
<ul><li>frowning</li><li>little or overlong eye contact</li><li>moving away</li><li>yawning</li><li>sneering</li><li>picking at teeth</li><li>shaking head</li><li>cleaning or filing fingernails</li></ul>	<ul><li>a good handshake (firm but not wrist-breaking or the 'wet fish' hand shake)</li><li>keep body language open; don't cross arms, legs, fingers!</li><li>lean forward when the client is talking to show interest</li><li>subtle mirroring (i.e. copying the client's body language) often comes naturally but don't overdo it as this can be off putting</li><li>direct eye contact (no more than 60 per cent otherwise this will be seen as threatening or intimidating)</li><li>smile (using the eyes not just the mouth!)</li></ul>

Listening techniques

Before we address questioning skills, first you must realize that being able to listen is just as important in communicating effectively as verbal communication.

Active listening demonstrates that you *are hearing* what is being said.

- Concentrate.
- Face the client and lean forward to show interest keep hands and arms opens.
- Acknowledge what is being said, keep eye contact, nod in agreement (beware of too much nodding as this is also an indicator for the person to keep talking!), raise eyebrows occasionally and smile (if appropriate).
- Make listening noises: Hum, Yes, Aha, OK.
- Acknowledge what is not said; watch NVC.
- Don't interrupt; pause before talking to leave time for the client to talk further.
- Don't fidget.
- Summarize and confirm what the client has said to demonstrate that you understand and that you have not made assumptions.
- Evaluate what is being said.

Work towards being a good listener. Encourage the client to talk and tell you about 'their' needs and life stories.

Questioning skills

There are two types of questions: open and closed.

Choosing the right type of question can help you gain the information you require. It can also help you to lead the consultation and devise an effective treatment plan

Open questions are used to start a conversation and to gain information. They usually start with 'W'; What, Where, Why, When, Who, Which and How. You can also use *t*ell me, *e*xplain and *d*escribe (TED).

Tip

Funnelling technique
During the consultation it may be useful to draw on the funnelling technique.

- Think of the shape of a funnel. This is how you need your information – wide and broad, then narrow it down.
- Open – the conversation; keep it broad and light.
- Probe – narrow the information down to get the facts you need.
- Close – finalize the consultation.
- Check – summarize and confirm.

Probing questions are open questions which

- narrow down information
- gain specific information
- extract details.

Combining these open questions will help you lead the conversation and acquire the relevant information.

Closed questions are used when

- only a short response of one or two words is required
- you need to confirm or establish information, e.g. how often do you take your medication?
- you want to close down rambling and talkative clients, e.g. Is that comfortable?

Positivity and negativity

When you communicate do you speak positively or negatively? Is the glass half full or half empty?

Try to incorporate positive phrases when you talk to clients. Positivity is the key to good customer services and for motivating clients.

Tip

Positive words and phrases to use
Positive = 'expressing certainty or affirmation to emphasize what is good.'

Use the following:

What I can do is . . .'	'Me', 'I', 'We'	'Yes'
'Successful'	'Now'	'recommended'
'Challenge'	'You can be confident that . . .'	'Thank you'
'Immediately'	'Resolved'	'Money-saving', 'time-saving'
	'easy', 'new', 'safe', 'proven'	'I will'
'I can'	'now'	'It's quicker for you . . .'
'Powerful'	'I will investigate . . .'	'I am positive . . .'

Tip

Negative words and phrases to avoid
Negative = 'expressing a refusal or denial', 'lacking positive qualities such as enthusiasm or optimism', 'showing opposition or resistance'

Avoid the following:

'You must'	'It's not my job'	'No', 'Can't', 'Never'
'cheap'	'Sorry'	'Sadly . . .', 'I'm afraid . . .'
'problem', 'failure', 'wrong'	'I am not able to . . .'	'All I can do . . .'
'Them', 'They'	'It's salon policy	'Unfortunately . . .'
'Useless'	'won't'	
'I don't know'	'weak'	

Telephone skills

Effective communication skills are also important when using the phone. This is an aspect often neglected when addressing communication yet it is part of the day-to-day running of any business. Often the telephone will be the first point of contact with a business, and as such it provides an opportunity to make a professional first impression.

Telephone etiquette is of great importance. Always answer the phone with a proper salutation. Speak slowly and clearly, don't race, you are reciting important information. We usually don't hear the first words spoken, which is why many salutations start with 'good morning/afternoon'. Once the caller has tuned in, follow with the name of the business. Then state who you are so that the caller knows with whom they are talking too: e.g. 'Good morning, The Holistic Clinic, Helen speaking – How may I help you?' As silly as it may seem, try to smile when you are on the phone. When you smile it changes the tone of your voice.

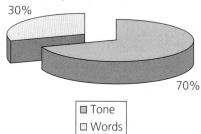

Telephone communication

- 30% Tone
- 70% Words

Challenging customers

There will always be challenging customers whether you are dealing with them face to face or over the phone. The challenging customer comes in a variety of packages, lacking in manners, treating their therapist with contempt, hard to please, generally awkward or angry.

Reasons why a client might find fault include:

- poor personal or salon hygiene
- being shown a lack of courtesy and/or good manners
- uninterested service, therapist not paying attention
- therapist's hands in poor condition
- being given unsuitable treatment.

Why are they angry?

Customers rarely get angry without a reason. Anger is associated with people not getting their own way. Dissatisfaction with a situation being poorly managed often makes customers become angry.

When you encounter a challenging client always keep in mind the following.

- Move them away to a quiet area.
- Encourage a client to sit down if they are angry. It's much harder being angry if you are sitting down. Think: what is often the first thing you do when you get angry? You stand up!
- Do not interrupt.
- Apologize – quite often a simple apology for the inconvenience or misunderstanding will calm an angry customer down, but don't pass the blame, e.g. 'I am sorry that the services did not meet your expectations' rather than 'I am sorry Jo isn't very good at that treatment, she is new'.
- Empathize and acknowledge their emotions – 'I appreciate you are angry/upset/disappointed'.
- Manage your emotions, speak slowly, clearly and calmly, the calmer you stay the more quickly it will be resolved. Don't get angry: remember customers will react to how you behave.
- Physically, take deep breaths, count to ten, stand or sit up – it makes you feel more in control.
- Always thank the client for drawing an issue to your attention – no matter how you feel. If there has been a genuine error there is always room for improvement.

Tip

When clients get angry it may not be your fault so remember that you are simply listening to someone who is in an 'attacking mode'.

Tip

Think of a bottle of fizz that's been shaken up. When you open the lid it will be uncontrollable, but eventually the fizz will die down. Angry people are the same. Let them get their problems out, have a good moan, and then they will simmer down.

Counselling skills and the therapist

> Counselling is the skilled and principled use of relationships to facilitate self-knowledge, emotional acceptance and growth, and the optimal development of personal resources. . . . The counsellor's role is to facilitate the client's work in ways that respect the client's values, personal resources and capacity for self-determination.
>
> (British Association of Counselling 1989)

Counselling is a person-to-person form of communication. It is a process designed to help people make choices and take appropriate actions, free from authoritarian judgements or coercive pressures.

Counselling is a broad and diverse activity that increasingly reaches into all aspects of people's lives.

During a consultation you counsel the client, but this is only to gain information and offer the client options and choices – that is as far as it goes. No matter how familiar you are with a client, they must make their own decisions, no matter how obvious the solution.

If counselling is needed to resolve personal issues the client should be directed to practitioners with training to meet the client's need. Credentials of counselling practitioners is a matter of public debate and so referral should be made through the client's General Practitioner or through a recognized organization such as 'Cruise' (bereavement counselling) or Relate (relationship counselling).

Ethics, boundaries and confidentiality

Ethics

Ethics are the guidelines that the therapist works to. They ensure good professional practice.

It is not a legal requirement that you follow the guidelines but they can be used if something goes wrong or if you are negligent in your practice.

Different organizations will issue you with their own professional codes of practice should you decide to join their organization. Ethics and codes of practice generally state

- expected standards professional conduct
- what is expected from you to maintain good working practices
- stipulate that you only carry out those treatments you are qualified to do so
- respect confidentiality
- refrain from slandering other businesses
- comply with legislation and local by-laws (includes hygiene practices).

Boundaries – friend or foe!

One of the hardest ethical boundaries is the distinction between the 'client' and the 'friend'. Clients often develop a great trust in their therapist, telling them information that they wouldn't tell their best friend. Others are lonely and develop one-sided bonds with the therapist. There are few who can comfortably cross these boundaries without problems; but for others the relationship can become strained. The client may feel that, as

Tip

Formal address
When you first greet a new client always address them formally. Do not use first names unless the client refers to themselves by their name or invites you to do so. Always use the client's name when addressing them or giving them instructions.

your 'friend', they should have preferential treatment or discounts. These boundaries can become a particular problem for therapists who work at home. It must be clear to the client that it is not just your home it is your business also.

Remember these points:

- Keep information confidential, both yours and theirs.
- Don't discuss clients with other clients or refer to clients by name in public areas.
- Only write on a record card the information necessary to perform their treatment, keep the rest in your head. Let the client lead the conversation so that they choose the topic for discussion.
- Try as much as possible to keep the conversation centred on the client. As the professional relationship develops you may find conversation becomes more relaxed. You should not be discussing your personal details with the client. You should still remember that the client is there for a reason and not so that you can unburden your problems onto them.
- Clients often ask for advice. It is also important to remember that you should never tell the client what to do, you can make suggestions and offer choices but the client should make the decision. Avoid the catchphrase 'If I were you I'd . . .'. You must remain objective and non-judgemental.

Working on the opposite gender

For some therapists the option of working on the opposite gender may be one they choose not to undertake. Some have religious restrictions which forbid them from doing so while others just feel uncomfortable at the prospect.

There is a tendency to think that only female therapists are at risk while working on men, but the situation can become problematic for those of any gender. Remember to

- behave and dress professionally
- maintain the client's modesty (as with any client)
- make sure that the doors cannot be locked and leave the door ajar while you are working on a member of the opposite sex
- if possible ask another therapist to discreetly keep an eye open if you are nervous
- alternatively have a panic button installed for emergencies
- avoid any situation where you are on your own if you feel at risk, especially if you do not know the client.

Protecting yourself

For some it may be bizarre, for others it comes naturally. You need to protect yourself, not from physical harm, but from negative energy. Remember our chemistry: molecules are leaving our bodies all the time as water, sweat, dead skin, etc! Nervous responses and emotions revolve around molecules too.

Your aim is to avoid picking up these negative atoms during a treatment. Always make sure you wash your hands at the beginning and end of a treatment. There are some practitioners who believe you should wash up to the elbows after treatment. While you wash your hands, think about the negativity from the treatment washing down the drain. Wash with cold then hot water.

Other strategies for protection work on a similar theme and involve sealing your body in an imaginary protective shield. This may be an energy ball, a bubble, cloak or an imaginary protective suit.

The important lesson from protecting yourself is to approach your treatment in the right frame of mind. Clear your thoughts and focus on what you are doing. Keep your mind uncluttered. Step back from your client when you have finished (literally and mentally), wish them well and tell yourself the treatment is over.

Preparing for a treatment

Be prepared for each client. Before taking the client into the treatment room, make sure you have everything to hand that you will need during the treatment.

Preparing the couch

Your couch should be set up with clean linen for each treatment. For hygiene reasons any sheets/covers should be covered with couch paper, which can be disposed of at the end of treatment. Protect supports and pillows and have these ready and within reach

There are several options as to how to set up the couch:

- towels only: the couch is covered with towels and towels are used to cover the client
- couch covered with a towelling cover and towels used to cover client
- a blanket lies over the couch, covered with a cotton sheet and the client is wrapped in the sheet and blanket (a warm option and good for facial or reflexology).

For some treatments a 4.5-tog duvet can be used to keep the client warm.

Whichever method you use, you need to be able to access the client easily without fumbling about. Remember that as the client relaxes during treatment the body temperature drops slightly and the client can begin to feel cold. Keep a check on them at intervals during treatment.

Tip

Cover towels and undergarments with couch paper as you work to reduce the amount of contact with oil. This can also be used to blot the oil should the client wish you to do so.

A nice touch is to have a heated towel rail or warming facility (or place towels on radiator) to keep towels and blankets warm prior to use (in the summer and hotter countries the reverse may be necessary).

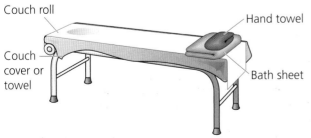

Couch roll
Hand towel
Couch cover or towel
Bath sheet

Couch set up

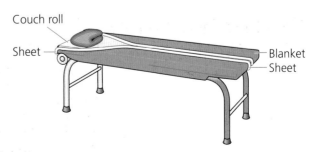

Couch roll
Sheet
Blanket
Sheet

Alternative couch set up

The consultation process

A consultation must be performed at the start of a treatment to:

- gather information about needs and expectations
- assess clinical diagnosis (i.e. is the client suitable for the treatment or is further assessment required, e.g. medical; before any treatment commences?)
- establish a rapport
- explain the way a treatment works and other related information and give the client the opportunity to discuss the treatment plan and to ask questions
- create the opportunity to devise a treatment plan for the client taking into account suitability for treatment, frequency, availability and any cost implications
- motivate the client (be positive).

Realistic or unrealistic – be honest

Are the client's expectations from the treatment they have booked in for realistic or unrealistic? If they are unrealistic then you need to address this early on. Explain tactfully why the treatment will not meet their expectations and offer an alternative.

The client will respect your honesty and you do not want a dissatisfied client who has had an unsuitable treatment.

Consultation techniques

Carrying out the consultation

When you first meet a client remember to introduce yourself; it's a nice gesture to shake their hand.

The consultation is often carried out in the room in which you are working and should be carried out before the client gets undressed in case there is any reason that they cannot be treated.

There are three skills required as part of the consultation.

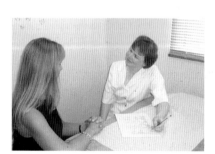

Side-by-side consultation

1 *Observation*. What can you observe about the client? Are they nervous, extrovert, holding their body in such a way that might give indication for treatment?
2 *Verbal questioning*. Gain the information required.
3 *Physical examination*. What can you physically see and feel on the client? This third part is only carried out once you have assessed that, so far, the client is suitable for treatment.

Approximately 15 minutes should be allocated to carry out the initial consultation to ask the client questions and it should be in a private area free from interruptions. Ideally you should be sitting face to face or next to your client to create an open atmosphere. Avoid any barriers such as couches or a table coming between you.

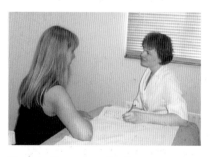

Face-to-face consultation

If you are performing the consultation in a communal environment this may create barriers and inhibit the client's responses. Keep your voice low throughout to avoid personal details being overheard.

What to record and why

Holistic treatments treat the individual as a whole, taking into consideration general well-being, i.e. health, emotional, physical and mental states. You need to explain carefully to the client why you are carrying out a consultation.

Use open questions to tactfully encourage the client to give you information that you need rather than interrogating them and asking lots of direct and often personal questions. Use the record card as a prompt rather than a list to be ticked off.

If your client has trouble accepting the reasons for obtaining information about their health and lifestyle it may be that there is an underlying question of what do they feel they have to hide! While you are not in the position to challenge the client you may be able to err on the side of caution. Effective communication should reassure the client that your only motives are to offer a safe and effective treatment.

Options for recording information

- One comprehensive record card for all treatments.
- Alternatively you may have a basic generic information card (i.e. personal details) with a different additional sheet for each treatment as the information will vary.

Only the relevant information for the treatment you are giving needs to be completed. You can always add to it at a later date if additional treatments are undertaken.

Not all the information needs to be verbal – remember to use your observational skills where appropriate. Additional details can be added while the client is relaxing at the end of their treatment.

Record keeping

Records must be maintained for a number of reasons:

- they provide contact details in case you need to alter or cancel an appointment
- so that you can monitor the client's progression
- another therapist should be aware of what treatment and products the client has had should the need arise
- to track any after care advice that you have given the client
- to monitor samples given to the client or products that the client has bought (useful in prompting for further sales and ensuring stock is available)
- as a back up in case the client has an adverse reaction to a treatment.

Important information

The following general information should be recorded for all clients.

- *Personal details*
  Full name (family name or surname), address, contact number, GP's name and address. You will also need for most treatments a detailed medical background of the client including the following information.

- *Specific contra indications* (see below)
  These should all be noted accordingly. You will probably find as you go through that the client will lead you rather than you having to read off a list, as this can be quite unnerving for the client.
- *Medication*
  What medication are they taking (and for what condition)? If a client is taking medication it will give you clues to their health.
- *Are they consulting their GP or a consultant and if so, for what condition?*
  If they are consulting their GP on a regular basis or under a consultant you may need to check further their suitability for treatment.
- *Have they had recent surgery?*
  You will need to consider scar tissue and there may be post-operative precautions you need to take. Many people find it takes a while to get anaesthetic out of their system and may feel low.
- *Life-changing illnesses*
  Includes: arthritis, cancer, any disablement, AIDS, epilepsy, diabetes, stroke and depressions.
- *Accidents*
  What implication do these have? Have they had to have surgery? Do they need referral to other professionals? Will your treatment plan need adjusting?

Tip

It is useful to keep a medical encyclopaedia and check details of any medication that the client cannot explain.

Other information

- *Physical fitness*
  How fit is the client? A client may think they are fit and many will say they are fitter then they really are. A resting pulse will give you a guide.
- *The client's occupation and lifestyle*
  These factors will give you a rough indication of free time and budget to consider before negotiating a treatment plan. This information will give you clues as to where the client may have stress and muscular tension. This information will also give you an insight into their level of activity.
- *Life-changing conditions*
  Includes: puberty, pregnancy, menopause, retirement, bereavement, divorce and any illness.
- *Hobbies*
  You may choose not to include this but it is useful to find out the client's interests; this will also give you an idea of levels of activity and spare time.
- *Personality, temperament and emotional state*
  Not the sort of question you can ask but you can make a mental note of these points as you carry out your consultation. These factors will help to indicate which oils or zones to work on further.
- *Disclaimer*
  Always add a disclaimer and the client's signature to verify that the information the client has given you is to the best of their knowledge true and correct.

Tip

Level of fitness
Maintaining a good level of fitness involves increased cardiovascular efficiency. The aim is to do at least three sessions of a minimum of 20 minutes during which one should be slightly out of breath, i.e. breathing faster, but still able to hold a conversation.

Consultation during consecutive treatments

On consecutive treatments a shorter consultation should always be carried out prior to commencing treatment. The person you are today is not the person you will be tomorrow. An individual's health and well-being will vary from day to day and records must be kept up to date and adjusted accordingly.

Contra indications

A 'contra indication' is something that will prevent you from performing a service – contra means against, i.e. an indication against treatment. Contra indications can be:

- *general*, and you will be unable to treat the client, or
- *specific*, which will prevent you working over or on an area.

It is advisable that you are familiar with the list below. You need to be aware of what the condition is, how it is caused and why it is contra indicated, i.e. what adverse effect could your treatment have on the condition.

General contra indications

- Diabetes
- Cardiovascular conditions, including hypertension, hypotension, thrombosis, embolism, phlebitis, angina, pacemakers
- Any dysfunction of the nervous system, e.g. anaesthesia (loss of sensation), epilepsy
- If a high temperature or fever is present (pyrexia)
- Recent operations (as applicable)
- Any unexplained swellings and swollen glands
- Pregnancy (first 12 weeks and where applicable)
- Post-natal (6 weeks)
- Any general infection whether viral (e.g. flu), bacterial (e.g. impetigo), fungal (e.g. tinea) or infestations (e.g. head lice)
- Blood diseases, including HIV (unless under specialized supervision) and hepatitis

Err on the side of caution and consider any condition which is being treated by a medically qualified practitioner, e.g. cancer.

Anyone who is unwell must be questioned tactfully. If in doubt do nothing.

Contra indications specific to an area

- Open wounds, cuts and abrasions
- Acne rosacea
- Acne vulgaris, pustulant skin
- Focus of sepsis, boils, bites, stings
- Dilated arterioles, telangiectasia (where applicable)
- Varicose veins (only work above affected area)
- Warts
- Moles
- Over the abdomen during the first 2/3 days of menstruation
- Be cautious with clients fitted with an IUD (intrauterine device – coil) over the abdomen
- Eczema
- Psoriasis
- Bruising

- Recent fractures
- Recent scar tissue
- Sunburn

To ensure you are familiar with contra indications, review Chapter 4.

Seeking professional guidance

Contra indications can put you in an awkward position during consultation because many clients with long-term conditions manage them well and their treatment is established and effective, e.g. diabetes, high blood pressure, hyperthyroidism. They may feel victimized, especially if they have not had problems for a number of years. However, do not be bullied into giving an unsuitable treatment. If you are concerned about losing a client remember these points.

- Could you cope with an adverse reaction?
- Are you prepared to be sued if something goes wrong and you are found to be negligent?
- If you were found to be negligent your insurance may not cover you.

Reassure yourself that you are doing the right thing and that you only have their interests at heart.

The worst-case scenario is the client who chooses to lie. Clients are in control of the information and may choose to tell you only what they want you to know. You must create an environment which will give them the opportunity to be honest so that you can treat them safely.

There are occasions when medical guidance will be necessary before treatment and General Practitioners are unhappy about getting involved. GPs will charge a fee even if it is just for a signature to acknowledge a response and clients will find this off putting. However, if a prospective client genuinely wishes to be treated, it is in their interest to gain the necessary information. They will also appreciate the reason why it is being requested.

The following points should also be considered when seeking medical guidance.

- The client should contact their doctor.
- Remember you are not asking for approval or permission to carry out your services. Some physicians will not want to get involved and this arises when they are asked for approval and as such do not have direct control over the treatment. By giving their approval they may also be accountable for any adverse results.
- Many doctors are unaware of what the treatments involve and so an information leaflet is a useful addition.
- You are enquiring as to whether in their medical opinion there is any medical reason why their patient is unsuitable for treatment. Clients are often unaware of the implications of their condition. I have had clients who are taking medication and they are not sure what for!
- If you need to contact the client's doctor do not refer to the client's condition by name, even if the client has discussed this openly with you.
- If you are unsure of a condition but suspicious that it needs medical treatment again do not state the condition by name. Remember that only a doctor is medically qualified to offer a diagnosis.

Tip

Professional working relationships
Develop professional working relationships with local doctors. Promote your treatments with them. Tell them

- what qualifications you have
- how many years you have been practising
- which professional organization you are registered with
- that you have current indemnity insurance.

- You may feel more comfortable referring clients with some illnesses to clinics that specialize in treating them. There are many centres now attached to hospitals and hospices etc. where specialized treatments are offered under the supervision of medical staff.

There are some alternative practices.

- Where a client demonstrates an understanding of their condition, the client can consult with their doctor who can then discuss with them their suitability for treatment. The doctor can then advise the client directly of any restrictions or precautions.
- You could write to the doctor citing the information above. Give the details of the client you are intending to treat and with what treatment. You could then state that if you do not hear within a specified number of days you will presume that there are no objections to the treatment commencing.

In both cases the information is then noted on the client's records which the client signs to verify the content.

What you need to know

The following is a guideline for a general consultation sheet.

Remember, in depth information is usually only required in detail for reflexology and aromatherapy.

Note: those entries given in bold may be general contra indications.

Website

Visit the companion website at www.thomsonlearning.co.uk/ beckmann where you will find a copy of a general consultation sheet.

About the circulation

- **High blood pressure**
- **Low blood pressure**
- **Heart valve disorder**
- **Thrombosis**
- Cellulite
- Thread veins
- Cold hands/feet
- Varicose veins

About the muscular or skeletal system

- **Rheumatism**
- **Arthritis** (depending on severity)
- **Recent fractures**
- **Recent whiplash**
- Stiff joints
- Recent sprains
- Tension
- Backache

- Sciatica
- Headaches

About gynaecology

- Caution over related points if using **coil/IUD**

During *pregnancy*

- (reflexology and aromatherapy) **over abdomen**/reflexology

Menstruation

- Menstrual cycle
- Irregular
- Painful
- Heavy
- PMT
- Trying to conceive
- History of miscarriage
- Number of pregnancies (only if applicable)
- Contraceptive pill
- HRT
- Thrush

About nervous and stress-related problems

- Any dysfunctional disorders, e.g. **multiple sclerosis**
- **Epilepsy**
- Mood swings
- Panic attacks
- Depression
- Irritability
- Anxiety

About the digestive system

- **(over abdomen) Hiatus hernia**
- Indigestion
- Constipation
- Candida
- Heartburn
- Irritable bowel syndrome
- Allergies

About diet

- Eat regularly?
- Type of diet
- Taking supplements?
- Dieting?
- Amount of caffeine consumed (tea, coffee, cola)
- Water intake

About the kidney/ urinary system

- Fluid retention
- Cystitis
- **Kidney disease**

About the respiratory system

- Asthma
- Smoker
- Catarrh
- Bronchitis
- Prone to chesty coughs
- Sinus problems
- Hay fever

About the endocrine system

- **Diabetes**
- Hyperthyroid
- Hypothyroid

About the immune system

- **Unknown swellings**
- Glandular fever
- Prone to illness
- ME
- Sore throat
- Tiredness

About sleeping patterns

- Insomnia
- Awake early
- Dreamer
- Difficulty getting to sleep
- Periods of wakefulness
- Amount of sleep needed

About the condition of the skin, hair, nails

- **Hair**
- **Nails**
- Skin condition – face
- Skin condition – body
- **Eczema (if weeping)**
- Psoriasis
- Sensitivity
- Stretch marks
- Scar tissue
- Loose skin
- Acne
- Dry
- Oily
- Imperfections
- Moles
- Allergies (especially nut)

Observations before treatment

Once you are happy with the information you have gathered from your oral questions and that there is nothing that you have ascertained which may contra indicate the client can be prepared for treatment. Always check the client for visual contra indications. There may be skin blemishes that need an explanation or scar tissue that the client has lived with for so long they have forgotten to mention or blemishes of which the client is unaware. Even at this stage you are perfectly within your rights to refuse treatment. Do it tactfully however, and where possible offer an alternative treatment.

After care and advice

Contra actions and adverse reactions

The client should be made aware of any adverse reactions that they may experience without alarming them. It is a good idea to have a leaflet detailing advice and after care for the client to take home. After treatment your client will be relaxed and may forget what you have told them.

Some reactions may occur both during and after treatment. While changes are a positive step to the body re-establishing equilibrium, these need to manageable and symptoms should not persist. See table on pp.142–3, for further details.

The healing crisis

The 'healing crisis' is the name given to noticeable 'adverse' reactions.

- A client could experience a return or increase in symptoms before they notice an improvement. This should only be temporary. Where there is a long history of imbalance or illness this is more likely.
- It may also be an indicator that instead of having a healing reaction the client has been 'over treated' and the body has been thrown into a crisis.
- It may be a reaction between treatment and medication that the client is taking.

If an adverse healing crisis occurs during treatment it should be stopped immediately and the treatment re-evaluated.

Additional after care and home care advice can be found in the various treatment chapters.

Non-effective treatments

It may be evident on the completion of a treatment that it has not been effective. The client may not be relaxed and may even seem agitated. You need to address the reasons straight away. These could simply be that the client has never had the treatment before and was nervous or just generally finds it difficult to relax. Hopefully this will be resolved on consecutive treatments. However, it could be your fault. Did you carry out a consultation, consider the client's needs, communicate with your client and create the right environment?

Tip

Evaluation
Upon completion of each treatment spend a few moments evaluating it. Next time would you change anything? Even if you were really pleased with the results, was the client?

Tip

Booking the next treatment
Offer to book the client's next treatment before they leave. They can always phone to change arrangements. They are more likely to do this than phone to make an appointment at regular intervals.

You should also advise the client when they should return for further treatment and if appropriate discuss any suitable products they should be using at home – hopefully this will become a retail opportunity.

General after care

The client will be in a relaxed and more emotional state after treatment and any further questions should be carefully phrased.

It is not only useful to record what products you have chosen to use but it is also a good idea to record any sales you have made so that these can be followed up. The following is a simple sheet that can be added to the client's record sheet/card.

Date	Treatment/products used	Sales (samples)	Therapist
Comments			

Contra actions (positive and negative)

Reaction	***Reason***	***Treatments***							
		Applies to all treatments	Aromatherapy	Indian head massage	Massage	Reflexology	Holistic facial	Reiki	Thermal auricular therapy
Feeling of tiredness	the body's natural way of making you slow down so that it can heal		✓	✓	✓	✓		✓	✓
Feeling of thirst	increases fluid intake to encourage excretion of toxins		✓		✓	✓		✓	
Aching muscles	due to the release of toxins from the muscle fibres as a result of the massage		✓	✓	✓				
Increase in the feeling of well-being	due to release of endorphins	✓	✓	✓	✓	✓	✓	✓	✓

Reaction	Reason	Applies to all treatments	Aromatherapy	Indian head massage	Massage	Reflexology	Holistic facial	Reiki	Thermal auricular therapy
Relief from muscular tension and stress	increased circulation into tissues during massage removal of metabolites		✓	✓	✓	✓	✓	✓	
Tingling or twitching in the limbs	stimulation of circulation and nervous system		✓		✓	✓		✓	
Clearer mental awareness	increased circulation to the brain		✓	✓	✓				
Heightened emotions	natural process of healing – includes uncontrolled laughter, giggling, weeping, tearfulness		✓	✓	✓		✓		
Increase in urination	stimulation of system, body getting rid of toxins being released during treatment; urine can be darker and have a stronger odour		✓		✓	✓			
Increase in bowel movements, movements, wind and/or motions	relaxation encourages efficient gastric activity stimulation through treatment		✓		✓	✓			
Cold sweats, clammy hands	anxiety					✓		✓	
Increased mucus secretions (vaginal, nose, throat, chest)	stimulation through treatment, clearing process					✓			✓
Change in sleep patterns	a result of the general changes in the body the client may sleep deeply or be more aware of vivid, colourful dreams		✓	✓	✓	✓		✓	
Light-headedness	a result of deep relaxation blood pressure drops during deep relaxation *Slowly sit the client up and let them take their time*		✓	✓	✓	✓		✓	✓
Feeling faint	drop in blood pressure or oxygen to the brain *Raise client's legs above head if lying down or place head between knees* could be the result of getting up to quickly or a general adverse reaction to treatment	✓	✓	✓	✓	✓	✓	✓	✓
Nausea	common where there are digestive disturbances the smell of certain oils may cause nausea		✓			✓			
Skin irritation	sensitivity to product *Rinse with lukewarm water until all traces of the product have been removed. For larger areas, recommend a lukewarm shower*		✓	✓	✓		✓		

General after care advice

Reaction	Reason	Applies to all treatments	Aromatherapy	Indian head massage	Massage	Reflexology	Holistic facial	Reiki	Thermal auricular therapy
Allow the client to **rest** for at least five minutes. This can be in a quiet area away from the treatment room	To gain the maximum benefit from the treatment	✓	✓	✓	✓	✓	✓	✓	✓
Offer the client a **drink of water**. Encourage them to drink it (don't simply ask if they want one). The client should **drink plenty of water** to flush the system; toxins will have been released from the manipulation of the soft tissues where applicable or as a result of the body relaxing and releasing tension	Toxins and waste will have been released during treatment. Drinking water will help to encourage the urinary system to flush these toxins out. If these are allowed to build up the client may feel 'hung over'		✓	✓	✓	✓		✓	✓
Advise the client to **avoid strenuous activity** for a few hours; ideally the client should go home to rest and relax	To have maximum effect, the client needs to allow the body to continue to balance itself after treatment. Resting will give the body the opportunity to do this	✓	✓	✓	✓	✓	✓	✓	✓
Avoid alcohol and stimulants, including any drink with caffeine in it, e.g. cola. The client may drink herb/fruit teas or infusions	Alcohol and stimulants will put stress on the urinary system which will be working hard to eliminate toxins released during treatment If you are encouraging the body to relax you need to avoid chemicals that will stimulate it		✓	✓	✓	✓		✓	
Avoid heat treatments for a few hours as this will speed up the absorption of the oils (if used as part of the treatment); this includes sunbathing, sunbeds, hair dryers, saunas, steam baths, hot baths, etc.	Heat will speed up the absorption of essential oils and may cause an adverse reaction Some essential oils will increase skin sensitivity to ultra violet rays	✓	✓	✓	✓	✓	✓	✓	✓
Where oils have been used advise the client to **leave the oils on the skin/hair** for as long as possible	The oils will have an emollient and conditioning effect on the skin. Where essential oils have been used these should be left to continue their therapeutic work for some time after the treatment has completed (ideally 24 hours)		✓	✓	✓		✓		
If driving **keep a window open**	The client may be feeling drowsy and should get fresh air to keep them alert. Some essential oils have particularly relaxing effects. If the client is very dopey get them to wait a while. Ideally get someone else to drive!		✓	✓	✓	✓		✓	

Reaction	Reason	Applies to all treatments	Aromatherapy	Indian head massage	Massage	Reflexology	Holistic facial	Reiki	Thermal auricular therapy
Follow a simple skin care routine at home	To continue the effects of the facial treatment. As an ongoing process this will help to slow down the effects of ageing. Also to boost body treatments and keep the skin of the body in good condition	✓			✓		✓		
Advise the client of any possible contra actions/adverse reactions	The client should be aware of any changes that may be experienced, as these are part of the treatment process. However, there are occasions when the client may want to seek further reassurance and as such they should be given the opportunity to know they can call you for advice	✓	✓	✓	✓	✓	✓	✓	✓
Discuss with the client further treatments	Many therapists fail to follow up their treatment. Make sure you advise the client when to return for their next treatment	✓	✓	✓	✓	✓	✓	✓	✓

Knowledge review

1   What is NVC? Give some examples.

2   What are the two main types of question? State briefly when you would use these during a consultation.

3   Make a list of all the different methods of communicating that are used in the salon; include both verbal and non-verbal (including written).

4   Why are telephone skills essential?

5   Write a brief explanation of how you might handle different types of client; include the following clients – nervous, introverted, extrovert, reserved, pushy and angry.

6   Why would it not be ethical to offer a client professional counselling?

7   List all the factors you would consider when preparing your working environment.

8   List the potential contra actions a client might have.

9   What are the benefits of recording product information on the client's record card?

10 What factors would you consider when preparing your working environment?

6 Nutrition

Learning objectives

This chapter covers the following:

- **the macro-nutrients – carbohydrates, proteins and lipids**
- **the micro-nutrients – vitamins, minerals and trace elements**
- **anti-nutrients, enzymes and water**
- **the balanced diet**
- **the nutrition consultation**
- **identifying current diet**
- **body mass index and hip-to-waist ratio**
- **making meaningful recommendations**

Nutrition is an important subject for all therapists, as many of the problems clients have can be helped nutritionally. Skin problems including acne, stretch marks and cellulite as well as problems with weight, stress, anxiety, fatigue and digestive problems can all be helped nutritionally. Nutrition can largely determine how we look, feel and work; whether we will be nervous, tired and pessimistic, or joyful, comfortable and happily active. Nutrition can also determine whether we will age prematurely or enjoy our lives to the full. By studying nutrition you will be able to promote healthy eating to your clients.

The macro-nutrients – carbohydrates, proteins and lipids

Nutrients are the absorbable components of the food we eat and are necessary for good health, energy, organ function and cell growth. Nutrients can be divided into two main categories – the macro-nutrients and the micro-nutrients – both equally important to good health.

Macro-nutrients – which are needed in quite large quantities in the body – comprise the following:

- carbohydrates
- proteins
- fats.

Micro-nutrients – needed in much smaller amounts – are no less important.

- vitamins
- minerals
- trace elements.

The carbohydrates, proteins and fats provide energy and the vitamins, minerals and trace minerals are the substances required to release the energy.

Carbohydrates

The main function of carbohydrate foods is to provide energy for all body functions and muscular exertion. The term carbohydrate includes a variety of dietary compounds varying from simple carbohydrates (one sugar molecule also known as *monosaccharides*), to more complex carbohydrates (*disaccharides*), to still more complex carbohydrates (many sugar molecules lined, together also known as *polysaccharides*).

The energy provided from simple carbohydrates such as those in fruit and honey are very quickly absorbed. Double sugars such as sucrose (table sugar) take a little longer to be absorbed, but complex carbohydrates – the polysaccharides – require prolonged action by digestive enzymes in order to be broken down into simple sugars ready for absorption.

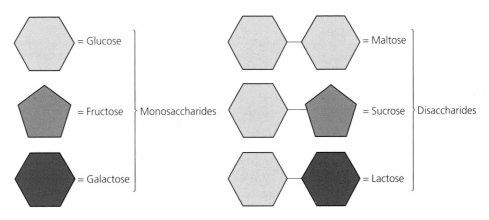

Carbohydrate molecules

The main difference between them is that the simple carbohydrates are water-soluble. This means they are readily absorbed into the body through the stomach, giving a burst of energy. The complex varieties, on the other hand, need digesting through the small intestine and therefore provide a more steady energy burst for a longer period of time. It is the complex carbohydrates (the polysaccharides) that are needed for sustained energy and to keep blood glucose levels steady.

Fibre

Fibre can be classified as soluble or insoluble but both are largely indigestible by human beings. They are important in our diets for different reasons. Fibre is only found in plant foods.

Soluble fibre is soluble in water and include pectins found in apples and gums found in beans, some fruits, vegetables, oats and barley. Soluble fibre takes up bile acids, cholesterol and toxins and carries them out of the body. They therefore lower harmful cholesterol levels and reduce the risk of cardiovascular disease. Soluble fibre absorbs many times its volume of water, soothes the intestinal tract, eases bowel movements by making stools slippery and also provides food for beneficial bacteria in the intestines.

Insoluble fibre is not soluble in water. It helps combat weight gain, colon cancer and gallstones. However, an excess of insoluble fibre can irritate the delicate lining of the intestinal tract. Insoluble fibre such as wheat bran is a harsher type of fibre and adds bulk to our stools. By bulking the waste, it can move more rapidly through the system, thus preventing constipation. It also helps against irritable bowel syndrome (IBS), haemorrhoids, diverticulosis, varicose veins and cancer of the colon. Cellulose and hemicellulose are other kinds of harsher, insoluble fibre and can be found in foods such as wholewheat flour, bran, cabbage, green beans and broccoli.

Eating enough fibre may also help guard against breast cancer, either directly or indirectly. Women who eat more vegetables and fruit and starchy whole grain cereals have a lower incidence of breast cancer, whereas a high intake of red meat and fried or browned food may increase the risk.

Vegetables and fruit

Fruit is the ultimate convenience food, requiring little or no preparation. It is easy to carry and enjoyable to eat any time, anywhere, making it a versatile snack. Vegetables are an integral part of all healthy meals. For optimum nutrition, five portions of vegetables and fruit per day are highly recommended – and there is additional benefit in consuming more, if you want to. Because most fruit can be eaten raw and many vegetables can be eaten raw in salads, or lightly cooked, they retain most of their vitamins and minerals, which in other foods are depleted or destroyed by cooking. Vegetables and fruit include all fresh, frozen, chilled and canned varieties (with the exception of potatoes, which are a starchy food). Also included are dried fruits and fruit juices, but not fruit-flavoured drinks, which contain very little, if any, fruit juice and a lot of added sugars or sweeteners and other non-nutritious ingredients.

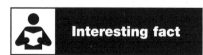

Interesting fact

The Greek for protein is 'protos', which means 'of prime importance'.

Proteins

Proteins have two main functions: one structural, for the growth and repair of body tissues; the other metabolic, for the production of enzymes, hormones, antibodies, neurotransmitters and energy.

Proteins are the most complex of all food compounds, the key factor of protein being nitrogen, the crucial ingredient in the formation of amino and nucleic acids (both nitrogen-containing compounds).

Without protein we would be unable to rebuild body cells, tissue, muscles and organs, and synthesize many important enzymes, neurotransmitters (used in the nervous system like serotonin), the important structural proteins that make hair and nails and the all-important hormones of the endocrine system. Proteins inactivate foreign invaders in the form if antibodies, thus protecting the body against disease. Protein also helps to maintain the volume and composition of body fluids.

- *Non-essential amino acids*. More than half of the amino acids are non-essential, meaning that the body can synthesize them for itself. Proteins in foods usually deliver these amino acids, but it is not essential that they do so. The body can make any non-essential amino acid by a process called transamination, which takes place in the liver.
- *Essential amino acids*. There are eight amino acids that the human body either cannot make at all or cannot make in sufficient quantity to meet its needs. These eight amino acids must be supplied by the diet and are essential for life itself. As the body is unable to synthesize these amino acids, we must actually ingest them on a daily basis.
- *Conditionally essential amino acids*. Sometimes a non-essential amino acid becomes essential under special circumstances. For example, the body normally uses the essential amino acid phenylalanine to make tyrosine (a non-essential amino acid). But if the diet fails to supply enough phenylalanine, or if the body cannot make the conversion for some reason (as happens with the inherited disease phenylketonuria), then tyrosine becomes conditionally essential.

When we think of protein foods, we tend to think immediately of meat, poultry, fish, eggs and cheese and indeed about 30 years ago these protein foods were called 'first class protein' as they contain all the 'essential' amino acids needed for human growth and health.

Protein foods can be described as 'complete' and 'incomplete' foods; the latter have a 'limiting' amino acid.

A limiting amino acid is an amino acid that is present in relatively small amounts but below the recommended essential amino acid requirements. Examples would be quinoa and wheat, both of which are short in the amino acid lysine. Lysine would therefore be called the limiting amino acid. A vegetarian would have to 'top up' with lysine by eating foods high in the amino acid, which would include soybeans, pinto beans and other legumes. These foods would then be called complementary foods.

A complete protein is therefore any food substance that contains all eight essential amino acids in the correct proportions. Eggs (organic) are an excellent example of a complete protein, with all its essential amino acids in the correct proportions. Other complete protein foods are fish, meat and cheese.

The essential amino acids

There are eight essential amino acids and two additional ones for children:

- isoleucine
- leucine
- lysine
- methionine
- phenylalanine
- threonine

- tryptophan
- valine

plus

- arginine
- histidine.

Synthesis by the body requires vitamin A. High protein intakes require concomitant vitamin A intake. Vitamin B6 (pyridoxine) is also required for protein synthesis.

The liver needs particular nutrients to convert and rebuild amino acids. Vitamins A and B6, as mentioned above, together with vitamins K and B12, are the important nutrients needed for this function.

How much protein do you actually need?

Children need more protein than adults. Most nutritionists agree that after the age of 19 protein requirements stop increasing and remain at approximately 2 oz per day (55 g) for an average-sized man and 1.5 oz (45 g) per day for an average-sized woman. So while vitally important to our diet, we do not need very much of it – it comprises only around 15 per cent of our total daily calorie intake. So, if you were consuming 2000 calories per day, your protein requirement would be approximately 300 calories. Choose low-fat protein sources such as turkey, chicken, cottage cheese, fish and tofu. A more accurate way of evaluating how much protein you actually need is to make a calculation using body weight.

How to calculate protein requirements

1 Find out the client's body weight in kilograms, or calculate weight in pounds and convert to kilograms (pounds divided by 2.2 equals kilograms).

2 Multiply kilograms by 0.8 to get your RDA (recommended daily average) in grams per day
Age adjustments:
Males age 11–14 multiply by 1; males age 15–18 years multiply by 0.9.
Females age 11–14 multiply by 1; females age 15–18 multiply by 0.8.

Example:
For a female weighing 150 lbs
150 lbs divided by 2.2 lb/kg = 68kg (rounded up)
68 kg × 0.8 g/kg = 54 g protein (rounded up)
54 g protein at 4 kcals per gram = 216 kcals protein

Fats

Many people are surprised to learn that fats have many virtues. It is only when there is either too much or too little fat in the diet that health problems may arise. The fats important in nutrition can be divided into three classes: *triglycerides*, *phospholipids* and *sterols*. Additionally, dietary fats may be divided into saturated or unsaturated fats, which refers to the saturation of hydrogen.

Fats provide a highly concentrated source of energy, which can be stored and used instead of carbohydrates when necessary. Fats provide us with insulation and protect delicate body organs. Fats also produce highly active biological substances that are vital for the normal working of the body – these substances are known as *prostaglandins*. Fats also assist in the conversion of sugars to fats.

Triglycerides

Triglycerides are the main class of food fats. They make up about 95 per cent of all the fats we eat as well as most of the stored fat we carry around in our bodies. They are a major way of storing energy for future use.

- *Storage*. We store triglycerides as adipose tissue and this is used as a reserve of energy to be called upon between meals, while asleep, during increased exertion, during pregnancy or during famine.

- *Protection*. The adipose tissue (stored triglycerides) also acts as a shock absorber to protect the body's delicate organs while we are carrying out our daily activities – walking, jumping, running or bumping into things.

- *Insulation*. Triglycerides form a layer around the body, which conserves heat to keep the body temperature constant.

Triglycerides also serve as the body's reserve of the valuable essential fatty acids, LA (linoleic acid) and ALA (alpha linoleic acid) which are required for the structure and functions of the membranes and which are the precursors of prostaglandins.

An important function of triglycerides is to convert excess sugar to fat should this be necessary. The brain needs glucose to function, but sugars in excess are toxic and are converted to triglycerides that are less harmful in large quantities. Thus triglycerides provide a safety net for the body by converting a potentially toxic substance (excess sugar) into neutral ones (triglycerides). It is for this reason that it is so easy to become overweight without actually consuming large amounts of fat.

The triglycerides are thus divided into the three familiar groups known as saturated fats, mono-unsaturated fats and polyunsaturated fats.

- *Saturated fats* are the most damaging to health. They clog up the arteries and are one of the main causes of obesity, which itself brings a host of other health problems. They are recognized as a factor in hypertension and heart disease and are responsible for inflammatory actions in the body. Saturated fats are hard at room temperature, for example butter, margarine and lard. There are many 'hidden' fats in foods such as biscuits, cakes and all confectionery.

- *Mono-unsaturated fats* are the fats that should be used in cooking. As a result of their chemical make-up they remain stable at high temperatures. The best oil for this purpose is cold-pressed virgin olive oil. As it is unrefined it is more beneficial than any refined vegetable oils.

- *Polyunsaturated fats* are 'liquid' at room temperature. Any oils that come in bottles, for example walnut, corn and sesame, are classed as polyunsaturated. These oils should not be used for cooking but for salad dressings, or to put directly on vegetables instead of a saturated fat such as butter. Polyunsaturated fats are responsible for anti-inflammatory actions in the body. As natural anti-inflammatories they are essential in the maintenance of eczema, allergies, asthma, arthritis and many other inflammatory responses in the body. Polyunsaturated fats can also be described as essential, meaning human beings cannot synthesize them in the body and so they should be ingested as part of our daily food intake.

One reason many people are deficient in essential fatty acids is because these foods are usually high in calories and as such have been demonized by the weight-loss industry. Avocados for example are a highly nutritious food, high in essential fatty acids, vitamins and minerals, but because of their high calorie value, many people on calorie-restricted diets will not eat them.

Nuts too suffer from the same bias – high in essential fatty acids but also high in calories they are nonetheless an excellent health food source of protein.

The polyunsaturated fatty acids can be divided into two groups:

- omega-6 fatty acids
- omega-3 fatty acids.

The omega-6 group of fatty acids

We obtain the omega-6 group of essential fatty acids from the food we eat by way of linoleic acid which is obtained exclusively from seeds and their oils. We then convert this LA to GLA – gamma linolenic acid – which you are probably familiar with if you take evening primrose oil. This in turn is converted to DGLA – di-homo gamma linolenic acid – and from there to prostaglandins. Prostaglandins are hormone-like substances which are very short-lived but which have important functions in the body. They help keep the blood thin, have anti-inflammatory influences on the joints, prevent fluid retention, help to lower blood pressure and assist insulin in working efficiently.

Many people are deficient in the omega-6 group of fatty acids. Women in particular shy away from any type of oil or fat because of the calorie content, in the misbelief that all fats are bad, resulting in a state of deficiency.

Even if we consumed enough seeds and their oils, there are many obstacles hindering the conversion from the original LA to GLA. These include smoking, drinking alcohol and stress in its many forms (chemical, emotional, physical, mental) and vitamin and mineral deficiency. Consequently, without the GLA we cannot go on to make the DGLA or the all-important prostaglandins. Omega-6 deficiency signs are high blood pressure, inflammatory problems such as arthritis, difficulty in losing weight, dry eyes and skin disorders including eczema. Good sources of the omega-6 essential fatty acids are hemp, pumpkin, sunflower, safflower, sesame, corn, walnut, soya bean and wheatgerm oil where as much as 50 per cent of the fats in these oils comes from the omega-6 family.

The omega-3 group of fatty acids

We obtain the omega-3 group of essential fatty acids from the food we eat by way of linolenic acid found in oily fish. We convert LA into two substances known as EPA (eicosaopentonic acid) and DHA (docosahexaenoic acid) and from there again to substances called prostaglandins.

Whereas with the omega-6 group of fats the prostaglandins are known as series 1, with the omega-3 group they are known as series 3 prostaglandins.

Omega-3 deficiency signs are dry skin, poor co-ordination and impaired vision, high blood pressure, inflammatory health problems, tendency to infections and fluid retention.

Still short-lived hormone-like substances but with different functions in the body, the series 3 prostaglandins are essential for proper brain function, co-ordination and mood, for reducing the stickiness of the blood, controlling blood cholesterol and fat levels, improving immune function and metabolism, reducing inflammation and maintaining water balance.

An excellent way of including these vital nutrients in your diet is by eating oily fish such as herring, salmon, sardines and tuna at least 3–5 times each week. By eating oily fish you are bypassing the first conversion stage and taking into your diet directly the EPA and DHA. The best seed oils for the omega-3 group of fats are flax (also known as linseed), hemp and pumpkin.

Maximum recommendations for fat intake (based on a daily intake of 2000 kcals from all food groups)

10% saturated fats (non-essential)	Butter, lard, margarine Any fat hard at room temperature	200 cals
10% mono-unsaturated fats (non-essential)	Olive oil for cooking or for making salad dressings	200 cals
10% polyunsaturated fats (essential)	Seeds, seed oils, oily fish Essential balance	200 cals

Note: Of the lipids in foods, 95 per cent are fats and oils (triglycerides) and 5 per cent are other lipids (phospholipids and sterols). Of the lipids stored in the body, 99 per cent are triglycerides.

As part of a balanced diet, the maximum you should be consuming in fats is 30 per cent; 25 per cent would be even more beneficial and the 5 per cent would be deducted from the saturated fats column. This can be broken down as shown in the table above.

Phospholipids – lecithin

In addition to the triglyceride family of fats there are the phospholipids, which are compounds with a unique chemical structure that allows them to be soluble in both water and fat. The fatty acids make phospholipids soluble in fat and the phosphate group allows them to dissolve in water. Such versatility enables the food industry to use phospholipids as emulsifiers to mix fats with water in such products as mayonnaise and sauces. Lecithin is the best known of the phospholipids. The phospholipids are important constitutes of cell membranes. Because they can dissolve in both water and fat, they can help lipids move back and forth across the cell membranes into the watery fluids on both sides. They thus allow fat-soluble substances, including vitamins A, D, E and K and hormones to pass easily in and out of cells. The phospholipids also act as emulsifiers in the body, helping to keep fats suspended in the blood and body fluids.

Sterols – cholesterol

The most famous sterol is chole*sterol*, which over the years has received a bad press. However, like the triglyceride family of fats, cholesterol has many virtues. Cholesterol is essential for physical health, even though it is not required in our food supply since our bodies can manufacture it. The body makes 80 per cent of the cholesterol it needs so there is no need to add cholesterol in the form of saturated animal fats through our diet.

Cholesterol has four essential functions in the body:

1   it is a constituent of cell membranes
2   it is a precursor of bile acids
3   it is a precursor of steroid hormones
4   vitamin D, the sunshine vitamin, is synthesized from cholesterol.

As cholesterol (and other fats) do not dissolve in blood, they are carried around by proteins. The combination of a fat and a protein becomes a lipoprotein. There are two types of cholesterol: harmful cholesterol known as LDLs (low-density lipoproteins) and beneficial cholesterol known as HDLs (high-density lipoproteins). A high ratio of HDL to LDL is desirable to protect against atherosclerosis, arteriosclerosis and cardiovascular disease. Increasing the intake of polyunsaturated essential fatty acids in favour of the harmful saturated animal fats can increase the levels of HDLs.

Exercise is vital in reducing high levels of the harmful LDL cholesterol and increasing the HDLs. It is important for you to explain to your clients the benefits of exercise and that a single 30-minute walk, three times a week, could make all the difference in reducing high cholesterol levels.

Many foods can assist in reducing high harmful cholesterol levels and preventing them becoming high in the first place. Regular daily fibre in the diet such as fruit and vegetables and complex carbohydrates will help remove harmful LDL cholesterol. Apples and other foods high in the soluble fibre pectin can also reduce high cholesterol levels.

Vitamins C and E and other anti-oxidants can be described as anti-cholesterol supernutrients. They earn this title by virtue of the fact they destroy harmful free radicals that would otherwise turn the harmful LDL cholesterol toxic and even more dangerous. The anti-oxidants block free radicals and make LDL unable to infiltrate artery walls.

Anti-nutrients, enzymes and water

An anti-nutrient is any substance that stops the beneficial nutrients being absorbed and used by the body, or any substance that promotes the excretion of a beneficial nutrient.

Alcohol, cigarettes, manufactured chemicals, pesticides, antibiotics and synthetic hormone residues can all be described as anti-nutrients. Even tap water in some areas may be described as an anti-nutrient. Tap water may contain nitrates, lead or aluminium, all of which are anti-nutrients in their own right. Fried food, foods cooked on a BBQ and burnt food can all be classed as anti-nutrients as they cause free radical damage to our cells. Many common medicines can also be described this way: for example, aspirin, irritates the gut wall, making it more permeable.

Enzymes

Interesting fact

In general, a word ending –ase identifies an enzyme (maltase), and the stem word identifies the molecule that the enzyme works on (maltose). Stem words ending with –ose are usually sugars. e.g. sucrose, lactose, maltose.

Enzymes are a delicate life-like substance found in all living cells whether animal or vegetable. Enzymes are complex protein molecules that perform specific biochemical reactions vital for life. They can be described as protein catalysts. Enzymes do more than just break down the foods we eat ready for absorption. Enzymes also build substances (such as bone) and transform one substance into another (amino acids into glucose for example).

There are three classes of enzymes: digestive, metabolic and food enzymes. The main function of digestive enzymes is to break down food into particles chemically simple enough and physically small enough to be absorbed. Every day we produce an average of ten litres of digestive juices containing various enzymes to break down the food we eat. The liver, pancreas, stomach and intestinal wall produce these juices.

Enzymes change one substance into another, without actually changing themselves. They carry out millions of chemical activities in our bodies every second to keep us alive. The liver alone produces over 1000 different enzymes. The lack of even one enzyme can break the chain of biochemical reactions causing imbalances, which manifest themselves as allergies, nutritional deficiencies and illness. For example, the lack of a stomach enzyme known as 'intrinsic factor' can lead to pernicious anaemia unless the diet has sufficient vitamin B12 intake. This maybe a problem for vegans and vegetarians as the best source of B12 comes from animal foods.

Natural enzymes are found in abundance in fresh, unprocessed, natural foods. Their main function is to trigger food digestion.

The majority of digestive and metabolic enzymes are dependent upon vitamins and minerals to activate them. Our bodies produce 25 per cent of the enzymes we need for digestion; the other 75 per cent is expected to come from our diet in the form of natural, raw, unprocessed sources in fruit, vegetables, grains, nuts and seeds. These natural enzymes cannot be stored in the body, so fresh vegetables and fruit should be eaten with every meal, every day.

Examples of foods that contain significant amounts of enzymes are

- *apples* and *mangoes*, which contain peroxidase and catalase and whose job it is to disarm free radicals
- *pineapple*, *wheat* and *kidney beans*, which contain amylase to digest sugars, and protease which digests protein
- *mushrooms*, which contain amylase, protease, peroxidase and catalase
- *bananas* and *cabbage*, which contain amylase.

Water

Water is essential for life. A fit, healthy adult can survive many weeks without food but only a few days without water. Water is inorganic as it contains no carbon and while it is not a nutrient as such, it is often described as an essential nutrient as it necessary in large amounts on a daily basis. Water makes up about two-thirds of our body weight. How much water do we really need? It depends upon age, weight and activity levels. Children need more water, more frequently, than do adults as they have faster, more hard-working metabolisms, are very active and have a small stomach capacity.

The main sources of water for the body are food and drink, although some is produced when nutrients are oxidized to produce energy. For example, when glucose is oxidized it breaks down to form carbon dioxide and water. A kilogram of glucose produces just over half a litre of water on oxidation. The balance between input and output must be maintained at all times.

Water is unlike the other essential nutrients in that most of it does not undergo chemical changes within the body. Whereas proteins for example are broken down to amino acids during digestion, most water passes through the body unchanged. The table below outlines our daily recommended intake.

As a rule of thumb a healthy adult should drink at least two litres of water every day – as *water*, not an accumulation of coffee/tea/soft drinks and alcohol! However, fruits and vegetables have a high water content so if five servings are being taken every day, water intake can be reduced.

Water participates in many metabolic reactions and supplies the medium for transporting vital materials to cells and waste products away from them.

A general guide to water requirements

Age	ml water per kg body weight
1–3 years	95 ml/kg
4–6 years	85 ml/kg
7–10 years	75 ml/kg
Adults	35 ml/kg

Other vital functions of water are to:

- enable the formation of cells and tissues
- regulate body temperature
- protect the central nervous system
- form a lubricant for joints and membranes
- carry enzymes and support the digestive system
- transport nutrients around the body
- carry oxygen and carbon dioxide around the body.

The body cannot store water and so it needs to be replenished regularly throughout the day. The body loses water through sweat, urine, faeces and exhalation.

The micro-nutrients – vitamins, minerals and trace minerals

Micro-nutrients are needed to *release* energy from food. They are needed in much smaller amounts than the macro-nutrients but are no less important. The organic vitamins and the inorganic minerals have vital roles to play in the health of a human being. Hundreds of metabolic activities in the body rely on enzymes, of which many are vitamin- and mineral-dependent. Vitamins give us vitality and are needed not only to support all our body systems, but also to be used as co-enzymes to allow other chemical reactions to take place in the body.

Vitamins are organic substances obtained from food or dietary supplements. There are 13 vitamins known to date, and we need every one of them for good health. They are required in tiny amounts to perform specific functions that promote growth, reproduction, or the maintenance of health and life. The first vitamins were discovered only in the early 1900s when researchers first recognized that there were substances in foods that were 'vital to life'. Vitamin A was the first vitamin to be discovered (in 1913).

Vitamins are components of our enzyme systems which, acting like the spark plugs in your car, energize and regulate our metabolism, keeping us tuned up and running at high performance. Although taken in minute amounts compared to the macro-nutrients a deficiency in even one vitamin can endanger the whole human body.

For metabolism, for example, we need good supplies of the B vitamins or our metabolism will be unable to efficiently turn our food into energy. For carbohydrate metabolism vitamins B1, B2, B3 and B5 are needed; biotin is needed in fat metabolism; and B6, B12 and folic acid are needed for protein metabolism. Vitamin B6 and the mineral zinc are needed to make the enzymes that digest food.

Vitamins can be classified into two groups:

- *water-soluble vitamins:* the B complex group of vitamins and vitamin C
- *fat-soluble vitamins:* vitamins A, D, E and K.

The main difference between these two groups of vitamins is that the water-soluble vitamins need to be ingested every day as the body cannot store them whereas the fat-soluble vitamins are stored in the body and need not be ingested every day. The storage of the fat-soluble vitamins is one of the many functions of the liver.

The fat-soluble vitamins

The four fat-soluble vitamins are vitamins A, D, E and K. Fat-soluble means they dissolve in fat but not in water. They play many specific roles in the growth and maintenance of the body. Their presence affects the health and function of the eyes, skin, gastrointestinal (GI) tract, lungs, bones, teeth, nervous system and blood; and their deficiencies become apparent in these same areas. We store these fat-soluble vitamins in fatty tissues and in the liver so you don't have to have a daily intake of them. However, the fact that we store these vitamins means toxicity is possible, especially when supplements are being taken.

Vitamin A (retinol, beta-carotene)

Vitamin A is an anti-oxidant and is available to us in two forms. Pre-formed vitamin A, known as retinol, which is found only in foods of animal origin, and pro-vitamin A, which is obtained from fruits and vegetables and is also known as beta-carotene.

Main functions include: an essential vitamin for promoting vision, supporting reproduction and growth, for the maintenance of the skin and for supporting the immune system.

Main deficiency symptoms include: poor night vision, dry flaky skin, acne, frequent colds or infections and mouth ulcers.

Main food sources include: the richest sources of the retinoids are foods derived from animals. Fish liver oil, liver, eggs and dairy produce – especially margarine, which is usually fortified. As vitamin A is fat-soluble, it is lost when milk is skimmed. Other good sources are all yellow fruits and vegetables, which contain beta-carotene that the body converts to vitamin A as needed.

Vitamin D (calciferol, viosterol, ergosterol, sunshine vitamin)

Known as the sunshine vitamin, vitamin D is an anti-oxidant and promotes absorption of calcium and phosphate from food. It is also necessary for strong bones and teeth; for the correct function of thyroid and parathyroid glands; promoting release of calcium from bones and ensuring proper distribution in the body as well as increased uptake of mineral by bone. A fat-soluble vitamin, we do not need it every day as it is stored in our liver. Vitamin D (calciferol) is different from all other nutrients in that the body can synthesize it, with the help of sunlight, from a precursor that the body makes from cholesterol. Therefore, vitamin D is not classed as an 'essential' nutrient; as given enough time in the sun, you need no vitamin D from foods. All you need is 10 minutes a day in the sun, exposing just your arms and legs while walking around. There is no need to actually 'sunbathe'. After the 10 minutes you will then need to apply your usual sunscreen to protect yourself against sunburn, sun-damaged skin and skin cancer.

Main deficiency symptoms include: joint pain or stiffness, lack of energy, rheumatism or arthritis, hair loss, osteoporosis, rickets in children and osteomalacia in adults.

Main food sources include: fish liver oils, sardines, herring, salmon, tuna, fortified milk, meat and eggs.

Causes of deficiency include: lack of meat, fish and dairy products in the diet and lack of exposure to sunlight. With vitamin D deficiency, production of the protein that binds calcium in the intestinal cells slows. Thus, even when calcium in the diet is adequate, it passes through the GI tract unabsorbed, leaving the bones undersupplied. Consequently, a vitamin D deficiency creates a calcium deficiency.

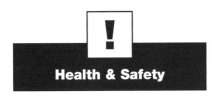

Vitamin A
Excess vitamin A during pregnancy can cause birth defects. Check vitamin A content in supplements and restrict your intake of liver to once a fortnight. There is no need to restrict beta-carotene (fruit and vegetables).

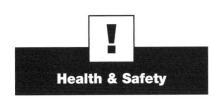

Vitamin D
Too much vitamin D from supplements is dangerous. Do not exceed 25 µg daily.

Vitamin E (alpha-tocopherol)

Four different tocopherol (tuh-KOFF-er-ol) compounds have been identified and are designated by the first four letters of the Greek alphabet: alpha, beta, gamma and delta. Alpha-tocopherol is the only one with vitamin E activity in the human body. Vitamin E was originally called tocopherol from the Greek words *tokos* meaning 'offspring' and *pheros* meaning 'to bear' after researchers found vitamin E improved fertility in rats.

Main deficiency symptoms include: easy bruising, exhaustion after light exercise, slow wound healing, lack of sex drive, varicose veins and loss of muscle tone.

Main food sources include: soya beans, unrefined corn oils, broccoli, Brussels sprouts, green leafy vegetables, sunflower seeds, sesame seeds, peanuts, whole grain cereals, wheatgerm, tuna and sardines.

Vitamin E is readily destroyed by heat processing (such as deep-fat frying) and oxidation, so fresh or lightly processed foods are preferable sources.

Vitamin E is a fat-soluble anti-oxidant and one of the body's primary defenders against the adverse effects of free radicals. It protects the cardiovascular system, prevents thrombosis, arteriosclerosis, thrombophlebitis, increases HDLs, maintains healthy blood vessels, reduces the oxygen needs of muscles and promotes white cell resistance to infection. Vitamin E enhances the activity of vitamin A and selenium and is important as a vasodilator and an anti-coagulant.

Causes of deficiency include: fat malabsorption (for example, a very low-fat diet or gallbladder removal); high intake of refined oils; alcoholism; intestinal surgery; cirrhosis of the liver and coeliac disease.

Vitamin K (phylloquinone)

Like vitamin D, vitamin K can be obtained from a non-food source. Bacteria in the GI tract synthesize vitamin K that the body can absorb. Vitamin K acts primarily in blood clotting, where its presence can make the difference between life and death.

Main deficiency symptoms include: excess bleeding (nosebleeds), abnormal blood clotting, fall in prothrombin content of blood.

Main food sources include: cabbage family, lettuce, beans, peas, watercress, potatoes, tomatoes, asparagus and corn oil provide the best sources. Milk, meats, eggs, cereals, fruits and vegetables provide smaller but still significant amounts.

Also synthesized by gut flora, vitamin K can be made in the GI tract by the billions of bacteria that normally reside there. Once synthesized, vitamin K is absorbed and stored in the liver. This source provides for only about half of a person's needs.

Main functions include: the formation of prothrombin (a blood-clotting chemical) and normal liver function. It helps in preventing internal bleeding and haemorrhages and aids in reducing excessive menstrual flow, as well as promoting proper blood clotting.

Vitamin K also participates in the synthesis of bone proteins. Without vitamin K the bones produce an abnormal protein that cannot bind to the minerals that normally form bones. An adequate intake of vitamin K may help protect against hip fractures.

Causes of deficiency include: birth – before sufficient intestinal flora is present to produce vitamin K, anti-coagulant therapy, cirrhosis of the liver and viral hepatitis.

There is an abundance of natural vitamin K generally in the diet. However, antibiotics destroy the vitamin K producing bacteria in the intestine so

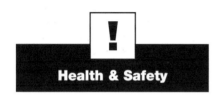

Health & Safety

Vitamin E
Extremely high doses of vitamin E may interfere with the blood-clotting action of vitamin K and enhance the effects of drugs used to oppose blood clotting, causing haemorrhage. Do not use high doses if taking warfarin or other anti-coagulant drugs.

Interesting fact

One cup of green tea, made from leaves, provides approximately 16 µg of vitamin K. As well as being an effective antioxidant, green tea is a healthy alternative to coffee or tea.

foods containing vitamin K should be increased after taking antibiotics. If taking the Pill or HRT supplementing vitamin K should be avoided as vitamin K is involved in blood clotting and the risk of blood clots are increased by synthetic hormones. There is never any need to restrict dietary forms of vitamin K from cauliflower and other vegetables.

The water-soluble vitamins

The B complex group of vitamins helps the body to use the fuel (food) the body has taken in through carbohydrates, proteins and fats.

The B complex group of vitamins works as a family – synergistically. A shortage of any one of the B complex group of vitamins can hinder many metabolic processes, which is an excellent reason to have as varied a diet as possible to incorporate all the vitamins and minerals needed for optimum health.

The B complex group of water-soluble vitamins include:

- vitamin B1 (thiamin)
- vitamin B2 (riboflavin)
- vitamin B3 (niacin)
- vitamin B5 (pantothenic acid)
- vitamin B6 (pyridoxine)
- vitamin B12 (cyanocobalmin)
- folic acid (folate)
- biotin
- choline
- inositol
- PABA.

Main food sources of the B group of vitamins include: all protein foods (eggs, fish, meat, poultry, organ meats, cheese, dairy foods, nuts and soya products); whole grains, Brewer's yeast, legumes, mushrooms, watercress, cabbage, bananas, avocado, asparagus and many other foods.

Causes of deficiency include: diets high in refined foods, low in fruit and vegetables, poor absorption, stress, alcohol, infections, ageing, drugs (aspirin and barbiturates), contraceptive pill and antibiotics.

Main deficiency symptoms include: fatigue, depression, irritability, nausea, sleepiness, smooth pale tongue, loss of appetite, muscular pains, fluid retention, poor dream recall and allergies. There are many other symptoms of deficiency but these are the main ones.

Vitamin C (ascorbic acid)

Main functions: an anti-oxidant which protects other nutrients, prevents cellular damage, detoxifies heavy metals and carcinogens, makes collagen and keeps skin, bones, joints and arteries healthy. Vital for supporting the immune system and for antibody production, it is a natural 'anti-histamine', reduces cholesterol levels, aids absorption of iron, produces anti-stress hormones and activates folic acid.

An anti-oxidant is a substance in foods that significantly decreases the adverse effects of free radicals on normal physiological functions in the human body.

Main food sources include: all fruits and vegetables, especially guava fruit, yellow peppers, cantaloupe melon, pimientos, papaya, strawberries, Brussels sprouts, grapefruit juice and sprouted seeds and beans.

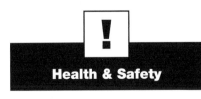

Health & Safety

Vitamin C
Taking too much vitamin C in supplement form (over 1 g) may have a laxative effect in some people. If you experience loosening of the bowels when taking vitamin C supplements, decrease dosage and increase fruit and vegetables consumed.

Main deficiency symptoms include: frequent colds and infections, lack of energy, allergies, bleeding gums, easily bruised, nosebleeds, slow wound healing, anaemia, premature ageing. Deficiency disease is *scurvy*.

Main causes of deficiency include: a diet high in refined foods, low in fruit and vegetables, poor absorption, stress, alcohol, infections, ageing, drugs (aspirin and barbiturates), contraceptive pill and antibiotics.

Minerals and trace elements

Minerals and trace elements required by humans

Macro-minerals	Trace minerals
Calcium	Boron
Magnesium	Chromium
Potassium	Copper
Sodium	Iron
Phosphorus	Manganese
	Molybdenum
	Selenium
	Sulphur
	Zinc

Minerals and trace elements are inorganic substances mined from the earth, which is why they are found abundantly in foods that are grown in the earth – vegetables.

Until recently the way that minerals affected our bodies was very poorly understood and as such they tended to be ignored in favour of other nutrients. It is now clear that without them there would be no life at all.

About 60 different minerals have been identified in the body, of which 21 are considered 'essential'. Essential minerals, as with essential amino acids and essential fatty acids, are minerals that must be supplied in the food daily, as they cannot be manufactured in the body. Some minerals are required in substantial amounts, often referred to as the gross minerals or the macro-minerals; these include calcium, magnesium, sodium, potassium and phosphorus. Others are needed in minute or trace amounts but are equally important to health, these are known as the trace minerals and include boron, chromium, copper, iron, manganese, molybdenum, selenium, sulphur and zinc. Four minerals tend to be particularly low among Western people: calcium, magnesium, zinc and iron.

Calcium (Ca)

Calcium is an essential element for living organisms, being required for normal growth and development.

Main functions include: builds and maintains healthy bones and teeth, controls nerve and muscle excitability, controls conduction of nerve impulses, controls muscle contraction, aids blood clotting, controls cholesterol levels, aids B12 absorption and reduces menstrual cramps.

Main food sources include: ricotta cheese, parmesan cheese, milk, mackerel, salmon and sardines, dried figs, tofu, low-fat yoghurt, sesame seeds, oats, millet, almonds, kelp, green leafy vegetables, parsley and pumpkin seeds.

Main deficiency symptoms include: rickets (in children), osteomalacia (in adults), bone pain, muscle weakness and cramps, delayed healing of fractures, tetany (twitches and spasms), tooth decay, brittle nails, insomnia or nervousness, joint pain or arthritis, high blood pressure, fragile bones, menstrual cramps, eczema and rheumatoid arthritis.

Magnesium (Mn)

Main functions include: strengthens bones and teeth, promotes healthy muscles so helping them to relax, beneficial for PMS, heart muscles and nervous system. Involved as co-enzymes for many functions in the body and essential for energy production.

Main food sources include: wheatgerm, almonds and cashew nuts, soybeans, whole grains, green leafy vegetables and sesame seeds, potato skins and crab meat.

Main deficiency symptoms include: depression, muscle tremors or spasms, muscle weakness, insomnia or nervousness, high blood pressure, irregular heartbeat, constipation, fits or convulsions, hyperactivity, poor memory, irritability and calcium deposits in soft tissue, e.g. kidney stones.

Tip

Avoid taking calcium supplements which are not combined with magnesium. Always choose a supplement containing calcium and magnesium in a 2:1 ratio.

Sodium (Na)

Main functions include: maintaining intra- and extra-cellular water balance, in nerve impulse transmission (with potassium), in all muscle contraction, especially heart muscle, involved in control of acid/alkaline balance in body, active transport of amino acids and glucose into cells.

Main food sources include: table salt, sea salt, yeast extract, bacon, smoked fish, salami, sauces, cornflakes, processed cheese and cheese spread, olives, pickles, many meats, especially the smoked variety, ready-made meals and most other refined and processed foods (consumption of which should be kept to a minimum).

Main deficiency symptoms include: low blood pressure, rapid pulse, dry mouth, mental apathy, loss of appetite, muscle cramps and twitches, dehydration, 'sunken' features and sagging skin.

Potassium (K)

Main functions include: essential for healthy nerves and muscles, maintains fluid balance in the body, relaxes muscles, helps secretion of insulin for blood sugar control, enables nutrients and waste products to enter and leave cells, maintains heart functioning and stimulates peristalsis to encourage proper movement of food through the digestive tract.

Main food sources include: kelp, Brewer's yeast, raisins, peanuts, dates, vegetables and fruits, wheatgerm, bananas, avocado, dandelion coffee, prunes, grapes, whole grains and nuts, blackstrap molasses, baked potatoes, cantaloupe melon, dried peaches and prunes, tomato juice, low fat yoghurt, salmon, apricots and herring.

Main deficiency symptoms include: muscle weakness and loss of muscle tone, fatigue, constipation, mental apathy, poor reflexes, nervous disorders, arthritis, irregular heartbeat, and low blood sugar.

Phosphorus (P)

Main functions include: forms and maintains bone and teeth, needed for milk secretion, builds up muscle tissue and is a component of DNA and RNA, helps maintain pH of the body and aids metabolism and energy production.

Main food sources include: carbonated soft and 'diet' drinks, red meat and all junk food, Brewer's yeast, wheat bran, cheddar cheese, brown rice, nuts and eggs.

Main deficiency symptoms include: calcification causing 'spurs' and imbalances such as osteoporosis, loss of muscle control and strength, trembling, convulsions, high blood pressure, arteriosclerosis and heart disease.

The trace elements

These comprise:

- boron
- chromium
- copper
- iron
- manganese

- selenium
- sulphur
- zinc.

Boron

Boron helps absorb calcium into bones and keeps it there. There is usually no problem getting the daily requirements from food. Good food sources are fruits, especially apples, pears, peaches, grapes, dates and raisins. Nuts and beans are also high in boron.

Chromium (Cr)

Main functions include: forms part of Glucose Tolerance Factor (GTF) to balance blood sugar, helps to normalize hunger and reduce cravings. Essential for heart function and protects DNA and RNA.

Main food sources include: Brewer's yeast, whole grains especially rye, oysters, green peppers, eggs, liver, beef, mushrooms and molasses.

Main deficiency symptoms include: excessive or cold sweats, dizziness or irritability after six hours without food, need for frequent meals, cold hands, need for excessive sleep or drowsiness during the day, excessive thirst and addiction to sweet foods, arteriosclerosis, improper glucose metabolism, hypoglycaemia, diabetes, heart disease, decreased growth and improper fat metabolism.

Copper (Cu)

Main functions include: essential for life but in small amounts – only 2mg daily is required. It is involved in many enzyme systems including one which protects us from free radicals and is needed to help iron carry out its functions of oxygen transfer to the cells. It helps manufacture a thyroid-stimulating hormone, assists protein manufacture, helps iron to form red cells and assists in the formation of the pigment melanin. Copper helps relieve rheumatism and assists in the metabolism of cholesterol. It is also used for the formation of insulating the myelin sheath around the nerves.

Main food sources include: shellfish especially oysters, organ meats, cereals, dried fruit, almonds, beans and green leafy vegetables. We also take it in by absorbing excess copper from water pipes, water softeners, fungicides and metal utensils. Oestrogen-containing birth control pills and HRT may also elevate blood copper levels.

Main deficiency symptoms include: general weakness, anaemia, osteoporosis, arthritis, atherosclerosis, heart damage, skin sores, hair loss, digestive problems and diarrhoea.

An excess of copper is more likely to be a problem than deficiency. Symptoms include: hardening of the arteries, high blood pressure, kidney disease, psychosis, early senility and other signs of early ageing. It is also said to be linked to post-natal depression.

Iron (Fe)

Main functions include: iron is an essential nutrient, vital to many cellular activities, but it can pose a problem for many people who simply do not get enough iron from the food they are eating. There are between 3 and 4 grams of iron in the body and more than half of this is used in the blood as a substance called haemoglobin. Iron transports oxygen and carbon dioxide to and from cells, is a component of enzymes and is vital for energy production.

Main food sources include: meats, fish, pumpkin seeds, parsley, almonds, brazil and cashew nuts, dates and prunes.

Main deficiency symptoms include: anaemia, poor vision, insomnia, pale skin, sore tongue, fatigue or listlessness, loss of appetite or nausea, heavy periods or blood loss, breathlessness, difficulty in swallowing, general itching, nail deformities, cramping, depression, palpitations and an underactive thyroid gland.

Manganese – (Mn)

Main functions include: co-factor in over 20 enzyme systems involving growth, health of the nervous system, energy production and health of joints, female sex hormones, production of thyroxin. Co-factor for vitamins B, C and E, and important for maintenance of healthy bones and stimulation of glycogen storage in liver.

Main food sources include: seeds, nuts and grains, green leafy vegetables, beetroot, pineapple, bran, wheat, egg yolk, kelp, nuts, tropical fruit and black tea.

Main deficiency symptoms include: muscle twitches, childhood 'growing pains', dizziness or poor sense of balance, fits or convulsions, sore knees and joints.

Selenium (Se)

Main functions include: protects the body against toxic metabolites and cancer as an anti-oxidant and co-factor of glutathione peroxidase. Protects against toxic minerals, aids the maintenance of normal liver function and production of prostaglandins, supports male reproduction, maintains health of eyes, hair and skin, is an anti-inflammatory agent, maintains health of heart, potentiates action of vitamin E and helps produce co-enzyme Q.

Main food sources include: organ meats, fish and shellfish, muscle meats, whole grains, cereals, dairy produce, fruit and vegetables, brazil nuts, puffed wheat, sunflower seeds, Brewer's yeast and garlic.

Main deficiency symptoms include: no specific symptoms yet established but appear to be related to liver disease, cancer, cataracts, heart disease, ageing, and growth and fertility problems.

Sulphur (S)

Sulphur is an essential element in living organisms, occurring in the amino acids cysteine and methionine and therefore in many proteins. It is also a constituent of various cell metabolistes, e.g. co-enzyme A. Sulphur is absorbed by plants from soil.

Main functions include: joint protection and repair, anti-oxidant/ free radical scavenger, protection and strengthening of skin, hair and nail tissue, detoxification, heavy metal removal and general connective tissue repair. Helps maintain oxygen balance necessary for proper brain function.

Main food sources include: eggs, onions, garlic, seafood, milk, cabbage, lean beef, dried beans.

Main deficiency symptoms include: joint aches and pains, frequent infections, poor nails, hair and skin, back pain.

Zinc (Zn)

Main functions include: essential for bone growth, sexual development, energy production, maintenance of blood sugar levels (as it is needed for insulin production). It is needed to use B6 and vitamin A efficiently and carries carbon dioxide from the cells to lungs. It maintains acid–alkaline balance in the body and is an essential component of the prostate, ovaries and testes.

Main food sources include: oysters, beef, lamb, sardines, crab meat, calf's liver, dark turkey meat, brazil nuts, egg yolk, yeast and pumpkin seeds.

Main deficiency symptoms include: poor sense of taste or smell, white marks on more than two fingernails, frequent infections, stretch marks, acne or greasy skin, low fertility, pale skin, tendency to depression and poor appetite.

Causes of mineral deficiency

Low dietary intake is the most obvious cause of mineral deficiency. Other causes include taking the contraceptive pill; malabsorption due to low stomach acid; coeliac disease; lactose intolerance; pregnancy and breast feeding (with the minerals diverted to the baby); dehydration due to high temperatures; hard exercise; heavy bleeding (iron); alcohol intake and some antibiotics.

A balanced diet

A guideline for a 'balanced' diet should be 55 per cent of your daily calories coming from good sources of carbohydrate (potatoes, bread, pasta, all unrefined), 15 per cent of your dairy calories coming from good sources of protein (chicken, turkey, lamb, fish, dairy foods and nuts, organic is possible). Lastly, 30 per cent of your daily calories should come from fats, which can be broken down into three distinct groups: 10 per cent from saturated fats (these you can really forget about as they are 'hidden' in so many foods, sweets for example); 10 per cent from mono-unsaturated fats, the best example of which is olive oil, which you should be cooking in; and 10 per cent from polyunsaturated fats – the most important group – which are anything liquid at room temperature, for example sunflower oil which would be used in salad dressings.

To give an example, if your diet was 2000 calories per day, you should be having:

- 1100 from carbohydrates
- 300 calories from protein
- 600 calories from fats:
    200 calories from saturated fat
    200 calories from mono-unsaturated oils such as olive oil
    200 calories from the liquid polyunsaturated oils.

'Fat-free' and other diet foods

These foods may be low in fat, but they are usually high in sugar, and as you now know, the body will convert excess sugar, which could be harmful, into fat, which although potentially harmful is a safer alternative. It is no wonder that many unsuccessful dieters become depressed and anxious.

You should discourage clients from using these products and encourage their going back to what nature intended by eating plenty of vegetables, fruit and whole grains.

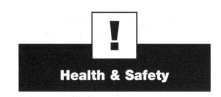

Health & Safety

Dieting
It is unwise to go on a weight-reducing diet without the guidance of your GP, a qualified clinical nutritionist or a dietician. Losing weight and/or not receiving sufficient nutrients to meet daily requirements may result in menstrual problems, skin problems such as acne, impaired growth, infertility or even osteoporosis later in life.

The nutrition consultation

To be able to recommend a more beneficial diet to your clients, you need first to ascertain their existing diet. The best way to do this is to ask them to keep a food diary for at least three days. One of these days should be a non-work day, as we tend to eat differently when we are not at work. As well as knowing what the clients are eating you also need to know what they are drinking and also the times of these activities. Below is an example of a sheet you could hand your client for completion.

A three-day food diary

	Day 1	*Day 2*	*Day 3*
Time	Breakfast	Breakfast	Breakfast
Time	Lunch	Lunch	Lunch
Time	Dinner	Dinner	Dinner
Time	Snack	Snack	Snack
Time	Snack	Snack	Snack
Time	Drinks	Drinks	Drinks
Time	Other	Other	Other

Specific questions to ask during a nutrition consultation

1 You need accurate weight, height and body measurements so you can calculate body fat ratio and hip and waist ratio.
2 You need to ascertain they have no contra indications to nutritional therapy. Check with your awarding body, as contra indications differ (due to age etc.).
3 You need to ascertain the reason for the consultation – weight loss, to improve skin condition or reduce cellulite, for stress relief or they may just want to be healthier. You need to know at the outset of their expectations of the consultation. If you feel unable to meet their expectations, you can refer to someone with more experience in this field.

Contra indications for nutritional therapy

- Clients under 18 and over 70.
- Clients undergoing medical treatment.
- Clients on a medically prescribed diet.

- Severe obesity.
- Severely underweight.
- Suffering from eating disorder.
- Pregnancy.
- Medically identified food intolerances/allergies.

Timing

As you can see, there is a box available in the diary for the client to include *when* they ate. It is very important to establish the time of eating. Natural and healthy eating is regulated by feelings of hunger and satiety, but many people no longer tune in to these internal signals, or they confuse them with other feelings. For example, they may interpret anxiety or thirst as hunger. Or they may confuse feeling full with being fat. Encourage the client to complete the 'time' box. This will give you valuable information as to eating patterns – whether they are regular or erratic – which may indicate an underlying problem.

Establishing weight parameters

Body mass index

Your body mass index (BMI) gives a good indication of whether you are a healthy weight. You work out your BMI as follows.

Height chart

Feet and inches	Metres	Feet and inches	Metres
4'10"	1.45	5'9"	1.74
4'11"	1.5	5'10"	1.78
5'	1.52	5'11"	1.8
5'1"	1.55	6'	1.82
5'2"	1.57	6'1"	1.85
5'3"	1.6	6'2"	1.88
5'4"	1.62	6'3"	1.9
5'5"	1.65	6'4"	1.92
5'6"	1.68	6'5"	1.95
5'7"	1.7	6'6"	1.98
5'8"	1.72	6'7"	2

1 Work out your height in metres (see the height chart) and multiply the figure by itself.
2 Measure your weight in kilograms.
3 Divide the weight (step 2) by the height squared (i.e. the answer to step 1). For example, you might be 1.6 m (5'3") tall and weigh 65 kg (10 stone). The calculation would then be $1.6 \times 1.6 = 2.56$. Your BMI would be $65 \div 2.56 = 25.39$.

The table below gives the standard ratings for BMI.

Body mass index

Category	Range
Underweight	Less than 20
Ideal	20–25
Overweight – advisable to lose weight if you are under 50	25–30
You should lose weight	30–40
Clinically obese – seek GP assistance	Greater than 40

If your BMI falls within the ideal range and you are the right weight, that's great, but it is still important to eat healthily to receive all the nutrients needed to stay healthy, fit and well. It is also important not to put on weight. People aged 30–74 with BMIs at the lower end of the normal range have the lowest death rates. And people who stay the same weight in middle age as they were in their youth live longer, are generally healthier and therefore more able to enjoy themselves.

Hip-to-waist ratio

While the BMI is a good general indicator of whether you are overweight or not, the hip-to-waist ratio is probably a better indicator. The risk of heart disease doesn't only depend on how much fat you're carrying, it's also where you are carrying it that matters. Our genes determine our basic shape – whether fat is deposited around hips, breasts and upper arms making us 'pear-shaped', or whether fat is deposited around abdomens making us 'apple-shaped'.

It may seem unfair but if apple-shaped people become overweight they are at greater risk of heart disease and diabetes than pear-shaped people.

To make the calculation:

1   Measure your waist and hips.
2   Divide the waist measurement by the hip measurement to get your waist–hip ratio.

For example, if your waist is 86 cm (34 inches) and your hips 102 cm (40 inches), your waist–hip ratio will be 86 divided by 102 = 0.85. If the ratio of your waist to hip measurement is more than 0.95 as a man and more than 0.87 as a woman you are apple shaped.

There is another rule of thumb as far as waist measurements are concerned. If a man has a waist that measures more than 94 cm (37 inches), or a woman's is more than 80 cm (31 inches), they are categorised by some doctors as overweight. Waists do thicken with age, a phenomenon often referred to as 'middle age spread'. If you are younger and already have a 'spare tyre' – act now. It is this abdominal fat that increases the risk of heart disease. Now calculate your own hip-to-waist ratio.

Knowledge review

1   What is the difference between macro-nutrients and micro-nutrients?

2   What is the main function of carbohydrate foods?

3   Give five reasons why fibre is important in the diet.

4   What are the two main functions of protein?

5   How many essential amino acids are there? Name them.

6   What are the three main divisions of dietary fats?

7   What are the main functions of dietary fats?

8   What are the three main divisions of triglycerides?

9   What are the four main functions of cholesterol?

10 Vitamins are divided into two main divisions. What are these?

11 Define an anti-nutrient and give five examples.

12 Define an enzyme.

13 What foods contain natural enzymes? Give some examples.

14 What are the main causes of mineral deficiencies?

15 What are the recommendations for a 'balanced diet'?

16 What is the main concern with low-fat diets?

17 What is the connection with a high-protein diet and osteoporosis?

18 What are the contra indications to nutritional therapy?

19 Why is the hip-to-waist ratio probably a better indicator of being overweight that the body mass index?

Posture and figure analysis

7

Learning objectives

This chapter covers the following:

- **the value of figure analysis**
- **the process of a figure analysis**
- **body shapes**
- **posture and postural faults/weaknesses**
- **examination of muscular condition**
- **simple postural exercises**
- **concluding a figure analysis**

Performing a figure analysis is important if you are offering remedial or more advanced massage techniques, and some of the knowledge can be equally beneficial when used within other treatments. This chapter explains the importance and the benefits of figure analysis including:

- **assessment of the client's figure problems and faults so that you can decide where to concentrate or apply specific techniques**
- **recognizing faults requiring referral for specialized attention**
- **indicating a course of action for an effective treatment and, where applicable, a course of treatments for the client.**

The process of a figure analysis

Activity

Checking posture

To check posture stand with feet slightly apart and slightly inverted. In this position the weight goes from the point in front of the ankles through the feet, partly down to the heel and partly spread down the feet to the toes.

Note how the body changes as you do the following movements

- move the chin back and forth
- lean back and then forwards
- roll the shoulders back and forth
- rock the pelvis back and forwards.

Now find a comfortable standing position and practise the good posture points listed in the table on p.173.

Tip

If the client has low self-esteem and feels embarrassed standing in front of a mirror or finds this inhibiting and feels uncomfortable, stand them with their back to the mirror.

1 Initial observation

Observe your client carefully as you take them to the treatment area. Ask yourself the following questions.

- What is their overall posture like, is it good or poor?
- How do they move, carry themselves?
- What is the client's disposition – does the client appear nervous, anxious or confident and relaxed?

Assess the client while both in a standing and a sitting position.

2 Verbal consultation

To ensure you are familiar with consultation techniques, go to Chapter 5, p.134.

Carry out your consultation. Complete as much of the consultation card as possible before asking the client to undress. Record all the client's personal details and discuss with the client their expectations. Record your findings on a record card. It is a good idea to have a pictorial card on which you can make notes (see figure on p.171). Symbols or codes are useful to save lots of writing.

3 Physical assessment

The degree to which you carry out a figure assessment will depend on the type and extent of the treatment you intend to carry out. With more advanced massage techniques analysis is vital for devising a treatment plan.

The figure analysis should be performed with the client in their underwear. However, make sure that you only expose the client as and when you need to, otherwise keep them robed. The room should be warm and private so that the client can relax. Stand the client in front of a full-length mirror so that you can discuss your findings with them.

Your aim is to observe the following points considering each part of the body.

- body shape
- good posture and postural faults/weaknesses
- general tone of muscles
- fat distribution, cellulite (or lack of)
- condition of skin – good, dry, oily, scars, stretch marks, scaly, evidence of skin disease
- evidence of circulatory problems, blue tinges, excessive redness, varicose veins, bruises
- personal hygiene.

Palpation

This is the use of touch or pressure to examine the body. It is essential to develop good palpation skills to help assess the condition of the body tissues both before and during treatment. You will be feeling for warmth, swelling, tenderness, tension, firmness and grittiness.

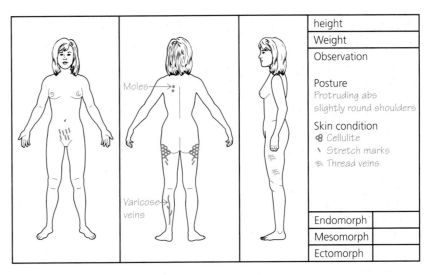

			height	
			Weight	
			Observation	
			Posture	
			Protruding abs slightly round shoulders	
			Skin condition	
			✪ Cellulite	
			＼ Stretch marks	
			✿ Thread veins	
			Endomorph	
			Mesomorph	
			Ectomorph	

Consultation card

Body shapes

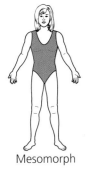

Ectomorph

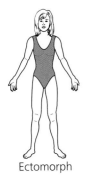

Mesomorph

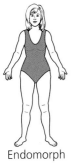

Endomorph

There are three main body shapes. Realistically, many of us are a combination of body types.

The *ectomorph* has

- narrow shoulders and hips
- a long thin torso
- long bones
- average muscle bulk
- low percentage of body fat
- a lack of curves.

The *mesomorph* has

- athletic build
- inverted triangular shape
- well-developed or broad shoulders
- slim, boyish hips
- well-toned, defined muscles
- low percentage of body fat.

The *endomorph* has

- rounded shoulders
- heavy build with a higher percentage of body fat to muscle bulk
- body contours padded, with a tendency to be overweight
- movements may be slow and deliberate.

Posture and postural faults/weaknesses

Activity

Look at the muscle diagrams on pp.88–9 in Chapter 4. Locate the anti-gravity muscles. Try to locate each muscle on your own body.

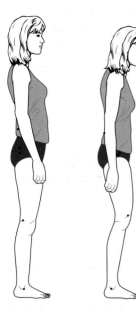

Posture

Posture

Posture is concerned with body alignment, the relationship and placement of the body segments with each other, all of which are balanced over the feet.

Posture gives others an outward non-verbal impression of how you regard yourself, either as a person who is positive, confident and assured, or someone who is shy, reticent or lacking in self-confidence.

The postural mechanism

Posture is maintained or adapted as a result of 'neuromuscular co-ordination'.

The groups of muscle most frequently used are those required to maintain the upright position of the body. These work to counteract the effects of gravity and are therefore known as the anti-gravity or postural muscles.

The postural reflex

Our posture is maintained in response to a variety of stimuli from all over the body. The most important postural stimuli come from the muscles, eyes and ears. Impulses from all these receptors are conveyed and co-ordinated in the central nervous system (CNS) and then suitable messages are sent to maintain balance. The incoming messages do not reach the conscious brain as they are too quick; however, the mechanism for maintaining posture does requires practice.

Centre of gravity

This is the point of balance of an object, the imaginary point about which the surrounding masses are equal. In the standing position it is usually thought to be above the pelvis on average level with the second sacral vertebrae. Additional weight above this raises the centre of gravity; additional weight below makes the centre move lower.

Good posture

A good posture is one that allows every part of the body to function well with maximum efficiency and minimum effort. It relies on the interaction of groups of muscles, which work more or less statically to stabilize the joints and in opposition to gravity and other forces. Our posture is changing all the time although we are usually unaware of it. The slightest shift of our body weight produces reactions all over the body to adjust the line of our centre of gravity and keep us stable. Posture is affected by the position of the feet, head, shoulders and tilt of the pelvis.

Good posture is of great importance. It helps:

- the internal organs to function properly
- increase endurance
- reduce fatigue
- increase body co-ordination and control
- increase speed in physical tasks
- increase balance and body flexibility

Good and bad posture

Good posture	Indicators of a postural problem
• Body weight evenly distributed • Feet slightly apart, facing forwards, weight even over balls and heels of both feet • Head erect (suspended on a string pulling up from the centre of the crown), the chin neither overextended or retracted • Eyes looking straight ahead, ears and eyes should be level • Rib cage should be symmetrical, neither hyperexpanded nor sunken • Shoulders square, chest slightly forward • Arms hanging evenly at each side • Pelvis tilt balanced at midpoint, stomach pulled in, buttocks tucked under – gluteal folds should be level • Knees relaxed, not locked	• Body weight visibly uneven • Feet turned in or outwards, body weight shifted onto balls of foot, or weight carried predominantly on one foot (scoliosis, tilted pelvis, back, hip or leg pain) • Chin pushed forward, or head held backwards, head cocked to one side (neck or back pain, spinal deviation) • Level of eyes and ears uneven (spinal deviation, hearing or sight problems) • Rib cage prominent (anorexia, breathing problems, hyperextension) • Round shoulders (kyphosis, dowager's hump, back pain, lack of confidence) • Arms hanging unevenly (scoliosis) • Pelvis uneven – weight uneven on feet, buttocks sticking out, gluteal fold even (lordosis, spinal deviation) • Knees touching (knock knees) or hyperextended in a relaxed position

Tip

Assessing posture

The use of a hanging plumb line (a decorator's tool comprising a long cord with a weight on the end to make it hang straight) is an excellent guide for assessing body alignment. Fix the plumb line in a position so that it can hang straight and is easily accessible; a door frame is ideal.

• Hold the line down the centre of the back and look at the line of the spine and pelvis.

• Hold the line down the side of the body from the ear over the shoulder and check for body rotation and pelvic tilt.

• Check the body from the front.

• Place one hand on each hip and compare to check they are level.

• prepare your body and muscles for sudden energy spurts and resist accidents and injury
• reduce menstrual pain and facilitates childbirth
• contribute to self-confidence.

The golden rules are:

• keep your back straight
• keep your feet flat on the floor, whether you are standing or sitting.

Poor posture

Poor posture is inefficient as an extra amount of energy is used by the muscle to maintain the balance of the body. Compensatory mechanisms throw the body out of alignment placing strain on muscles and ligaments. The result is aches and pains, cramping of abdominal organs and reduced movement. This inefficiency prevents the body from working to its best advantage and often results in fatigue.

Re-education of posture

This can be a lengthy process and will depend on the cause of poor posture. The client will need to work on strengthening weakened muscles and increasing mobility. Relaxation and practice of the good postural positions are essential in the re-training process.

Postural faults/weaknesses

As a therapist your aim with a postural weakness is to loosen and stretch tight, shortened muscles.

There may be evidence of scar tissue in the muscle which will need to be released.

Interesting fact

Antagonistic muscles are muscles that work in opposition to one other, e.g. the bicep relaxes while the tricep contracts and vice versa.

With any condition there will be muscle that will be shortened causing restriction; the opposite or antagonistic muscle will be stretched or lengthened to compensate. In the long term the client needs to exercise to strengthen the weak muscles.

Pelvic tilt

Pelvic tilt is the key to all posture. Movement in the vertebral column and at the hip joints makes it possible for the pelvis to be stabilized in a variety of positions. Tilt may be anterior, posterior, lateral or rotated.

The angle of the pelvic tilt when in a standing position is stabilized by either the

- tension of the structures which lie at the front of the hip joint preventing the pelvis tilting backwards
- the action of the abdominal muscles and the hip extensors preventing the pelvis from tilting forward.

Scoliosis

This is a sideways (lateral) deviation of the spine, which is always accompanied by rotation of vertebra, usually the thoracic. The main curve (primary curve) may vary in degree and location. A secondary curve develops below the primary curve, so that upright posture can be maintained. The condition is usually progressive. There are two categories of scoliosis.

- *Reversible scoliosis* due to a postural fault. Commonly seen in developing teenage girls. It may be as a result of bad posture, a disc prolapse or as a result of a ligament sprain.
- *True scoliosis* is an irreversible condition as a result of a congenital abnormality or spinal injury.

Symptoms: apart from the obvious 'S' spinal curve, there may be muscular aches and pains and the symptoms of sciatica.

Muscles:

- shortened: one side of the body
- lengthened: opposite side to shortened muscles.

Treatment guidance: deep massage to alleviate stress and strain in the affected muscles.

Home advice: postural awareness in different positions (standing, sitting); balancing and strengthening exercises including crawling.

Kyphosis

This is an exaggerated backward curve of the thoracic vertebra resulting in a rounded back. It may be caused by several factors including weak back muscles, osteoporosis and spinal disorders.

Symptoms: pronounced curve of the thoracic region causing round shoulders; in larger breasted women the breasts may droop.

Muscles:

- shortened: pectoral muscles
- lengthened: upper back muscles.

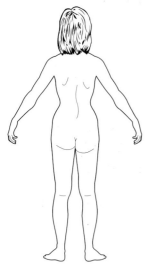

Scoliosis

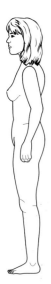

Kyphosis

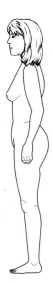

Lordosis

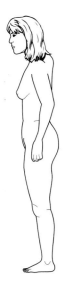

Dowagers hump

Tip

Check the client whilst they are lying supine and prone. Stand at the bottom of the couch and look up the body. How straight are they lying? Are they comfortable? If the body posture is comfortable but the body alignment is crooked in any way this will indicate shortening and muscle weaknesses. It may also indicate some injury for which the body is compensating.

Treatment guidance: deep tissue massage to affected muscles.

Home advice: exercise to strengthen the long back, gluteals and abdominal muscles and awareness of pelvic tilt.

Tip

Kyphosis
Changes in the body due to kyphosis include:

- narrowing anteriorly of inter-vertebral discs
- shortening of pectorals
- stretching of the longitudinal and transverse back muscles, resulting in weakness and possible some fibrous tissue (individual may develop scar tissue as a result of inflammation).

Backache may be associated with the condition and is localized to the thoracic region. Exaggeration of the curve causes the shoulders to be brought forward and the chin extended.

Lordosis

Lordosis is an increase in the lumbar curve formed to compensate a forward tilt of the pelvis. In more extreme examples the knees may become hyper-extended. The condition is sometimes referred to as hollow back and is caused by weakened muscles, osteoarthritis or a prolapsed disc.

Lordosis may appear in association with kyphosis and these two together result in kypho-lordosis.

Muscles:

- shortened – back extensors
- lengthened and stretched: abdominal, hamstrings.

Treatment guidance: as for kyphosis, i.e. correction of pelvic tilt, strengthen the abdominal and back extensor muscles, scapula retraction.

Flat back

The lumbar region of the back has a flat appearance with no natural curve, giving an erect military stance. The pelvis is tilted forward.

Dowager's hump

A condition generally associated with older ladies but can also be congenital. (Similar symptoms can occur as a result of degeneration of bone tissue caused by osteoporosis.) The head becomes tilted forward and there is extreme kyphosis and round shoulders.

Where the condition has developed over a period of time it is often caused by fatty deposits accumulating at the lower cervical and upper thoracic vertebra and as a result is accompanied with restricted mobility in the region.

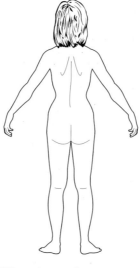

Winged scapulae

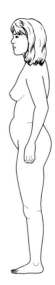

Protruding abdomen

Winged scapulae

Elevated scapular bones that stand out prominently giving a winged appearance. Caused by damage to the serratus anterior muscle and the nerve supply to it. The person is unable to raise the arm or to carry out pushing movements (attempts to do this may extend the scapula further).

Treatment guidance: exercises to maintain any position which takes the weight on the arms, e.g. stretching forward, interlocking hands behind the back, crawling, standing parallel to the walls and leaning forward on to hands, rowing, ball games, scrubbing, cleaning!

Protruding abdomen

There are three possible causes:

- lordosis
- fatty deposits
- weak abdominal muscles – especially noticeable after childbirth.

Treatment guidance: tapotement and/or pincemont massage that can be used at home to stimulate the circulation.

Home advice: exercises specific for the abdominal muscles and awareness of pelvic tilt.

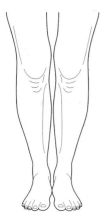

Knock knees

Knock knees – tibial torsion

The knees rotate medially due to slack tendons around the knee.

Home advice: exercises to strengthen the knee flexors, extensors and hip abductors and postural awareness.

Hyper-extended knees

The knee joint when locked gives a curved appearance to the leg. For many this is a natural position.

Home advice: advise against locking the knee joints and keeping the knee slightly relaxed.

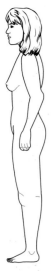

Hyper-extended knees

Body fat

Examine the body for evidence or lack of body fat and its type. Problems areas tend to be the gluteals, thighs, abdomen and across the latissimus dorsi. There are three types of body fat: soft, hard and cellulite.

- *Soft fat:* the fat is soft to the touch and can be easily mobilized.
- *Hard fat:* firm, even hard to the touch, and difficult to manipulate; difficult to treat and mobilize.
- *Cellulite:* dimpled lumpy fatty tissue common around the thigh and buttocks; loose cellulite will be obvious while more compacted cellulite can be seen by gently squeezing the skin.

To ensure you are familiar with cellulite, go to Chapter 4, p.50.

Muscle tone

To ensure you are familiar with muscle tone, go to Chapter 4, p.87.

Remember that naturally there is always a certain amount of normal tone in the muscle fibres. What we tend to associate with muscle tone is in fact muscle definition or bulk. Are the muscles defined or poor with loose muscle tone?

Skin condition

Make observations about the condition of the skin. Check for evidence of any contra indications of which the client may be unaware, such as fungal infections (athlete's foot), verrucae and other skin infections.

Look at the overall condition of the skin and skin type – is it good, dry, oily? This may affect the medium you work with. For example a client with an oily skin would benefit from a light carrier oil.

- *Scaly skin* will benefit from friction movements to slough off the dead skin.
- *Loose crepe skin* can be more delicate and benefit from tapotement to stimulate the tissues; avoid unduly stretching the area with friction or harsh kneading.
- *Gritty skin* texture can be an indication of excretory problems. On close inspection these are tiny pimples giving a gooseflesh appearance (triceps, tensor fascia latae, gluteals, hamstrings). May be an indicator of too much acid in the system.
- A *congested skin* may indicate a congested body.
- Are there any *scars*? What are they from and how old are they?
- *Stretch marks*, also referred to as striations. The skin has become thin across the mark as a result of a loss in elasticity in the dermis. These marks are not always caused by weight gain and then weight loss; they often occur as a result of hormonal changes and can be seen on naturally slim clients too (usually around the buttocks and thighs). When there has been a sudden weight gain and loss, particularly after childbirth the skin does not have time to adjust to the changes resulting in excessive stretching of the collagen and elastin fibres.

Skin colour

Check the overall tone on the skin you are working on for system weaknesses.

- Are there any signs of poor *circulation*, e.g. cold extremities, puffy knees and ankles, chilblains in winter.

Tip

Stretch marks
Initially stretch marks appear as pink or discoloured lines. If the skin is paler than the surrounding area it indicates that the stretch marks are old.

Tip

Skin colour
Tones of the skin could indicate system weaknesses. These include:

- *grey skin* and *pallor:* may indicate excessive fatigue, nervous exhaustion
- *yellow-tinged* or *dirty looking skin:* may indicate poor digestion (particularly linked to liver congestion)
- *reddish tone:* may indicate a possible tendency to increased blood pressure and congested organs.

- Check the skin for *bruising*.
- *Thread veins*: apply gentle effleurage, kneading and drainage movements will be beneficial; avoid tapotement movements over areas where there are several visible arterioles however.
- *Varicose veins*: remember to work above the vein to drain and avoid pressure from below.

Examination of muscular condition

With any postural problem the muscles will be affected. There will be muscle fatigue; some muscles will have shortened or tightened fibres while the antagonistic muscles will be lengthened or stretched.

The following are simple tests that you can ask the client to perform to assess the client's muscular condition, i.e. strength, muscle shortening and mobility. Observe the following:

1   range of movements, i.e. how much movement is there

2   whether there is any discomfort during movement.

- **Pectorals**
  Have the client lie on couch on their back, hands behind the head. Do elbows come down flat on the couch? Inability to do this indicates a shortening of the pectoral muscles.

- **Arms**
  Biceps: Client places their hand on their shoulder and resists therapist's attempt to bring arm down.
  Triceps: Repeat but this time the client resists the therapist's attempt to hold the hand up to the shoulder.

- **Abdomen**
  Strength of rectus abdominis, obliques: Therapist places hand on abdomen while client to attempts to sit up from prone position, (knees bent if necessary), note trembling and muscular strain. For older clients or those with known weak muscles, reverse the position so that the client lies down from a sitting position with knees bent.
  Ligament connection: Client lying in supine position. Grasp flesh firmly. Ask the client to contract their abdominal muscles to pull away from hand. If this can be done ligament attachment is good.

- **Legs**
  Mobility of the spine and hamstring shortening: Test for shortening by making the client stand then leans forward to touch toes.
  General strength in legs: Client lies on one side, raises upper leg slightly and brings lower leg up to join it. Repeat for other side.
  Gastrocnemius and soleus shortening and strength of quadriceps: Ask the client to bring the toes up while holding foot down to full extension with even pressure. Feel calf muscles to assess strength.
  Achilles tendon shortening: Foot will not fully extend if this is present.
  Hip mobility, adductor shortening: In a sitting position place feet together and drop knees down. Restricted ability will indicate muscle shortening.

Simple postural exercises

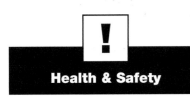

Health & Safety

Exercising

- Before doing exercises, especially stretching, make sure the body is warm. After a bath or shower is ideal.

- Never stretch further than is comfortable.

- If a stretch hurts, stop!

Tip

Exercising

- Encourage the client to exercise.

- It is more important to do the exercises correctly even if the movement or stretch is small, otherwise muscular strain may result.

- Squeezing the muscles to contract them helps to sculpture their shape, particularly the abdominal muscles.

Beneficial exercises are those which will improve mobility, and which stretch and strengthen the muscles. Below are a few simple postural exercises that can be suggested to the client to improve posture. The client should be encouraged to perform the exercises regularly and to be patient.

Back stretch

- Stand straight; place hand on base of back. To enhance the stretch raise arms above head and lean back.

- Kneel on the floor, buttocks on heels, head on floor, arms straight above the head on the floor.

- Supine, raise knees to chest and gently rock knees backwards and forwards.

Forward bend stretching the hamstrings and back

- Arms above head, knees unlocked; bend forward and bring the arms down to the floor as you go. Keep the head in line with the spine. Relax head and let arms hang. Hold; with the elbows crossed to add weight.

- To come back up, bend the knees, place the hands on the knees and slowly roll the spine up until standing.

Seated forward bend stretching back and hamstrings

- Sit with legs outstretched and toes flexed. Bend forward keeping the back straight and touch the toes. If you find this difficult keep the knees bent slightly or use a towel or belt around the feet to support you.

Side flexion

- Stand with feet together, arms to the side. With abdomen tucked in, gently reach with one hand down one side. Repeat for other side.

Progression

- Stand with feet together one arm above the head, the other with the hand on the hip. Reach over the head to the opposite side keeping the back in line, abdomen pulled in. Repeat for other side.

Lying pelvic tilt

- Lie on the floor, knees bent. Rock the pelvis and pull in the abdomen to push the back to the floor.

- Kneel on the floor. Pull in the abdominal muscles and raise the back up into an arch. Repeat several times.

Knee rotation side to side

- Lie supine. Bring the knees up to the chest and drop them to alternate sides. To increase the stretch extend the opposite leg and stretch the arms out on either side.

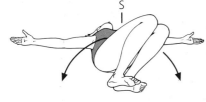

Knee rotation

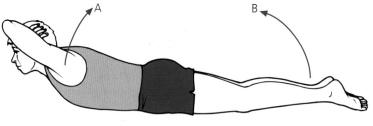

Prone stretch

Prone stretch

Stretches and strengthens the back and spinal muscles.

- Lie prone. Place the hands either by the side of the body or on the back of the neck.
- Raise the head and shoulder.

Progression

- Raise alternate legs; as strength builds raise legs together.
- Raise both the head and legs together.

Quadriceps stretch

- Standing with legs together, raise one leg behind you holding it by the ankle. Gently pull the leg back being carefully not to pull it to the side. Use a chair for balance if necessary. Repeat for other side.

Hamstring stretch

- Stand with one foot in front of the other. Resting on the heel of the forward foot lean forwards and gently extend the foot. Repeat for other leg.

Hip stretch

- Squat down and extend one leg out to the side; lean forward gently.
- Sit on the floor with the feet touching and dropped to the side, Gently push the knees down towards the floor.
- Squat down and hold. This is also good for stretching out the lower back and pelvis.

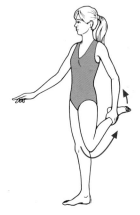

Quadriceps stretch

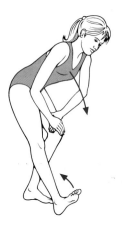

Hamstring stretch

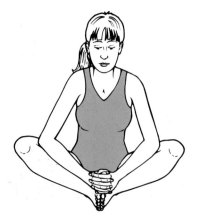

Hip stretch

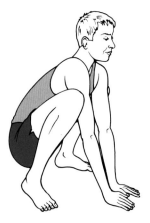

Squat

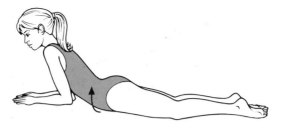

Abdominal strengthener

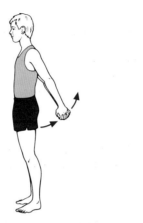

Shoulder and chest stretch

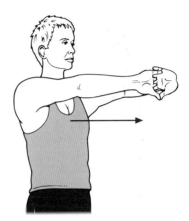

Shoulder and upper back stretch

Easy abdominal strengthener for very weak muscles

- Lie prone, raise the top up on to the elbows and contract the abdominal muscles. Repeat several times.

Shoulder and chest back stretch

- Stand or sit. Stretch hands behind back and hold.

Shoulder and upper back stretch

- Interlink fingers and stretch arms out in front of the body turning the hands so that the palms face outward. Stretch and hold.

Abdominal curl

- Lie supine with knees bent. Place hands behind the head and focus on a point above you. Lift the head and shoulder only, squeezing the abdominal muscle tight.

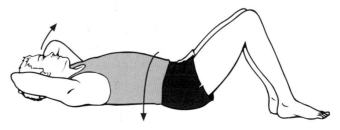

Abdominal curl

Concluding a figure analysis

Once you have completed your checks and observations, summarize your findings and discuss these with the client. Remember to make reference to positive points as well as areas for correction. Offer suitable advice and suggestions.

You may find it useful to have a specific after care leaflet with postural exercises that the client can follow.

 Knowledge review

1 What is the value of a figure analysis?

2 List the common postural faults.

3 Who might you refer the client to for additional treatment?

4 What are the three body shapes and how would you recognize them?

5 How would you recognize good posture?

6 What are the benefits of good posture?

7 What can your posture reveal?

8 List the anti-gravity muscles.

9 What is palpation?

10 What observations would you make with regard to the skin?

Classification of massage techniques

8

Learning objectives

This chapter covers the following:

- **definition of massage**
- **the benefits and effects of massage**
- **classic massage techniques**
- **preparation for massage**
- **additional techniques for massage**
- **other massage therapies**

This chapter aims to introduce the essential underpinning knowledge necessary for all treatments using any form of massage. It will guide you through the different types of movements, their benefits and effects. It will then introduce you to the use of more diverse massage skills.

The benefits and effects of massage

Interesting fact

The actual term massage is derived from the Arabic word *mas'h*: meaning 'to knead' and 'to press softly'.

Massage is the manipulation of the soft tissues of the body, with the aim of having a positive effect on the systems of the body.

There are many benefits to massage. Most of these are achieved through the systems it affects.

Blood circulation

- Massage improves the micro-circulation initially through the area being treated. The lifting and squeezing of the muscles particularly benefits the venous return which relies heavily on muscular action to pump blood back to the heart.
- Massage opens up the arterioles and capillaries improving the exchange of fluids in the tissues in a different way from exercise.
- Improved circulation brings nutrient-rich blood and assists the removal of waste products. This is of particular benefit to areas of the body that may have a sluggish circulation.
- Histamine is released making the blood vessels more permeable and improving micro-circulation (tiny capillaries).
- Increased circulation encourages cellular activity.
- Where more vigorous movements are used heat is generated in the tissues increasing suppleness and mobility.

Lymphatic circulation

- The flow of lymph in the lymph vessels is enhanced as the massage strokes move in the direction of lymph drainage to the nearest group of lymph nodes.
- Lymphatic circulation is assisted; the squeezing and pumping action encourages tissue fluid in and out of the lymphatic vessels.
- Pressure on the tissues will facilitate the transfer of tissue fluid across vessel walls. Fluid from the tissues will pass into the lymph vessels and will drain away more quickly; this will prevent or reduce oedema (swelling of the tissues).
- Larger particles of waste, which are able to pass through the lymphatic vessel walls, are removed more quickly.

Muscles

- Metabolism is improved by the increase in circulation and increased availability of nutrients.
- Vigorous massage such as percussion movements stimulate the stretch reflex in the muscle tissue. This causes a momentary involuntary contraction of the muscle fibres. Regular massage will help to improve muscle fibre elasticity.
- Promotes relaxation of the muscle tissue. This may be general or localized to a specific group of muscles.
- Tension over a period of time can lead to atrophy and fibrosis in the muscle tissue. This is a particular problem to those who stand for long periods, have restricted muscular movement or are immobile.

- Regular massage where there has been a long period of immobility helps to reduce the natural reduction in tissue elasticity. Tissues begin to waste and are replaced by less elastic components if not utilized.
- Scar tissue is formed within the muscular tissue as a result of old injuries. The tissue injury may be obvious with inflammation or through micro trauma to a section of muscle fibres. These scars may cause different tissues to adhere together resulting in a reduction in muscular flexibility which itself results in muscular tension. Massage helps to break down the tension and increase flexibility.
- Long-term restriction of movement due to pain, discomfort, bad posture or habit causes the elastic components of the soft muscular tissue to shrink and shorten forming inelastic fibrous tissue. Massage helps to improve the muscular inflexibility caused by the shortening of the muscle fibres.
- Prior to activity or exercise massage ensures an improved circulation is ready to supply the needs of the muscular activity. The muscles are warm and therefore more supple and mobile. This also helps to reduce the risk of muscular injury or damage.
- Following physical activity massage may be used to facilitate the recovery of the muscles.

The skin

- The condition of the skin is improved by the natural exfoliation during the massage resulting from the friction of the therapist's hand.
- The emollient effect of the medium applied to the skin leaves it soft and supple.
- Increase circulation helps to keep the skin nourished. Regular massage helps to improve the general appearance of the skin.
- Supple skin remains flexible and more resistant to damage and invasion by micro-organisms.
- With regular massage the skin's elasticity is maintained, reducing the visible effects of ageing.

Metabolism

- Cellular activity is increased.
- Excretion of nitrogen, inorganic phosphorous and sodium chloride are increased due to the increase in cellular activity.

The urinary system

- The stimulation of cellular activity when massaging particularly around the mid-back and abdomen increases elimination of toxins.

The skeletal system

- There is no direct effect, but the increased circulation indirectly benefits all the structures of the body.
- Mobility movements help to relieve stiff joints and improve the range of joint flexibility.

Endorphins
The word endorphin is derived from 'endogenous' meaning within and the chemical 'morphine', a painkiller. Endorphins are released from the central nervous system and pituitary gland.

Interesting fact

Dopamine
Dopamine, another neurotransmitter, may also be released from the limbic system, cerebral cortex and hypothalamus. It is thought to affect mood, emotional response and the ability to experience pleasure and pain.

The nervous system

- The sensory nerve endings may be soothed or stimulated according to the type and application of movement.
- The stretch reflex in the muscle fibres is stimulated.
- Applying pressure techniques to areas of sensitivity helps to release endorphins from the brain creating a sense of well-being.
- Pressure may also block some of the pain impulses resulting in a temporary numbing effect of the nerve impulses.

Digestion

- Massage of the abdomen helps to stimulate the peristalsis action of digestion. This is of particular benefit to anyone with a sluggish digestion or suffering with constipation.

The respiratory system

- Percussion movements performed over the ribs on the back help to loosen the mucus secretions of the lungs facilitating deep breathing.

Psychological benefits

- There is great psychological value in massage and touch. In today's stressed society the touch of massage does wonders for alleviating all kinds of symptoms.
- It is believed that the pleasure from massage helps to release endorphins preventing pain impulses reaching the brain.
- By generally increasing the metabolism the client will have an increased sense of well-being.
- The benefit of relaxation is often underestimated. In a relaxed state the body makes use of the time to rebalance and regenerate.

Classic massage techniques

There are five classic massage movements:

- effleurage
- petrissage (kneading)
- frictions
- tapotement or percussion
- vibrations.

Interesting fact

'Effleurer' is French and means to skim the surface of or to lightly touch and to touch upon.

Effleurage

Effleurage is a stroking movement. The pressure of the movement can be varied in line with the desired effect. Strokes are smooth, flowing and continuous. Effleurage is always performed with the pressure towards the heart. Effleurage may be applied with the palmar surface of one or both hands moulded to the shape of the area being worked. The fingers or the thumbs are used on smaller areas. For deeper effleurage over a large area the forearms can be used.

The uses of effleurage

- To introduce the therapist's hands to the client's body.
- To apply the medium to the client's skin.
- To begin the routine.
- To link movements together.
- To drain an area between movements.
- To complete a routine.

The benefits and effects of effleurage

- Stimulates the sensory nerve endings, yet has a calming, soothing effect.
- Assists venous return.
- Relaxes the muscle fibres.
- Aids desquamation.
- Increases cellular metabolism (increased blood supply).
- Effleurage creates a localized increase in the pressure in the tissue fluid causing the pores in the lymphatic capillaries to open. This allows a free exchange of tissue fluids and the removal of waste products.

Types of effleurage

Effleurage is defined by the method by which it is applied:

- *stroking* is slow and superficial
- *superficial* light effleurage
- *deep* for a greater effect
- *slow* to drain, calm and relax
- *fast* to stimulate.

Variations of effleurage

		Description	Area treated
Long effleurage		Hands parallel side by side or one in front of the other. Movement from the furthest point directed towards the heart	Limbs, back
Finger effleurage		Finger or thumbs used in a firm stroking action	Small areas, e.g. hand, feet, knees

	Description	Area treated
Superficial effleurage Feathering	Effleurage using the fingers with very light pressure, alternatively or singularly	Back
Circling	Slow broad circles drawn with the fingers, single or alternate hands with light pressure	Back
Deeper effleurage Reinforced 	One hand is place on top of the other to increase pressure and depth	Back, legs and buttocks

Tip

Palpation skills – feeling for tension
Tension within the muscle fibres can take different forms. Relaxed muscles are soft and mobile. Tense muscles are firm to the touch, sometimes even hard. Tension can be felt as crystals or firm nodules in part of the muscle tissue.

Petrissage

Petrissage movements generally incorporate a lifting action, moving the tissues away from the underlying organs and bones. Individual muscles or muscles groups may be manipulated.

The muscle is cupped between the hands, picked up, squeezed and released in repetition to form a kneading action. Several parts of the hand may be used to apply petrissage including: the whole palm, heel of the hand, fingerpads, thumbs, knuckles or the elbow. Movements should be performed with pressure towards the heart.

The benefits and effects of petrissage

- Compression and relaxation of the muscle tissues.
- Increase in vascular and lymphatic drainage, removing lactic acid and other waste from the tissues and bringing fresh nutrients. This will help to eliminate muscle fatigue.
- Mobilizing of fibrous tissue and localized muscle thickening.
- Stimulates the function of the abdominal organs.
- Desquamation.

Variations on petrissage

- **Kneading**
  Performed along the muscle length with the hands close together.
  Single-handed. Uses the palmar surface or the heel of the hand. The free hand supports the area being worked or is used to hold the muscle tissue into the working hand.
  Use: legs, buttocks, arms, back and abdomen.
  Double-handed. Alternate hands are used in succession, to knead and squeeze the muscles.
  Use: legs, buttocks, back.
  Reinforced. Sometimes referred to as *ironing*: Hands are reinforced with one hand on top of the other (ironing), to increase the pressure.
  Use: legs, buttocks, arms, back and abdomen.

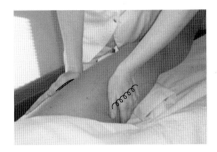

Single handed kneading

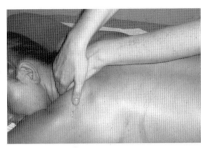

Reinforced petrissage

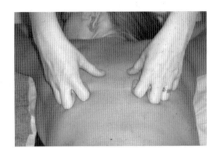

Picking up and squeezing

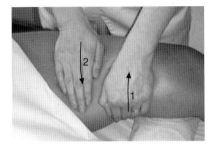

Wringing

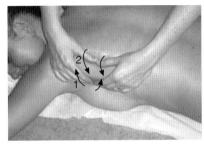

Skin rolling

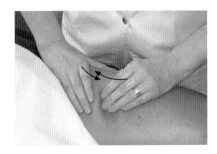

Knuckling

- **Picking up and squeezing**
  Two hands are used. The muscle is picked up with the fingers and thumb, squeezed and released into the other hand where the muscle is squeezed and released again.
  Use: legs, buttocks, arms, back and abdomen.

- **Wringing**
  Both hands are used, working in opposition across the fibres of a muscle. The muscle is lifted from the underlying structures using the fingers to push the tissue one way to meet the opposite hand using the palm working the tissue back. Contact should continuous between the exchange of hands. (Avoid friction, which can be achieved by speeding up the movement.)
  Use: legs, buttocks, back and sides of abdomen. Wringing is useful on large areas or muscle groups. It is good for maintaining tendon elasticity, e.g. Achilles tendon.

- **Skin rolling**
  The fingers from one hand roll the flesh to the thumbs which in turn roll the tissue back against the fingers. Do not pinch.
  Use: legs, buttocks, arms, back, abdomen. This movement is useful for mobilizing localized thickening especially on the upper back.

- **Knuckling**
  This is a deep movement using the flat surface of the 2nd phalanges. The fingers are moved up and down. The movement can be enhanced further by moving the hands in circles.
  Use: buttocks, back. This is excellent for areas of poor circulation, tension and where there is large muscle bulk.

Frictions

Some classify frictions as a separate movement. Frictions are small movements using the pads of the fingers or thumbs in a circular or transverse direction across the muscle fibres. Pressure is generally concentrated on a small area and penetrates into the muscles. Care must be taken not to over-irritate the skin or bruising may occur.

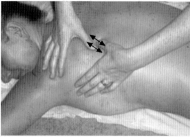

Thumb frictions

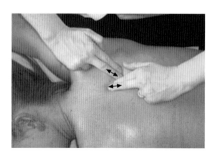

Finger frictions

The uses of friction

- To loosen fibrous adhesion caused by a build up in muscular tension.
- To break down localized fatty deposits.
- To mobilize scar tissue.
- To improve the appearance of stretch marks.

The benefits and effects of frictions

- Rapid increase in circulation – erythema.

Types of friction

- *Thumb:* the thumbs are placed onto the area and work against each other in a press and release action.
- *Fingers:* the pads of the fingers work into the soft tissue or between a joint using a rubbing action.

Tapotement/percussion

The hands are used alternatively. The wrists are used loosely producing a light springing movement. Rhythm is essential.

The benefits and effects of tapotement

- The muscle fibres contract, momentarily activating the 'stretch reflex' which has a toning effect on the fibres.
- Increase in erythema, hyperaemia and warmth.
- Frequent application of the heavier percussion movements may help in the dispersal of fatty deposits and to improve cellulite.

Variations on tapotement

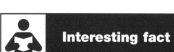

Interesting fact

Tapoter is French and means to tap, pat or strum.

- **Pincemont**
  Using the fingertips of both hands the skin is squeezed (almost pinched) and released in quick succession, with a flicking action.
  Use: legs, buttocks, arms, back, abdomen. Excellent over the back of the arms and smaller areas that need extra stimulation.
- **Tapping**
  Sometimes referred to as raindrops. The fingers are tapped in succession over the area as if playing a piano or typing quickly.
  Use: face, neck (décolleté), abdomen. Used on more delicate areas such as the face and head.
- **Hacking**
  The elbows are bent and abducted away from the body. Wrists are flexed and the fingers relaxed. The ulna border of the little finger is used to strike the tissue in rapid alternate succession, supplemented by the other fingers (it is not a karate chop). It should sound like raindrops. This movement is usually carried out across the muscle fibres. Bony areas should be avoided. Hacking can be performed deeply, lightly or gestured.
  Use: legs, buttocks, lightly on arms, back (avoid spine and caution over kidney area), abdomen.

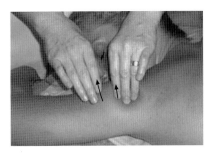

Pincemont tapotement

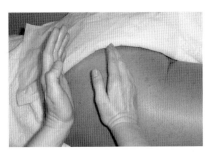

Hacking

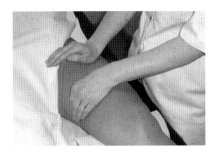

Cupping

Tip

Cupping

If you are cupping correctly the sound should be hollow. If your hands are not cupped enough you will slap the skin and the sound will reflect this.

☼ Activity

Hacking

When first attempting hacking it may be difficult to co-ordinate an even alternate movement between the two hands. To develop your skill, practise on a soft surface such as a couch or mattress. Try this on a partner (not too vigorously!) and ask for feedback.

With hacking it is important that the hands are relaxed and that the movement is from the wrists. Try alternating between relaxed, loosely cupped hands and hard-ridged straight fingers and notice the difference in both feel and sound.

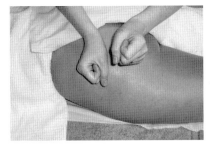

Pounding

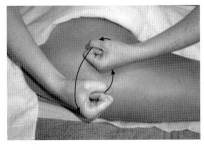

Beating

- **Cupping**
  The hands are lightly cupped and alternately strike the body creating a hollow clapping sound. The cupped hand has a vacuum effect appearing to draw the tissue up into the hand.
  Use: legs, buttocks, and lightly over upper back, abdomen.

- **Pounding**
  Lightly clench the hands to make a fist. Using alternate hands strike the body with the ulna border of the little finger.
  Use: only performed on bulky tissue; legs, buttocks.

- **Beating**
  Loosely clenched fists are used with the wrist flexed. The ulna border of the little finger strikes the tissue, rotating the hands around each other to lift the tissue.
  Use: only performed on bulky tissue; legs, buttocks.

Vibrations

A fine trembling action conveyed through the hand or fingertips, usually following a nerve pathway. There are two methods of application:

- *static*: the hand remains stationary and vibrates
- *running*: the hand travels along the skin whilst applying the vibration.

The uses of vibration

- To loosen scar tissue.
- For stretching adhesion.

The benefits and effects of vibrations

- Stimulates the circulation generating heat in the tissues. Histamine is released making the blood vessels more permeable.
- Loosens scar tissue.
- Vibrations can be stimulating or relaxing on the nerve endings depending on the manner in which they are performed.
- Encourages lymphatic flow.

Preparation for massage

Hand exercises

It is good practice when you first start to perform some hand exercises to increase mobility.

When you first start to massage your hands may get tired and ache. Your hands need to be flexible and supple as they will need to mould the client's body. The following are some simple exercises to improve suppleness and flexibility.

- Rotate the wrists clockwise and anticlockwise.
- Clench the fists and then release, point one finger at a time keeping the others closed in a fist.
- Place palms together at chest height (prayer position), apply slight pressure and release. Repeat several times.
- Interlock the fingers of both hands. Turn hands with fingers interlocked out so that palms face away from you and stretch out your arms with elbow joints locked.
- Place fingers on a surface and lift alternative fingers as if typing fast or playing the piano.
- Stretch the thumbs back towards the forearm.

Additional massage techniques

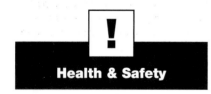

Health & Safety

Only mobilize a joint within its capability. Never force a joint, especially if it is stiff.

- **Assisted joint mobility**
  A limb is supported with one hand and rotated; flexed or extended. The client needs to relax the limb so that the movement can be performed passively without resistance. Care must be taken not to force a movement.
  Use: To improve or maintain joint mobility.

- **Squeezing and pumping**
  These are light movements used to stimulate the venous and lymphatic circulations and are always made towards the nearest lymph nodes.
  Squeezing: the tissues are supported between the thumbs, fingers or hands and squeezed.
  Pumping: uses the fingertips, which lightly pump the skin's surface in the direction of the nearest lymph nodes.

- **Rocking and shaking**
  Rocking: like rocking a baby this movement has a soothing action on the nervous system. The movement can be localized when a single hand holds the muscle or using both hands to shake the muscle. It is a wonderful movement for the lower back.

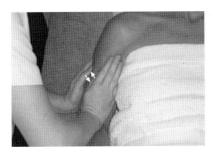

Squeezing

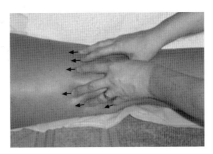

Pumping

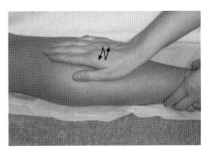

Rocking

Shaking: performed on the whole limb, this helps to loosen the joints. The wrist or ankle is raised, a slight contraction is applied and then the limb is shaken. The application of the shaking can be varied to create the desired response of either muscle relaxation – slow shaking – or stimulation – vigorous shaking.

Additional techniques for advanced treatment

Neuromuscular techniques – NMT

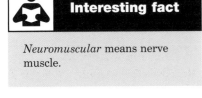

Interesting fact

Neuromuscular means nerve muscle.

These are techniques that can be used to enhance a massage. NMT uses a combination of pressure and deep friction. It is used to stimulate the nerve endings, muscle, tendons, ligaments and other connective tissue. The techniques used are less relaxing than classic movements as they may cause mild discomfort.

Uses of NMT

- To alleviate changes in the superficial and deep fascia of the muscles.
- To improving localized congestion in the muscle tissue.
- To preventing or reduce muscular adhesions caused by micro trauma.
- To improve the function of the nerve pathways (dermatomes).
- To increase joint mobility.
- For pain relief and to treat nerve injuries.

NMT works by dampening the response from a nerve. Pressure is applied to a sensitive spot, often the motor point of a muscle. This pressure may be very uncomfortable, but in a nice sort of way! The pressure squeezes the circulation out of the tissues under the pressure point which when released causes the blood to rush back into the vacant vacuum.

It is believed that stimulation of the pain receptors feeds back to the brain to release endorphins. These relax the body and create a feeling of well-being, hence relieving muscular tension.

NMT may be used in two ways.

Firstly, following the *dermatome* sensory areas. These are segmented areas of skin supplied by the sensory receptors from a single spinal nerve (dorsal root). Pressure is applied along the grooves along the spinal column but never on the spine itself. Reaction in the skin will give an indication of sensory status in that area. A lack of skin reaction will indicate poor circulation.

Pressure can be applied to a specific spinal nerve if you know that a specific area or organ need treatment.

Technique for dermatome. Apply the pressure using the thumb to the 'dip' for 20 seconds. Keeping thumbs stationary turn the side of the thumb and push away from the spine to release.

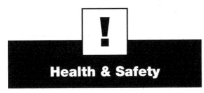

Health & Safety

When working near the spine never apply pressure to the spinal column itself as this may cause damage.

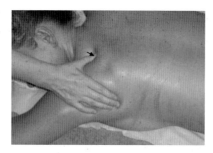

Neuromuscular technique

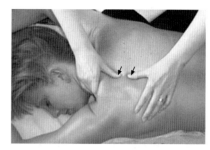

Neuromuscular technique

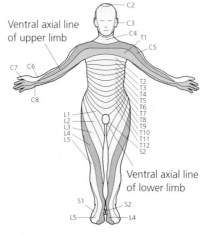

Ventral axial line
of upper limb

Ventral axial line
of lower limb

Dermatomes

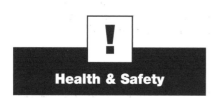

Health & Safety

If the area is very painful or the pain
becomes worse do not continue to
apply the technique – this will have
the opposite effect of causing tension
in the tissue.

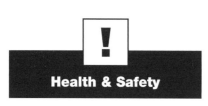

Health & Safety

The fingers may be used to avoid
strain on the thumb joints. On large
areas (not near the spine) the elbow
can be used.

The second method of application is on motor point sensitive areas. Good
palpation techniques need to be used. Whilst working generally on an area
feel for any changes in the muscular tissue. You are specifically feeling for
changes in firmness of the tissues. Where there are pockets of tension or
tightness check for level of pain.

Technique for motor point. Apply deep, firm pressure into the belly of
the muscles (tender area) using the thumb, elbow or fingers. Hold for up to
90 seconds. Release and repeat until the pain subsides. Movements may be
enhanced by rotating on the point, adding a slight friction with the thumb
or fingers.

Other massage techniques

These include:

- friction using the thumbs or fingers working opposite each other,
  or fingers working in a localized area in a sawing action.
- deep circular movements using the fingers, thumb or elbow.

Other massage therapies

There are several other classifications of massage therapies apart from
traditional Swedish massage. Many use similar techniques but work using
differing philosophies. Below is an introduction to lymphatic massage and
shiatsu.

Additional therapies to be summarized on the web are: No Hands, rolfing, Bowen technique, synchronized, and Ancient therapies (Tui na, Indonesian, Balinese, Kahuna, Thai). See www/thomsonlearning.co.uk/hairandbeauty/beckmann.

Lymphatic massage

There are many theories regarding lymphatic massage. Remember that lymph is a slow-moving fluid and as such the massage techniques should reflect this. The treatment aims to assist and encourage the flow of lymph. You cannot speed it up but you can make it more efficient. The techniques are often used as part an aromatherapy treatment and are more passive than those used in traditional Swedish massage.

The effects of massage on the lymphatic system

To ensure you are familiar with the lymphatic system go to p.71 above.

The pressure and squeezing movements of petrissage are the most effective in reducing oedema, followed by effleurage. This effect is enhanced if the part being treated is elevated whilst being massaged; gravity will then assist drainage.

You can use pillows or props to elevate the legs; alternatively the client can be placed with the legs elevated on the raised part of the couch. When working on the arms place the client's arm on your shoulder to increase gravity as this will assist filtration back to the node concerned.

Indications for lymphatic massage

A client may complain of swelling in the legs, knees and ankles, puffy areas or shoes feeling tight. This could be due to several factors including:

- non-medical oedema (medical oedema is contra indicated)
- lack of exercise
- having to stand around leading to gravitational oedema
- obesity
- poor/sluggish circulation
- weight reduction diets
- pre-menstrual tension
- long periods of immobility
- after exercise to remove accumulated metabolic waste (tension).

Technique

All movements during a lymphatic massage should be applied towards the nearest regional lymph node.

After initial effleurage, use movements to drain the area closest to the nodes first and gradually work further work away. Think of it as clearing a space or vacuum for the lymph to be drawn into.

- *Light effleurage* causes a cascade effect in the lymphatic circulation improving absorption of waste products.
- *Kneading by compression* and relaxation causes lymphatic vessels to be emptied and filled, thus hastening removal of metabolites.
- *Fingertips, thumbs or hands used in a pumping action* create an increase in the pressure in the tissues in front of the stroke and release the pressure in the tissue behind. This encourages the flow

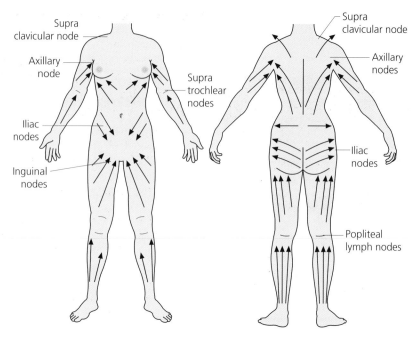

Lymphatic drainage

in venous and lymphatic vessels assisting the general movement of tissue fluid.

- *Vibrations* around the joints help to remove fluid.

For muscle stretching and energizing techniques (MST/MET) see Chapter 9, p.207.

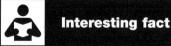

Interesting fact

'Shiatsu' means finger pressure. Shiatsu is a specialized form of massage, training for which can take up to four years.

Acupressure – shiatsu

What is acupressure/shiatsu

Acupressure is a treatment that manipulates the acupuncture points of the body using pressure instead of needles. Its roots lie in Traditional Chinese Medicine (TCM) and the Chinese system of healing.

A history of shiatsu

Shiatsu roots developed from TCM. Its history is so old that much of it is clouded and has achieved some degree of myth. The practice of acupuncture can be dated back before 2500 BC. Traditional theories spread to Japan during the sixth century and these were later mixed with European influences between the fifteenth and seventeenth centuries.

The development of shiatsu into a medical treatment continued in the early twentieth century. There are still today some variations in technique and these include Namikshi-style shiatsu, Zen shiatsu and Tsubo therapy.

Ensure you are familiar with Chapter 3, Understanding energy.

The treatment

The client often receives treatment fully clothed and pressure is applied to stimulate the local nerves and tissue. The muscles are also stretched and released.

During treatment pressure may be applied using:

- the thumbs
- by squeezing the skin in small delicate areas between the tips of the index finger and thumb (known as the 'dragon's mouth')
- the elbow
- heel of the palm
- the knuckles.

Pressure should be firm and even and applied with the therapist's body in a relaxed stance without locking the joints.

There are 365 pressure point or *Tsubos* located along the meridian lines. These can generally be located at points where it is easy for energy flow to stagnate. Primary points lie near the surface in fixed structures and depressions and bony prominences; others are located using reference to a specified distance. Extra channels lie deeper to carry Qi within the body (see Chapter 3, p.21).

Stagnated Qi may present as a variety of symptoms including tingling, stiffness, heat or pain. Shiatsu works to disperse the stagnated energy and encourage and stimulate the flow of positive energy (or Ki/Chi).

Interesting fact

Tsubos
When measuring the position of Tsubos the fingers are used for measuring distance. This can depend on the therapist's hands. The unit is called the cun or tsun.

1 cun = the width of the inter-phalange joint of the thumb

2 = the index and middle finger

3 = the four fingers.

Knowledge review

1 Define massage.

2 What are the psychological benefits of massage?

3 What are the effects of petrissage?

4 What is neuromuscular technique and how can it be applied?

5 What precautions would you take when applying tapotement/percussion massage?

6 Label the lymphatic nodes of the body on the following diagram and indicate the direction of massage movement.

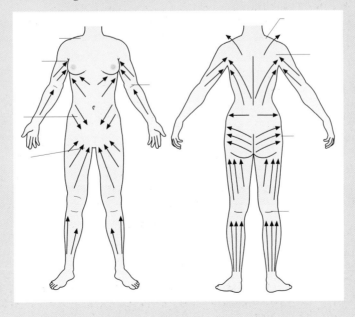

9

Body massage

Learning objectives

This chapter covers the following:

- **a brief overview of the history of massage**
- **preparation for massage treatment**
- **a sample body massage routine**
- **muscle stretching and energizing techniques**
- **after care for massage**
- **adaptations to massage**
- **the benefits and effects of body massage**
- **pre-heating treatments**

This chapter will build on Chapter 5, Client care, and Chapter 8, Classification of massage techniques, to encourage you to develop your massage into a complete treatment. It will explore treatments that can be used to enhance the effects of your massage as well as methods of adapting your treatment.

A brief overview of the history of massage

The existence of the use of massage is believed to date as far back as 5000 years. The Eastern Asians knew early on the therapeutic benefits. Many well-known therapies demonstrate the use of massage in varying forms and all have long established histories, such as shiatsu and Ayurvedic treatments.

Massage is mentioned in some of the earliest records and in the writing of philosophers, historians who make reference to the practices of rubbing and anointing. There was regular reference to the use of these practices for healing and anointing, especially as part of religious ceremonies and practices.

As human curiosity about the body grew massage techniques were developed. Hippocrates was one famous early doctor and philosopher who wrote of the benefits of massage.

Henry (Henrik) Ling, a Swedish physiologist, was responsible for bringing massage as we know it today to Europe. He discovered and developed techniques learnt during his travels to China and realized the necessity for adequate training coupled with an understanding of anatomy and physiology. He established the first massage system, hence the term 'Swedish massage', and was responsible for introducing many of the terms we associate with Western massage today.

Dr Mezger from Holland (1839–1901) finally achieved the professional recognition of massage when the Society of Training Masseuses was established in 1894. Its aim was to raise the standards and reputation of the profession. It amalgamated with the Institute of Massage and Remedial Exercise. In 1943 the organization changed again, becoming known as the Chartered Society Physiotherapies and achieving state registration in 1964. Training for physiotherapists continued to develop as did that for massage.

Massage started to become incorporated within the remit of the beauty therapist and courses were developed to train them in the techniques. Today, however, there are many who specialize as a masseur. The developmental possibilities for massage are vast, and we have already seen it extended to specialist massage treatments such as remedial, sports and baby massage and aromatherapy.

Preparation for a massage treatment

Preparation of the treatment area

To ensure you are familiar with this topic, go to Chapter 5, p.133.

Hygiene checklist:

- The area in which you are working should be clean and tidy.
- The bin should be lined and emptied when full.
- The trolley should be wiped with surgical spirit and covered with a clean sheet of couch roll.
- Remove cream from pots using a sterile spatula or disposable wooden spatula.
- The couch should be covered with clean couch roll for each new client.
- Check for contra indications.
- Cover any open wounds with a dressing.
- Remove jewellery.
- Wash hands before and after treatment.

Tip

Eau de cologne is useful for freshening the skin if the client is perspiring or has strong body odour and for wiping the feet before applying your massage medium.

Tip

What not to wear
Ideally the client should remove all their clothes, although it is recommended that a female working on a male client should request that the client keeps on his briefs. Some clients may feel uncomfortable with removing all their clothes and you need to give the client this option and respect their wishes. G-string panties are ideal

You will need the following equipment and resources:

- massage medium – oil (a suitable carrier or blended massage oil), cream, talc or talc subsitute
- surgical spirit or antiseptic wipe – this is for cleaning the client's feet
- cotton wool
- eau de cologne
- couch roll, folded – this is useful for protecting the towels and, if the client is modest, for protecting underwear
- record card and pen
- glass of water for the client.

Preparation for treatment

Carry out a full consultation (see Chapter 5, p.134). If it is a repeat treatment always review the consultation and update it if necessary.

Ask the client to remove their clothes. Be specific as to exactly which clothes you require the client to remove. If the changing area is the treatment room, leave the room while they undress. This is a good opportunity to excuse yourself if there is no hand basin in the treatment area to go and wash your hands. Knock to signal or tell the client you are returning. Once the client is ready, position them on the couch.

Ask the client to remove their jewellery. Ideally ask the client to store it (ladies could put it in their handbag) or place it in a bowl on the trolley within the client's eyeline.

Once the client is on the couch. Position your supports; make sure the client is comfortable and covered.

Wipe the client's feet with surgical spirit or cologne and check for contra indications.

Massage mediums

A massage medium is a product applied to the skin to facilitate the massage. A medium should be pleasant to use and have a soft, fluid feel (with the exception of talc). It should provide 'slip' and not be absorbed too quickly – the massage continuity may be broken if medium has to keep being reapplied. There are three main categories of massage medium:

Oil

Oil is the most popular medium for massage. It has an excellent emollient effect on the skin leaving it soft and smooth and is especially beneficial for dry or scaly skin. It gives slip to the hands and prevents excessive friction of body hair while giving smooth contact. Oil should not be used in excess, with only just enough oil used to maintain contact. Too much oil will weaken grip and tissue contact.

Oils may be manufactured, i.e. mineral oil, or natural, e.g. grape-seed or sweet almond. Natural oils are more preferable as they have better penetration of the skin; mineral oils form an occlusive layer on the surface of the skin but this does leave the skin feeling very silky and smooth.

It is common for oils to be ready blended for a specific types of massage such as relaxation or stress relief. These often contain essential oils.

To ensure you are familiar with carrier oils, go to Chapter 10, p.226.

Massage cream

The use of massage cream is not so common for a full body massage, although some masseurs prefer to use it. There are several different types of creams produced specifically for massage and, like oils, creams may have synthetic or natural ingredients. They may contain lanolin, petroleum or specialized active ingredients to enhance to effects of the massage. Many creams are quite thick in consistency but become more fluid when warmed so be careful not to use too much.

Talc

Unscented talcum powder is rarely used now although it has it benefits. Talc prevents irritation of the client's skin by perspiration from the therapist's hands. It provides good slip and gives great contact for deep kneading and stretching. Talc is simple to use but the necessity for frequent application may break the continuity of the massage. There are now talc subsitutes available which have the same benefits.

Some things to remember:

- Warm your hands before you start. The easiest way to do this is to rub them together to create friction.
- Maintain contact with the client's skin at all times during the massage sequence. Keep contact with one hand as you cover or uncover the client with the other.
- Check your technique with the client during at intervals during the massage. The most common adjustment is to pressure, which may need to be increased or decreased accordingly.
- When asking the client about their needs use open questions and give them a choice, e.g. 'How is the pressure, would you like it firmer or softer?' 'Are you warm enough, would you like another towel?'
- Check the pace of your treatment – are you relaxing or stimulating, slow or brisk?
- Monitor your rhythm – keep it smooth and flowing and not repetitive.
- Think about the amount of pressure you use – firm or superficial.
- Give your client your undivided attention at all times. Think about the effect you wish to achieve and focus on the muscles you are working on.
- Once you have begun your massage remember to encourage the client to rest. Keep conversation to the minimum.

Posture and stance

It is essential that you adopt good posture from early on to avoid muscle fatigue strain and eventually injury. There are two main working positions.

- *Walk standing*. Used when working longitudinally. The therapist stands with the hip nearest the couch just touching the couch, the other leg in front. The therapist can then shift their weight from one foot to other as they move the weight of their body.
- *Stride standing* (squat). When the therapist stands facing the couch with back straight and legs hip-width apart, the feet turned slightly outwards for balance. The therapist adjusts their height by bending the knees rather than leaning.

You may find on occasions that it is more comfortable to adopt other postures. For example, when working on the foot squatting or resting on the knees is more comfortable. If you are very tall a lunge can be adopted. Whatever the position, remember to keep the back straight.

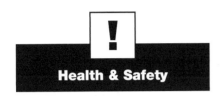

Health & Safety

Do not shake talc about. Avoid placing talc in a bowl that could be knocked over. There are respiratory hazards if the fine talc particles are inhaled so only use it in a controlled manner.

Tip

Watch your posture
You only have one back so it is important that you look after it.

- Avoid twisting unnecessarily – face the client and work transversely when you can.
- Keep your back straight (leaning over just gets you closer; it doesn't make your massage any better!)
- Keep your bottom tucked under and your tummy pulled in.
- Make the powerful thigh muscles take the strain.

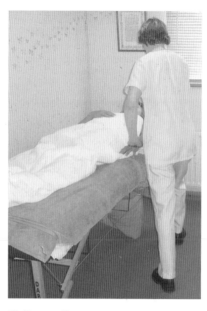
Walk standing

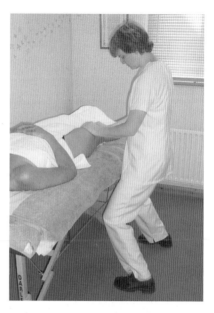
Squat/stride standing

A sample massage routine

Tip

Pace your routine. Perform each movement for either six repetitions or until the area has been sufficiently covered.

Sequence and timing

The commercial time for a full body massage is about 1 hour. The times given below are a guideline and will depend on the client's specific needs:

- left leg – 7 minutes
- right leg – 7 minutes
- right arm – 2.5 minutes
- left arm – 2.5 minutes
- abdomen – 2.5 minutes
- chest – 2.5 minutes
- back of legs – 7 minutes per leg, including gluteals
- back – 20 minutes.

Effleurage is used to link movements and where appropriate used between movements to assist drainage.

Supports should be placed as follows:

- if the client is *supine* – front of leg; under knees; under knees for abdomen
- if the client is *prone* – back of leg; under ankles; or feet should hang over bed.

The massage routine

Before you start, ask the client to take a few deep breaths with you. This will help to initiate relaxation and to bring in a good supply of oxygen for you both to focus and begin your treatment.

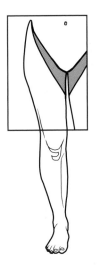

Femoral triangle

Femoral triangle

Interesting fact

The *femoral triangle* is the area around the top of the inner thigh and lower abdomen. It contains sensitive nerve endings, lymph nodes and is an erogenous zone.

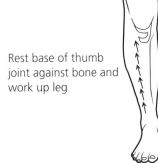

Rest base of thumb joint against bone and work up leg

Thumb knead tibialis anterior

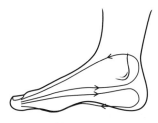

Medial effleurage

Legs

Start with the right leg.

Effleurage between movements and as necessary to drain the area you are working.

- Effleurage from the ankle to the top of the thigh, apply slight pressure and slide hands back to ankle.
- Effleurage from above patella over thigh.

Thigh/upper leg

- Single-handed palmar kneading.
- Alternate-handed kneading.
- Pick up and squeeze over upper thigh.
- Wringing across the thigh.
- Hacking.
- Cupping.
- Effleurage.
- Effleurage around patella with fingers.
- Finger knead around patella.
- Finger knead back of knee into the popliteal space.

Lower leg

- Effleurage lower leg from ankle to base of patella, divide hands and drain to back of knee into popliteal space.
- Thumb knead anterior tibialis from ankle to below the patella.

Turn foot out (laterally)

- Pick up and squeeze along the soleus and gastrocnemius.
- Hack lightly to soleus.
- Effleurage the leg from the ankle to the thigh.

One hand stays in contact while the other covers the leg, leaving the foot exposed.

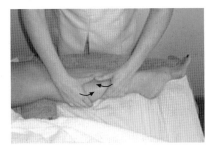

Picking up and squeezing to gastrocnemius and soleus

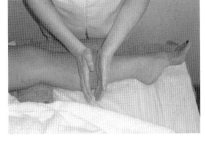

Hacking to soleus

Foot

- Effleurage from toes to top of foot, around ankle, sides of foot to toes.
- Effleurage medial foot up around ankle and back.
- Thumb effleurage dorsal foot.
- Slide thumbs into gap between each metatarsal, stroke up the foot.

Tip

Covering the feet
Feet are often a problem and are not always easily covered with the body towel, especially if the client is very tall. A useful tip is to extend the bottom towel covering the bed over the end of the bed. This can then be pulled up and over the feet to keep them warm. If you are using a couch cover, place a towel on just the bottom of the bed for the feet to rest on but extend it over the end of the bed so that it can be looped over to achieve the same effect.

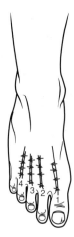

Thumb frictions between the metatarsals

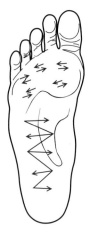

Thumb friction to the plantar surface

- Thumb frictions again in the gap between the metatarsals.
- Knead each phalange, concentrating on the nail plate and matrix area. Rotate the toe.
- Palmar knead plantar surface of the foot.
- Thumb frictions across plantar surface.
- Support the ankle with one hand and rotate ankle clockwise and anticlockwise.
- Flex and extend foot.
- Effleurage foot.

Repeat for the left leg.

Arm

Start with the left arm.

- Effleurage arm from the wrist to the shoulder (scooping).
- Thumb knead deltoid and top of the arm.
- Pick up and squeeze upper arm.

Place arm across chest.

- Pick up and squeeze triceps.
- Pincemont tapotement over upper arm (see Chapter 8, p.190).
- Light hacking to upper arm.
- Place arm back down and continue hacking.
- Slide to lower arm, pick up and squeeze extensor, brachioradialis of the lower arm using one hand.

Hand

- Effleurage around carpals using thumbs.
- Thumb effleurage back of top of hand.
- Thumb slide between metacarpals.
- Thumb frictions between metacarpals.

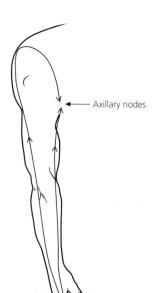

Axillary nodes

Effleurage to the arm

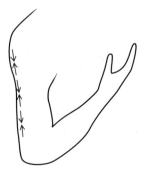

Pick up and squeeze to the triceps

- Knead each phalange, rotate clockwise and anticlockwise.
- Lift arm (elbow on couch).
- Knead metacarpals with thumbs.
- Thumb frictions to metacarpals.
- Palmar knead metacarpals.
- Rotate wrist.
- Flex and extend hand.
- Effleurage hand.
- Thumb frictions up tendons of inner wrist to halfway up arm.
- Effleurage arm to finish.

Repeat for right arm.

Chest

Stand at head of bed.

- Effleurage across chest from sternum (upper female, lower point male) around deltoids and upper trapezius.
- Thumb knead deltoids and upper trapezius.
- Knuckle across pectorals and trapezius.
- Deep stroking of upper trapezius using the fingers.
- Finger knead across occipital bone.
- Pick up and squeeze pectorals (male).
- Effleurage.

Abdomen

Stand on left side.

- Effleurage from pubis over abdomen, divide hands and take around to the back over the latissimus dorsi. Lift and return hands to pubis.
- Pick up and squeeze obliques.
- Wringing to obliques at sides of abdomen.
- Transverse wringing across abdomen.
- Finger knead ascending, transverse and descending colon, slide across lower abdomen without applying any pressure.
- Light hacking.
- Transverse vibrations using alternate hands across abdomen.
- Transverse effleurage across abdomen.

Back of legs

Expose all of the leg, including as much of the gluteals as possible. If the client has chosen to keep their underclothes on, tuck a tissue around them to protect them.

- Effleurage from the ankle, up the leg and over the gluteals.
- Single-handed palmar kneading to the thigh and gluteals.
- Alternate-handed kneading to thigh.
- Pick up and squeeze upper leg and gluteals.
- Wringing to thigh and lower gluteals.

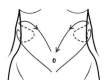

Effleurage to the abdomen

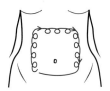

Kneading to the colon

Tip

When asking the client to turn over, hold up the towel in front of you and ask the client to turn away from you onto their back. This helps preserve their modesty.

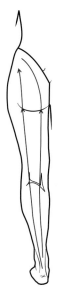

Effleurage to the back of the leg

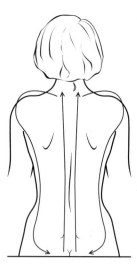

Effleurage to the back

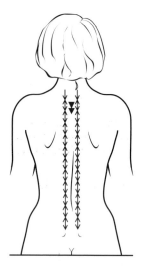

Frictions to erector spinae

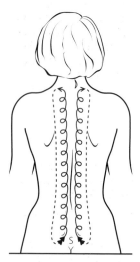

Thumb circles erector spinae

- Hacking and cupping to thigh and gluteals.
- Beating and pounding to gluteals and upper thigh (if there is excess adipose tissue).
- Effleurage thigh and gluteals.
- Effleurage from the ankle over gastrocnemius to popliteal space.
- Pick up and squeeze gastrocnemius.
- Light hacking to gastrocnemius.
- Using the fingers and thumb, knead along the Achilles tendon.
- Stroke down the plantar surface of the foot to the toes with the palm.
- Effleurage from the ankle up the thigh and over gluteals.

Back

Ensure you have exposed the back properly; you need to be able to work as low as the sacrum and so should just see the tip of the gluteal fold. (The lower part of the gluteals should have been covered while treating the legs so the top part will be treated during the back routine.) This maintains modesty and avoids embarrassment from overexposure.

- Effleurage from the sacrum up the centre of the back, over the trapezius, deltoid and down the side – latissimus dorsi, obliques, across the top of the gluteals.
- Transverse effleurage.
- Reinforced effleurage to upper back in a figure-of-eight movement. Keep fingertips pointing towards the head.
- Thumb knead around scapula.
- Thumb frictions around scapula.
- Knuckling to upper back (avoiding bony areas).
- Skin rolling to trapezius (see Chapter 8, p.189).
- Finger knead back of neck, trapezius (with neck straight).
- Pick up and squeeze back of neck, trapezius.
- Pick up and squeeze around perimeter of back (deltoids, latissimus dorsi, obliques).
- Effleurage (see opening movement).
- Thumb frictions down erector spinae.
- Circles with fingers up either side of erector spinae.
- Transverse effleurage.

Gluteals

- Deep wringing of gluteals, working with thumbs.
- Pick up and squeeze gluteals.
- Hacking, cupping, beating and pounding.
- Finger and thumb knead sacrum and across pelvis.
- Wringing around perimeter of the back.
- Wringing across back – change sides and repeat for other buttock.
- Effleurage to finish working from the centre of the back then reversing.
- Effleurage to go up the side of the back and down the spine.
- Waterfall: draw the hands lightly down the centre of the back, slowly reducing pressure until the hands lift off.

To complete the massage cover the client and place hands over the solar plexus, resting for a few minutes.

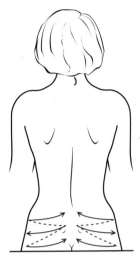

Wringing to the gluteals

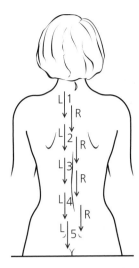

Waterfall

Muscle stretching and energizing techniques

Muscle stretching techniques (MST)

The stretching of a muscle draws it away from its attachments causing the fibres to lengthen. With this technique a muscle is stretched to just beyond its everyday capability to the point where resistance can be felt. This helps to pull out some of the tension within the muscle fibres.

Technique for MST. Stretch the muscle until resistance is felt, hold the stretch for 15 seconds then release, wait a few seconds and either repeat the stretch or apply effleurage.

Muscle energizing techniques (MET)

The therapist uses the contraction of the muscle to increase the stretch.

Technique for MET. The client contracts and relaxes the muscle to be energized. Stretch the muscles as above until increased resistance can be felt, then hold. Supporting the body (limb) firmly, ask the client to contract the muscle (isometric contraction), but do not allow any movement to take place. Hold the contraction for 10 seconds then relax. The muscle will undergo a short period of deep relaxation when the muscle can then be stretched further beyond its current range. Repeat until there is no further progress.

Uses for MST and MET

- During massage the muscle bundles are moved both longitudinally and transversely. This helps to break down muscle adhesions and generally improves intracellular circulation. MST enhances this.
- If deep massage is too uncomfortable or difficult to perform MST will achieve effective results.
- Often muscles in an area are unbalanced, some being weaker or stronger (postural problems fall into this category). Muscle may also become tight and weak in response to stress or an injury.

Interesting fact

Types of muscle work:

- *Isometric contract* is when the muscle is fixed but contracted without any movement taking place, i.e. static contraction such as pulling in tight the abdominal muscles. It should be applied for no more than 10 seconds at a time.

- *Isotonic (toning) exercises* are those in which the body works against its own weight or against external weight.

- *Isokinetic exercise* combines both isometric and isotonic principles.

MST and MET will help to compensate for some of the effects on the muscle tissue. Note: the tighter antagonistic muscle must be stretched first.

● Many muscles work antagonistically, i.e. to create movement one group of muscles contracts while another relaxes. By stretching and creating tension in a muscle the central nervous system relaxes the opposing muscle ready for movement to take place. This can occur naturally when a muscle becomes tense and tight. It causes a weakening in the opposing muscle.

Examples of stretch and release

Some of these stretches can be increased by combining them with isometric contractions. These are indicated with the symbol ISC.

Head and neck

Example 1
Supine position: Rest client's head in the crooks of your arms (your arms can either be crossed or straight with elbows bent) and gently raise head, tilting the chin towards the chest. Hold and release.

Muscles stretched: trapezius, levator scapula, erector spinae.

Example 2
Supine position: Place fingers along the base of occipital bone. Client has arms by their side. Gently pull the cranium towards you; do not raise it up off the couch. Hold and release.

Muscles stretched: trapezius, occipital, erector spinae.

Example 3
Supine position: Turn the client's face to one side, gently push the side of the head with one hand, push the shoulder down on the same side with the other.

Repeat on other side.

Muscles stretched: platysma, trapezius (on side being stretched), sterno mastoid deltoid.

Upper back

Example 1
Client lies on side: Bring top leg into a bent position to support the body. Place upper arm behind the client's back to raise scapula. Grip scapula firmly and lift up. Hold and release. (In this position you can also perform deep massage around the scapula.)

Repeat for other side.

Muscles stretched: rhomboids, trapezius, serratus anterior.

Example 2
Client supine: Raise one of the client's arms above their head and loosely hold it by the elbow so that the arm is at an angle. With your free hand grip the side of the scapula on the same side. Pull on the scapula and arm, hold and release.

Repeat for other side.

Muscles stretched: serratus anterior, teres major and minor, subscapulars, supraspinatus, infraspinatus, rhomboids, caraoc-brachialis, pectorals, deltoid.

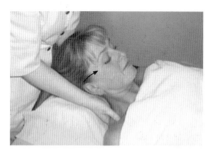

Neck stretch

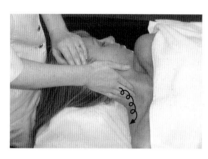

Sterno mastoid stretch

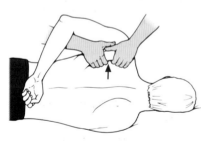

Lifting the scapula

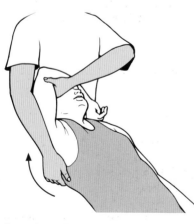

Scapula pull

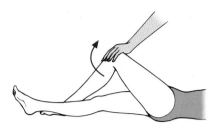

Gluteal stretch

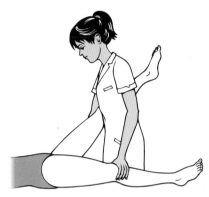

Leg adductor stretch

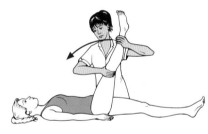

Gluteal and hamstring stretch

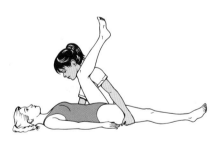

Lower back, gluteal, hamstring stretch

Lower body

Example 1

Supine position: Raise one leg into a bent position, leave the other leg straight. Standing at the side of the straight leg, lift the bent leg and pull it across the body towards you. Hold and release. A good stretch will lift the buttock off the couch. To increase the stretch further place your free arm on the client's shoulder above the bent leg to hold the body flat. (ISC)

Repeat for other side.

Muscles stretched: gluteals, obliques, latissimus dorsi.

Legs

Example 1

Supine position: Draw one leg out laterally, i.e. to abduct it away from the body. Your best position in which to do this is to stand at the side of the couch between the client's legs. (ISC)

Repeat for other side.

Muscles stretched: leg adductors.

Example 2

Supine position: Raise one leg straight and push up towards the client's head. Support the knee but do not apply pressure on the kneecap. Only extend to a comfortable stretch.

Be cautious with this movement. If there is sciatica it will be uncomfortable as the nerve will be stretched along with the leg. (ISC)

Repeat for other side.

Muscles stretched; gluteals, hamstrings.

Example 3

Supine position: Bend one leg leaving the other straight. Hook leg into the front of your shoulder and push up towards the head. Hold the straight leg flat. (ISC)

Repeat for the other leg.

Muscles stretched: gluteals and hamstrings, lower back.

Example 4

Supine position: Support the foot with one hand and hold leg down with free hand. Push the foot towards the body. (ISC)

Muscles stretched: gastrocnemius, soleus, foot extensors (hamstrings).

Example 5

Prone position: Raise the foot and lower leg up towards the hamstrings. Keep the other leg flat. Use your weight behind the lower leg to push it towards the body. (ISC)

Repeat for other leg.

Muscles stretched: quadriceps, tibialis anterior, foot flexors.

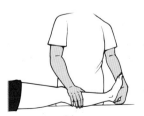

Lower leg stretch

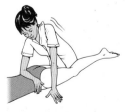

Quadricep, tibialis anterior and foot flexor stretch

After care for massage

Review Chapter 5, p.141 to ensure you are familiar with general after care.

Always follow up your treatment with some advice and guidance for your client.

Give the client an after care leaflet and go through the contents with them while they rest after treatment. Don't forget to recommend to the client when to have their next treatment.

Home care advice

It is always useful to suggest some general home care advice that the client can follow after massage: Some suggestions are:

- use an exfoliating product to remove dead skin cells and keep the skin smooth
- body brush: use a loofah, body brush or exfoliating mitt, this will not only remove the dead skin but help to stimulate the superficial micro-circulation
- use a pumice, hard skin remover or foot file to keep the feet clean and remove hard skin
- apply a body lotion, cream or oil daily to condition and nourish the skin
- in the summer remind the client about the dangers of the sun and to use sun protection products and after sun lotion
- where appropriate offer the client some postural exercises to do at home
- suggest some relaxation and/or deep breathing exercises.

Tip

Body lotion is most effective if applied to damp skin as it traps a layer of moisture on the surface. As moisture is lost from the surface this layer is the first to go, rather than a natural layer.

Adaptations to massage

Once a basic routine has been mastered, you will need to modify your knowledge and develop your skills. Each treatment ideally should be different as no two people are alike and their needs will be different.

During consultation and before commencing treatment you will have ascertained from the client their preferences, i.e. which area would they like you to concentrate on (if any), any problem areas, and areas that they may prefer to be omitted, e.g. the abdomen.

If a client is nervous or apprehensive during their first treatment take the time and care to explain procedures. This will help to reassure them and put them at ease. Never assume that a client is aware of what a massage involves. All instructions must be simple, clear and precise.

Massage and body fat

- Take precautions when massaging thin, bony clients. Avoid tapotement over these areas as it can be uncomfortable and may cause bruising.
- More padded clients will benefit from deeper movements as the circulation will be poorer through the adipose and cellulite areas.
- Obese clients sometimes experience sensitivity as cellulite seriously affects the functioning of the circulatory and sensory nervous

Tip

Communication
Be clear and concise with your instructions. There is an amusing yet genuine story of the therapist who told her client to take off their clothes and get on the couch. She gave the client time to carry out her instructions and on her return the client had done as she had instructed: the client was standing on the couch naked!!

systems. It is harder to access muscle tissue and so deep movements are required with particular emphasis on deep kneading and percussion movements.

Massage for the elderly

Remember that for elderly clients the rejuvenation process has slowed down. Use gentle pressure and always direct pressure towards the heart.

- Avoid heavy percussion movements.
- Concentrate on drainage and relaxation.
- Pay particular attention to the extremities (hands, lower legs and feet) where the circulation may be poor.
- Avoid pressure over bony areas as there is an increased risk of osteoporosis and fragile bones.
- Avoid elderly clients lying on their stomach for longer than 15 minutes as it becomes increasing difficult for them to get up from the prone position.

Massage during pregnancy

For many women, by the fourth month it becomes difficult to lie on the abdomen for any period of time. In the later stages it is generally not a good idea to lay the client flat on her back as this may make her feel light headed and the weight of the foetus can restrict circulation and cause tingling in the legs.

Despite this, massage is useful for a number of reasons.

- It is useful to massage the legs to counteract the effects of oedema, varicose veins and tired legs. These can be treated with the client in a semi-supine position or sitting in a comfortable chair. The arms can be massaged in the same position also.
- To massage the back the client can be seated, leaning forward with cushions for support. You can sit or stand behind the client to work the area.
- For a variety of ethical reasons is not a good idea to massage the abdomen other than to apply oil with light effleurage strokes. The client can massage her own abdomen should she choose.

Disabled clients

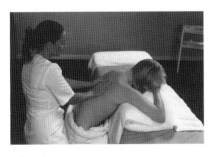

Adapting massage

With the introduction of the Disability Discrimination Act 1995 (final phase, 2004), access must be considered an issue. Some clients may not be able to get onto a couch or be able to lie down. Hydraulic or electric couches that can be lowered and raised are a good investment. Alternatively you may use some of the positions suggested above for pregnant clients.

Other disabilities are those that affect hearing and eyesight. The client who is visually impaired will need to be guided and to receive constant reassurance that you are there. With those who have hearing difficulties you will need to make sure you face them when you are speaking to them. If they are unable to lip-read you may even need to write down what you need to communicate.

Massage for males

Men generally have more defined muscle bulk. The skin has a different texture, being thicker and tougher with less adipose tissue. Male massage if often performed with greater pressure to give a firmer massage.

The following adaptations should be made:

- avoid the femoral triangle, i.e. top of inner thigh
- do not massage below the navel
- extend the chest massage right over the chest (an alternative is to extend the massage over the chest down to the upper abdomen rather than treat the abdomen separately).

If the client is very hairy, talc may be preferable to cream or oil to avoid friction with the hair.

General adaptations

- *General relaxation.*
  Speed will be slow and more rhythmical. Effleurage will be the prominent movement. Avoid percussion movements to keep the massage restful. Warm blankets and towels will help to increase the effect, as will appropriate music.

- *To help combat stress.*
  Stress is a common problem caused by modern lifestyles. It has many different physiological and psychological effects on the body. It is also responsible for tension in our muscles, which if left untreated can lead to postural problems affecting our general health. Treatment as for relaxation with specific kneading in areas where tension may be built up. Stretching of muscles will also be beneficial.

- *Muscular aches and pains.*
  It is important to assess that there is no underlying medical problem or injury as this will contra indicate treatment. Muscular tension can cause aches and pains and time will need to be devoted to particular problem areas. Deep kneading, neuromuscular techniques, and stretch and release followed by effleurage will help to drain away waste build up from the tissues once it has been released.

- *Massage for weight loss.*
  Massage alone can not reduce weight loss but it can help to mobilize fat deposits. It must be used in conjunction with other treatments such as G5, exercise and, most importantly, a calorie-reduced diet! Your massage needs to concentrate on deep petrissage and percussion movements.

- *Poor muscle tone.*
  Again this will need to be combined with other treatments, particularly exercise. Reasons for poor muscle tone might be a sudden weight loss, i.e. after dieting or pregnancy, natural ageing and lack of exercise. If the skin is very flaccid care should be taken not to stretch it unnecessarily. Stimulating movements such as petrissage and percussion movements are good for improving muscle tone if performed regularly.

- *To improve skin condition.*
  If there is poor circulation, friction will help to increase the superficial micro-circulation. This type of massage is very beneficial for improving the appearance of newly formed scar tissue.

Interesting fact

G5 is mechanical massage using a machine.

Pre-event massage

This massage aims to maximize both physical and mental performance. The massage is brisk and stimulating and usually includes deep kneading (skin rolling, wringing, squeezing, etc.), friction, percussion (hacking and cupping), joint mobilization and stretching. The massage is quite short, lasting between 10 and 20 minutes, and concentrates on particular muscle groups that will be used in the sports activity.

Benefits are:

- gently increases the circulation so that the body is prepared for physical activity
- improves joint mobility
- separates the muscle and connective tissue to maximize muscle performance
- movement is more fluid
- reduces the risk of sports injuries as the muscles are warm before the performance begins
- relaxes the body and mind, calms the nerves
- increases mental alertness
- ensures greater physical energy.

Inter-event massage

As its name implies this is massage applied during events. An athlete may be competing during the course of hours or days and this keeps the muscles in tip-top condition.

This massage is lighter, aiming more to improve circulation, drain and remove metabolic toxins, and incorporates stretching. Deep movements are avoided. It also aims to keep the athlete relaxed and focused.

Post-event

This massage is given within four hours of completion of an event.

Benefits are:

- prevents muscle fatigue.
- encourages venous blood flow back to the heart.
- facilitates the removal of metabolic toxins.
- increases the circulation, bringing nutrient to the muscle cells.
- assists the lymphatic system.
- speeds up recovery.
- where tissue has been damaged (micro trauma), massage encourages the formation of strong, mobile, scar tissue.

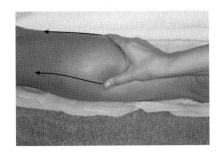

Finger and thumb palpation

Guidelines for post-event massage

Duration is approximately 10–15 minutes if close to the event or up to 1.5 hours if an hour or more after the event.

Begin with light effleurage over the muscles using palpation to feel for changes in the muscular tissue (tension, tightness, stiffness, pain). Gradually increase the deepness of the effleurage. Begin using techniques to facilitate balance in the muscular tissue and aid relaxation. Use a mixture of kneading and compression movements such as skin rolling, firm sliding strokes using the fingers and thumb, muscle shaking, joint mobilizing and stretching.

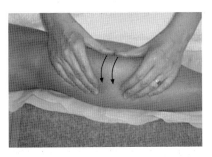

Muscle rolling

Once the muscle tissue has been relaxed continue with percussion movements. Complete the massage with deep effleurage and stroking.

Remedial massage

Remedial massage is more vigorous than Swedish massage and in some ways is similar to that given pre- and post-event. It works deeper on the muscle tendons and fascia using neuromuscular techniques. It is a more diagnostic massage tracing any ailments back to their original cause, working with scar tissue and muscular imbalance. Its aim is to reduce pain and improve mobility. The massage is often given as a course combined with an exercise programme to follow at home.

Pre-heating treatments (heat therapy)

Why pre-heat the tissues?

- The effects of massage are greatly enhanced if the muscles are warm. A visible hyperaemia indicates an active circulation and erythema indicates an increase in localized circulation.
- General relaxation.
- To alleviate muscular tension.

Pre-heat can be applied all over – i.e. general body heating using:

- warm shower
- warm bath including spa baths and hydro baths
- sauna
- steam bath or steam room
- thermal body mask, e.g. paraffin wax

or locally using

- infra red
- thermal body mask, e.g. paraffin wax applied to a specific area.

The physical effects of heat therapy

General effects include the following.

- There is an increase in the circulation causing the heart to work harder and pulse rate to rise (in some cases by up to 70 per cent).
- Vasodilation of the blood vessels caused by the heat.
- Body temperature rises.
- Blood pressure will fall because of the vasodilation.
- Lymphatic circulation is assisted by the general increase in circulation.
- Hyperaemia and erythema – heat will eventual be passed into the deeper tissues inducing relaxation.
- General increase in the metabolic rate.
- An increase in the sebaceous output in the skin.
- Sweating is increased causing a loss of body fluids (water and salts).
- General relaxation of the muscle tissues which will help to alleviate minor aches and pains.

Local effects include the following.

- Local heating will not have the same effects but there will be an increase in the local circulation and it will encourage relaxation in the muscle fibres.

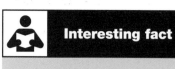
Interesting fact

Hyperaemia is a reddening of the skin caused by excess blood.

Treatments available

The simplest and easiest way to warm the tissues is to have a *hot shower*. Clients should ideally be offered the use of a shower before a massage. The following benefits should be spelled out to the clients:

- a clean skin will benefit from the oils and creams that are being applied
- a warm shower will help to relax the muscles and make the treatment more effective
- a power shower will further enhance the effects by stimulating the circulation.

Many clients get concerned if they are suddenly encouraged to have a shower; others will expect the facility. There are occasionally clients who have a problem with their personal hygiene. Always encourage every client to shower before a body treatment to prevent any embarrassing issues arising.

Baths are also a useful way of warming the tissues. Treatments include a normal bath, spa bath, foam bath and hydro baths.

Spa baths are large communal baths of hot water. Jets of bubbling water are produced from the base and sides of the bath, which have a massaging effect on the body. They contain chemicals to keep the water clean and these need to be monitored at regular intervals.

Hydro baths are usually enclosed bathing cabinets that the client reclines into. Water is squirted at the body through jets in the sides of the cabinet.

Sauna

The sauna is constructed from pine as this wood can withstand extremes of temperature. Pine is also used because it allows the transference of air so that the air flow does not become stagnated within the sauna. Dry heat is produced from electrically heated stones or coals. Once the wood has absorbed as much heat as it can the heat flows back into the sauna. Temperatures can reach up to 70°C.

Procedure

- Carry out a full consultation and check for contra indications, or review previous consultation records.
- The client should have a lukewarm shower before entering the sauna.
- The client should sit either on a towel or a piece of tissue for hygiene reasons. Suggest that the client starts by sitting at the lowest level and progresses up as their body becomes accustomed to the heat. The higher you go up in a sauna, the hotter it is.
- The client should stay in the sauna for a maximum of 10 minutes, leave and have a cool then warm shower.
- If returning to the sauna the client can move up a seating level to increase the intensity of the heat. Again they should stay no longer than 10 minutes.
- This process of sauna, shower, sauna be can repeated as required.
- On completion of a sauna treatment the client should rest for at least 15 minutes and drink plenty of water to replace that lost from perspiration. This helps prevent exhaustion and headaches.

Contra indications to sauna treatment

Alongside the general contra indications (see Chapter 5, p.137), the following issues need to be considered.

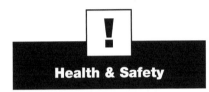

Interesting fact

After 12–18 minutes of heat treatment the blood vessels in the subcutaneous levels will be dilated to their maximum. The effect will recede after a time as the blood slowly spreads back into the core of the body. The process is known as vasodilation.

Health & Safety

Metal jewellery should be removed during heat treatment as when it is exposed it will heat up and cause burning to the skin through conduction.

Health & Safety

Always tell the client to leave the sauna if they feel unwell and call for assistance.

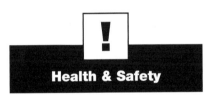

Interesting fact

Dry heat
Dry heat makes the sweat acidic, and it is thought that the body can thus shed certain toxins as it sweats profusely. The dry heat makes the sweat evaporate quickly leaving the skin dry. As the skin's pores are open any accumulated dirt is drawn out onto the surface.

- Do not allow a client to have a sauna or steam bath if they suffer with hyper- or hypotension.
- If they have eaten a meal, they should wait at least an hour and a half.
- If they have not eaten at all.
- If they have consumed alcohol – the heat will speed up the absorption and effects and the client may be sick.
- Kidney disease.
- Asthmatics and those with bronchitis.
- Any dry skin condition such as eczema, dermatitis, psoriasis as the heat will further dry the skin.
- During the first few days of menstruation as the client may feel faint.

Never leave the client. Stay within earshot just in case they become unwell or need assistance.

Steam baths and steam rooms

Steam treatments are produced by moist or wet heat and can be applied in two ways:

- steam cabinet
- steam room (Turkish bath).

The *steam cabinet* is a fibreglass cabinet with a door for access and a hole in the top (for the client's head). It has a heater in the bottom over which is placed a seat for the client to sit on. Distilled water is placed in the heater and the cabinet allowed time to heat up (about 20 minutes). The cabinet should be heated to around 35–40°C. The steam forms a barrier on the skin preventing sweat from evaporating. The metabolism is only mildly increased and so the cabinet can be used for some of the conditions contra indicated by the intensity of the heat of the sauna.

Procedure for a steam cabinet

- Carry out a full consultation and check for contra indications or review previous consultation notes.
- The client then showers.
- The door is opened and the client sits on a towel or tissue on the seat in the cabinet.
- The door is closed quickly to retain the heat.
- A towel is place around the client's neck to prevent any heat escaping from the top.
- The client remains in the cabinet for up to half an hour. There is a timer on the side of the cabinet to monitor the time.
- The client should have a shower to remove built-up sweat once their treatment is completed.

Contra indications for a steam cabinet

To ensure you are familiar with this topic, see the section above on sauna (p.215).

Asthma is *not* contra indicated as the client is not fully enclosed in the cabinet. Dry skin conditions such as psoriasis will also benefit from the treatment, as the heat is wet heat and therefore not dehydrating.

Steam rooms

Steam rooms are enclosed rooms where water is heated in a boiler and the vapour is circulated throughout the room. These also produce wet heat.

Tip

Only ever use distilled water otherwise the heater will be adversely affected by a build up of lime scale.

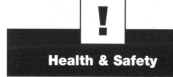

Health & Safety

The steam cabinet should be thoroughly cleansed after every client using either a disinfectant or a specially manufactured cleaning product.

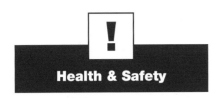

Contra actions to general heat therapy treatments

Feelings of faintness, feeling dizziness or nausea after a heat treatment can be all caused by

- excess treatment leading to heat exhaustion
- dehydration from a loss of body fluids
- a drop in blood pressure
- burns from exposure to metal jewellery (or interference with heating elements).

To ensure you are familiar with contra actions, see Appendix 1 on nosebleeds, fainting and cramp.

Other heat therapy treatments

Paraffin or thermal masks

This mask can be applied to a specific area or as a full body treatment.

- In addition to the benefits of pre-heating or warming the tissues these masks also soften the skin and aid desquamation.
- Paraffin masks are particularly beneficial for people with rheumatic or arthritic joints.

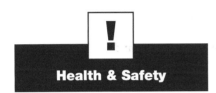

Paraffin wax

Paraffin wax is a mineral product that is solid when cold, but liquefies when heated. The ideal working temperature is 37°C. It is applied to the skin and allowed to cool. The initial heat of the wax causes an increase in vasodilation and sweating.

For the best results the body needs to be kept warm using a blanket (thermal if available) or wrapped in thermal foil sheeting. When the wax is removed it lifts off dead skin cells and surface debris. It leaves a layer of mineral oil on the surface of the skin leaving it feeling silky and smooth.

Some therapists do not like to use paraffin wax prior to massage as the mineral oil leaves a barrier on the skin through which other oils cannot penetrate; you will need to give this consideration.

To apply paraffin wax, follow the procedure outlined below.

- Pre-heat the wax to the required working temperature.
- Carry out a full consultation and check for contra indications.
- The client needs to undress fully if it is a full body treatment and to wear disposable panties.
- Put some wax into a bowl (disposable plastic or polystyrene cups are ideal for smaller areas).
- Always test the wax on the back of your wrist for working temperature then test a little on the client before application.
- Brush the wax onto the skin in several layers.
- Cover the client with foil and towels or a blanket.
- Leave on the skin for between 20 and 30 minutes.
- Remove the wax. It should lift or pull off in layers like a second skin.

(For hygiene reasons the wax should be disposed of and never reused.)

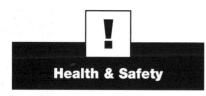

Contra indications for infra red
First review general contra indications in Chapter 5, p.137.

Other contra indications include:

- metal pins or plates – these will attract and hold the heat
- loss of skin sensation – anaesthesia
- sunburn.

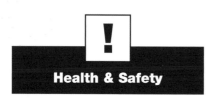

Health & Safety

Infra red
Never stare into the infra red rays and always protect the eyes. Overexposure can cause damage to the cataract tissue of the eye.

Tip

Infra red can be combined with the actual massage if time is short.

Infra red treatment

This treatment uses a special lamp which emits infra red radiation. Infra red light has longer wavelengths than normal daylight and rays penetrate into the epidermis where it is experienced as warmth.

Infra red treatment should be administered in the following way.

- Carry out a full consultation and check for contra indications.
- Test the skin for sensitivity.
- Cleanse the skin to remove any grease or ask the client to shower.
- Expose the area you wish to apply the infra red to.
- Protect the client's eyes either with goggles or by turning their face away from the lamp.
- Position the lamp at a right angle to the area on which you are working. The bulb should be between 40 and 55 cm away from the highest point exposed to treatment.
- Leave the rays on the skin for between 10 and 20 minutes, monitoring the heat on the skin constantly.
- On completion turn the lamp off and move to it a safe distance away from the client.
- Continue with massage if desired.

Positioning the lamp

The lamp should never be positioned over the client. It should always be placed so that if the bulb were to become loose and fall, it could never land on the client and burn them. It also needs to be positioned so that if the client suddenly attempts to get up they do not make contact with the lamp.

- Position the client so that the rays fall in a straight line on the body. You may need to prop the client up on pillows to make sure the angle is correct
- When the treatment is over move the lamp a safe distance away from the working area and warn the client that the lamp will be hot.

Knowledge review

1 List the contra indications to massage (see Chapter 5, p.137).

2 Name the three massage mediums and briefly explain when you might use each.

3 What are the benefits of pre-heating the skin before massage?

4 List four methods you could use for pre-heating.

5 Why do you use supports when massaging and where would you position them?

6 What is the sequence of the body massage routine?

7 What factors would you consider during your massage?

8 List the after care advice you would give to a client post-massage.

Aromatherapy

Learning objectives

This chapter covers the following:

- **a brief history of aromatherapy**
- **what aromatherapy is**
- **what an essential oil is**
- **the physiology of aromatherapy**
- **safety issues**
- **treating a client with pre-blended aromatherapy oils**
- **the aromatherapy treatment**

Aromatherapy is a complex art steeped in a long history of use; it should not be confused with Swedish massage. This chapter looks at the difference between the two treatments while exploring different techniques to develop a comprehensive service. It introduces the use of both pre-blended oils and blending and different ways of using aromatherapy.

A brief history of aromatherapy

Many religious practices for thousands of years have used plant materials to burn as incense to enhance spiritual experience and deepen meditation. There are recorded uses of balsams, oils, barks, resins and similar properties since the early Egyptians in 4500 BC. The Egyptians were particularly famed for their use of such products to preserve the body in life as well as in death. The use of aromatherapy in traditional Indian medicine can be traced as far back as 3000 BC. The use of plant extracts and essential oils for similar practices are also recorded.

The Greeks catalogued their knowledge of plants and oils in 400 BC and it was their knowledge that was passed on to the Romans (famous for their spa treatments) detailing the healing properties of herbs.

Avicenna, an Arabian living around AD 900, wrote several books on the healing properties of plants. Knowledge began spreading throughout Europe and herbs were widely used for their antiseptic and preserving properties. During the bubonic plague in the fourteenth century there were accounts of the use of pomanders and herbs to ward off infection.

By the eighteenth century essential oils were being used indiscriminately in medicines but by the nineteenth century the use of natural medicine had began to decline in the Western world as synthetic oils began to be produced.

Rene-Maurice Gattefoose, a French chemist, documents his accidental findings of the healing properties of lavender after badly burning his hand. He introduced the term 'Aromatherapy' and wrote the first book on the subject in 1937. In France aromatherapy is still viewed as a science.

Marguerite Maury developed the use of aromatherapy during the 1950s as the therapeutic treatment which is now used extensively today.

What is aromatherapy?

Aromatherapy is the use of smell in a therapeutic manner. It includes body treatments as well as the use of essential oils in a burner, for inhalation, in products and compresses.

During a treatment specific techniques are used; these might include adapted massage, acupressure and lymphatic massage to both the face and body. Treatment aims are to try to restore harmony and natural balance with an holistic approach considering physical, mental and emotional well-being. The client may be treated with pre-blended essentials oils or essential oils blended specifically for the individual client's needs.

What is an essential oil?

Essential oils are made up of tiny organic molecules; some may contain as many as 200 chemical constituents. It is these constituents that give the oil its therapeutic unique qualities and aroma. These can vary from year to year and from different regions as both soil and weather conditions have an effect on the therapeutic quality of the oil.

Essential oils are complex structures of different, naturally occurring constituents. Each contains several different chemical compounds, e.g. terpenes, alcohols, phenols, etc. (see Chapter 11, pp.241–3).

Methods used to extract essential oils

The extraction and refining of quality oils is a highly skilled practice and plays an important role in the therapeutic value of the oil produced. An essential oil is derived from a variety of sources including:

- leaves
- flowers
- seeds
- stalks
- bark
- roots/rhizomes.

Steam distillation

This is the most popular method used because it is very economical. The required plant material, which could be fresh or dried, is placed on a grid inside a distillation vat. Steam is then passed through the vat under pressure. The heat in the steam causes the cell walls in the plant material to break down, releasing the essential oils as a vapour. This vapour is passed through cooling tanks and as the vapour cools it condenses and the essential oils float to the surface, as they are lighter than water. The oils are then separated from the water.

Expression

Expression is used for extracting citrus oils. The peel is separated from the fruit and squeezed under pressure to press out or '*express*' the essential oils. Modern machinery has been designed to separate the juice that is also acquired from the essential oils. This method is also termed '*sacrification*'.

Expressed oils do not tend to last as long as those produced by distillation, usually only between six and nine months.

Solvent extraction

Solvent extraction was first used commercially during the 1890s. The product produced from this method is known as an 'absolute', a 'concrete' and/or a 'resinoid'.

The essential oil of fine flowers such as rose is obtained by solvent extraction.

The flower petals are placed in a sealed container on perforated racks. A liquid solvent (usually petroleum ether, hexane, liquid butane or liquid carbon dioxide) flows over the petals which must be kept continually immersed in the solvent. The solvent will dissolve the essential oils from the petals. The solvent is then distilled off and reused. A '*concrete*' is left which is a semi-solid liquid. This is shaken with alcohol, which is also distilled off. The coloured liquid that remains is called an *absolute*. It is not known as an essential oil because of the solvents used during the process.

When a resin is used (the solid or semi-solid substance obtained from bark when cut), a *resinoid* is created.

Other extraction methods

Before modern methods of extraction, oils were obtained by:

- *maceration:* whereby the plant material is placed in a vegetable base oil

- *enfleurage:* with this method flower petals are placed on purified animal fats.

For both methods the material is placed in trays with the oil or fat for several days. The material is changed regularly until the fat is saturated with plant extracts. These methods are still used for about 10 per cent of today's extractions.

The physiology of aromatherapy

The effect of the oils can be balancing, relaxing or stimulating to name just a few. Virtually all essential oils have some degree of antibacterial properties. The effect of essential oils is so diverse because they have three distinct actions:

- they initiate chemical changes in the body when the essential oil enters the bloodstream and reacts with hormones and enzymes
- they have a physiological effect on the systems of the body
- they have a psychological effect when the odour is inhaled.

How do essential oils work?

Remember that it is not the complete essential oil but the sum of its parts – the essential oil has many constituents and it is these that enter through the skin and nose, not the whole essential oil as applied. These chemicals achieve their effect in following ways:

- The *skin* is the largest organ and the most common route for application and absorption of essential oils. When applied diluted in carrier oil, or even in water, the now tiny molecules or constituents of the essential oils can penetrate the skin by entering the sweat glands, hair follicles and even through the intracellular network of the skin. Once through the epidermis into the upper dermis they have access to its expansive capillary circulation. The molecules are lipid-soluble and attach to similar carrier molecules enabling them to diffuse directly into the circulatory stream in minute quantities.
- Through the *respiratory system* via the nose. The delicate sensory cells located in the lining of the nasal cavity pick up a smell. The essence of the smell is carried to the limbic area of the brain via the bloodstream. The aroma given off has a direct effect on our emotions. Molecules are also carried deep into the lungs where they diffuse across the single-celled walls of the alveoli into the bloodstream.
- Via *psychological effects.* The sense of smell is a chemical sense stimulated by molecules of odour. The cerebral cortex in the brain integrates and interprets the smell. Particular smells associated with events in the past can evoke reactions by activating memories. As a result of stimulating the limbic system a response can be triggered resulting in a range of behaviour, e.g. the smell of a particular aftershave will remind you of a certain person.
- Through the *digestive system*. It should be noted that only those qualified should advise use of essential oils to be administered orally in case of the possibility of poisoning. In the UK this is not part of the training undertaken and is therefore should not be recommended.

Safety issues

Purchase and storage

Essential oils are volatile and should be treated with caution and care. Sadly there are many adulterated oils, but eventually you will develop a nose and eye to detect these.

Adulterated oils

An adulterated oil is one which has been altered in some way since it has been extracted. This may be a simple process or it may be one that is complex when only sophisticated equipment is able to detect the change. Adulteration may also be referred to as cutting, stretching, standardization, ennobling sophistication or rectification.

During adulteration

- alcohol may be added
- the product may be an isolate (collection of chemicals), which could be obtained from other extractions
- a synthetic product may be added to bulk out a product.

Alternatively, it may be a cheaper version, sold under another name.

Purchase

When purchasing essential oils consider the following points.

- Is it in a sealed bottle?
- Is the bottle made of smoked glass or sold in a specially prepared container? (Never buy or store oils in plastic containers.)
- As for a perfume, try before you buy. Smell using a testing paper (never apply to the skin). Never smell more than six oils at a time. Three is best to avoid a confused nose!
- When testing an odour, do so in an odour-free area, clear the nose before smelling, waft below the nose and inhale, but not too deeply. Once you are sure of a smell clear your nose (breathe to clear the odour).
- Buy in smaller quantities unless you are sure you will use the oil regularly. Oils deteriorate once opened (although special seals reduce this). Most oils have a shelf life of 2 years, with the exception of citrus oils, which have a shelf life of between 6 to 12 months.
- A 10 ml bottle is equivalent to 200 drops of essential oil.
- Be familiar with botanical names so that you know the source of the product you are buying.

Storage

When considering storage always consider the following points.

- Store in dark coloured bottles.
- Bottles should have an inserted stopper or a separate glass pipette rod (not rubber).

Tip

Synthetic oils
Avoid synthetic oils as they have no therapeutic value. Oils should ideally be organic but due to demand and expense this is not always possible. Most manufacturers specify when the oil is organic.

- Ensure the lids are tight and secure.
- Store in a cool, dark place away from light, heat, moisture and air.
- Due to the implications of COSHH (see Chapter 1, p.XX), oils should be stored away when not in use, in a secure place.
- Label all bottles clearly, particularly if oils are mixed or blended.
- Keep out of the reach of children (and animals).

Suitability for treatment

Go to Chapter 5 to ensure you are familiar with interpersonal skills (p.125), consultation techniques (p.134) and contra indications (p.137).

Patch testing

Several oils are known to be skin irritants and as a result should be used with caution. When dealing with a client who has sensitive skin, it is essential that you perform a patch test for possible irritation or sensitization to potentially hazardous oils.

Not all sensitive reactions occur straight away; sometimes they take a period of time to build up within the system.

Procedure for patch testing

Apply a couple of drops of essential oil to a moistened cotton bud and apply to the skin on the inside of the forearm. Alternatively, place drops on a piece of gauze and if possible use surgical tape to keep in place. Leave on the skin for 24 hours unless irritation occurs. Repeat if you suspect sensitivity.

Toxicity

Toxicity is a broad term that is used in aromatherapy to describe the hazardous effects associated with the misuse of essential oils. There are two main categories.

- *Acute toxicity* refers to the effects of short-term administration of a substance and usually involves a single, high lethal doses:
  1. *acute oral toxicity* is 'poisoning'
  2. *acute dermal toxicity* is excessive use of essential oil absorbed into the skin causing systemic toxicity – this could lead to damage to the liver and kidneys.
- *Chronic toxicity* refers to repeated use of a substance over a period of weeks, months and even years. It is used to describe the adverse effects both to the skin and other systems of the body. Symptoms include headaches, nausea, minor skin eruptions and lethargy. Citrus oils are a high-risk group due to their terpene content (the exception is bergamot).

The degree of toxicity will depend on the amount of essential oil used and the route of administration. Oral administration poses the biggest risk and for this reason aromatherapy oils should never be taken orally unless prescribed by a medically qualified practitioner.

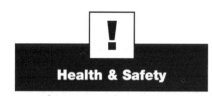

Health & Safety

Photosensitivity
Some oils increase the skin's photosensitivity, lowering the skin's resistance and increasing the risk of burning. All the oils listed below will produce a reaction when exposed to ultra violet light (natural and unnatural):

- bergamot
- lemon
- grapefruit
- lime
- orange
- verbena.

(Note that these are mainly citrus oils.)

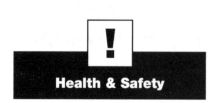

Health & Safety

How safe?
Aromatherapy is the use of essential oils in a controlled, sensible way. The majority of oils are quite safe provided they are treated with respect and used in low dilution. Some are highly toxic even in small quantities. It is the misuse of essential oils that causes problems. Oils when used in excess or over prolonged periods may lead to the body becoming immune to their effects.

Treating a client with pre-blended aromatherapy oils

NVQ qualifications and some other qualifications only treat the client working to a treatment objective or outcome. Ranges and performance criteria include the following: relaxation, stress relief and uplifting. After consultation with the client you may find that they have a single need or a combination.

Clinical aromatherapy

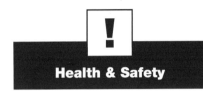

Health & Safety

Remember!

- Special care is required when treating babies or young children as they are much more likely to develop toxicity. For this reason essential oils should be more dilute and used sparingly.

- Elderly clients have thinning skin, which readily absorbs essential oils through its weakening structure. Again, essential oils should be used more diluted.

Tip

Support
Once the client is on the couch, carefully position your supports to make sure that they are as relaxed as possible. A flat couch is not particularly comfortable. If the muscles are relaxed the treatment will be more effective. Supports will be needed under the ankles while prone and under the knees while supine.

Taking aromatherapy further entails a more detailed look at the client's needs. The therapist will look at an holistic approach encompassing the general well-being of the client, i.e. health, emotional, physical and mental state. The therapist will then blend a choice of oils specifically to the needs of the client. Essential oils are chosen for their effect on balancing, specific problems or weaknesses.

You also need to consider the most appropriate carrier for your treatment as this can enhance the effects. Remember that the carrier oils and lotions have a therapeutic effect also.

Preparation for treatment

For an aromatherapy treatment you will need the following:

- a bath sheet, and two hand towels or cotton sheet or blanket
- couch roll
- massage props or supports
- a selection of carrier oils
- a selection of essential oils
- blending container with measure markers
- glass rod for blending
- glass pipette
- selection of pre-blended oils
- skin-sanitizing product to clean the skin where applicable.

The consultation process and preparing the client

To ensure you are familiar with consultation and preparation techniques, review Chapter 5, pp.133–4.

- Ask the client to remove their clothes. Be specific as to exactly which clothes you require the client to remove.
- If the changing area is the treatment room, leave the room while they do so. This is a good opportunity to excuse yourself from the client if there is no washbasin in the treatment area to go and wash your hands. Knock to signal or tell the client you are returning.
- Ask the client to remove their jewellery. Ideally ask the client to store it (ladies in their handbag) or place it in a bowl on the trolley within the client's eyesight.
- Once the client is on the couch. Position your supports and make sure the client is covered.
- Wipe the client's feet over with surgical spirit or cologne and check for contra indications.

Interesting fact

A *nut* is a fruit consisting of a hard tough shell around an edible kernel, or a pod containing seeds.

A *kernel* is the edible centre inside the hard shell of a nut, fruit stone or seed.

Selecting a carrier

Vegetable/base oils

The carrier makes application of the essential oils easier by

- diluting the essential oils so that they are more evenly distributed and therefore avoiding skin sensitivity
- providing a medium to work with on the skin.

There is a wide selection of carriers to use and each adds their own therapeutic value to the treatment.

Apricot kernel oil (*Prunus armenica*)

- Fruit seed.
- A pale yellow oil, high in vitamins and minerals, particularly vitamin A.
- Good for facials.
- Suitable for mature skin, prematurely aged skin, sensitive or inflamed skin.
- Shelf life, 2 years.

Avocado oil (*Persea americana*)

- Produced from dried fruit. Cold-pressed avocado oil is fairly viscous with a green tone and it may have a cloudy appearance with residue at the bottom.
- Contains saturated and mono-unsaturated fats rich in vitamins A, D and E.
- Excellent emollient and is used on dry or mature skins.
- Shelf life, 1 year.

Calendula oil (*Calendula officinalis*)

- Extracted by maceration from the flower heads.
- Beneficial as an anti-inflammatory, and very beneficial for skin problems (e.g. psoriasis).
- Shelf life, 1 year.

Carrot oil (*Dacus carota*)

- Extracted by maceration of the carrot root.
- High in beta-carotene, vitamins, B, C, D, E and fatty acids.
- Use to treat burns and is anti-inflammatory.
- Rejuvenating.

Evening primrose oil (*Oneothera biennis*)

- Extracted from the flower.
- Rich in linoleic acid.
- Suitable for dry skin conditions, in particular eczema. Accelerates healing.
- Shelf life, 6 to 9 months.

Grape-seed oil (*Vitis vinifera*)

- Produced by hot extraction of the seed.
- A fine-textured, yellow oil, rich in linoleic acid.

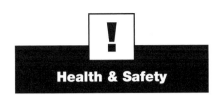

Nut allergies
Make sure that you check the client for known allergies. You will need to ensure that any oil you use is not nut-based and has not been contaminated during the production process.

- Good emollient, which does not leave the body feeling greasy.
- Shelf life, 1 year.

Macadamia oil (*Macadamia integrifolia* and *Macadamia ternifolia*)

- Produced by the macadamia nut.
- Refined oil is pale yellow with no aroma. Unrefined oil is more golden yellow with a hint of an aroma and a smooth texture. A warm pressed oil is also available.
- Contains high amounts of a mono-unsaturated fatty acid called palmitoleic acid, not found in other plant oils but found in sebum, giving this oil a natural affinity with the skin.
- Emollient, good for dry, mature and ageing skins.
- Do not use if there is a history of nut allergies.

Olive oil (*Olea europaea*)

- Pressed from the fruit.
- Has a slight green tinge (due to chlorophyll content) and a rich texture.
- Excellent emollient.
- Use for bruises and sprains.
- Best used in a blend of 50:50 with another carrier oil.

Peach kernel (*Prunus persica*)

- Extracted from the seed.
- Rich-textured oil, heavy in vitamin C.
- Ideal for the face, particularly dry skin.
- Shelf life, 2 years.

Rosehip oil (*Rosa canina*, *Rosa mollis*)

- Of plant origin.
- Has a rich, golden-red appearance.
- High in vitamin C and unsaturated fatty acids.
- Ideal for facial work.
- Ideal for mature skin as it is very nourishing.
- A tissue regenerator, good for scars, burns, wounds.
- Shelf life, 6 to 9 months.

Sesame oil (*Sesamus indicum*)

- Cold pressed from the seed.
- Pale yellow oil, rich in minerals and vitamins.
- Classified as very stable.
- Suitable for dry skin conditions, eczema, psoriasis and gives minor protection from ultra violet rays.

Sweet almond oil (*Prunus amygdalus*)

- Warm pressed from the kernel of the sweet almond tree; may also be cold pressed.
- Pale yellow in colour.
- One the most popular carrier oils used in aromatherapy as it has both high therapeutic and nutritive value.

- Soothing and calming, helps relieve itching, contains vitamins A, B1, B2 B6, E and is rich in protein. Contains a high proportion of fatty acids.
- Suitable for all skin types, especially dry, ageing and inflamed skins.

Sunflower oil (*Helianthus anuus*)

- Solvent or cold-pressed from the seed.
- Light in texture and non-greasy.
- Rich in vitamins A, B, D, E and high in unsaturated fatty acids.
- Use for bruises, skin diseases. Has an expectorant, diuretic quality.

Wheatgerm (*Triticum vulgare*)

- Derived from the seed.
- Dark orange in colour with a thick, rich texture and a distinct odour.
- Contains proteins, vitamins and minerals.
- Do not use on clients prone to allergies.
- Blend with grape-seed and or almond to improve texture (2–10%).
- Contains a natural preservative.
- Excellent for mature skins, scar tissue and stretch marks.
- Shelf life, 1 year.

Other carriers

Coconut oil – fractionated* (*Cocos nucifera*)

- Heat extraction of the white flesh of the nut.
- Clear oil, which is usually deodorized.
- Suitable for all skin types and a versatile carrier oil. Being fractionated, its wholeness and use within aromatherapy is often questioned.
- Shelf life, 2 years.

* may be adulterated/not pure as a result of the manufacturing process

Jojoba oil (*Simmondsia chinensis*)

- Extracted from the jojoba bean.
- Not really an oil, but a liquid wax.
- Colourless and odourless.
- Resembles sebum. Has the ability to dissolve sebum as it acts as an emulsifier, unclogging pores and freeing congestion. Useful for treating acne.
- Balancing and anti-inflammatory (contains myristic acid), rheumatism and arthritis.
- Good for dry skin and the scalp.
- Long shelf life; rarely turns rancid.

Creams

A base cream is an alternative to oil. The cream should be pure and made from plant extracts to complement the treatment. Products formulated for the purpose of blending should be used so that there is no conflict between ingredients. Base creams are usually oil-based products so that the essential oils will blend easily without separating. Creams often include carrier oils as part of their ingredients. Beeswax is another common ingredient.

Tip

Mineral oils
Mineral oils form an occlusive layer on the surface of the skin, i.e. they sit on the surface. This acts as a barrier and limits the therapeutic effect as the essential oils cannot penetrate effectively.

Creams have the benefit of staying on the surface of the skin longer than most carrier oils. This provides a good barrier on the skin surface and so is useful when treating many skin disorders.

Occasionally water-based creams can be found which have been formulated so that essential oils can be added. The ratio of cream to drops of essential oil is the same as for blending with oils.

Hydrolat/hydrosol

Hydrolats are the by-products of the distillation process; they are also known as *floral water*. Examples include, lavender, camomile, rose, tea tree, rosemary, melissa and orange flower (neroli) water. Hydrolats contain the water-soluble constituents of the plants and small amounts of the essential oil. They still have some diluted therapeutic value, although their properties may differ slightly from the essential oil itself. The product may be filtered to remove any microscopic remnants of the plant that may be floating in the water to refine its appearance. Hydrolats will not mix with carrier/vegetable oils. Hydrolats can be used in baths, sprays and for inhalations. Flower waters have been used in skin care for hundreds of years and are considered a gentle alternative for children.

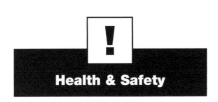

Health & Safety

Try to minimize the number of oils blended during a single day when working. Avoid using several different oils consecutively. Therapists often forget the quantity of oils that they are exposed to, both by direct contact and indirect contact, and by inhalation.

Selecting essential oils for treatment

Once you have made your selection, hold the bottles together and gently introduce the smells to your client by either wafting under their nose or, alternatively, put a drop of each on a smelling strip and let the client smell the result. It is important that the client likes what you are going to use as much as they appreciate therapeutic value. A client is not going to feel good if they find the blend sickly (or girly) and can't wait to wash it off!

Oils to avoid when blending

There are several oils which, by their chemical nature, are more toxic than others. It is suggested that these oils are not used during an aromatherapy treatment. General toxic oils include:

- camphor
- sage
- aniseed/anise
- hyssop
- pennyroyal
- wintergreen.

Blending essential oils

Once you have chosen your selection and the client has agreed with your choice the oils need to be blended.

Preparation and the blending process

- Always use a clean, dry, glass bottle (if you wish to store) or a measuring jar.
- Blend on a washable work surface.
- Have paper tissue handy.
- Measure the carrier into the bottle/jar. Do not overfill.
- Choose three essential oils suitable for your client's needs, remove the lids, hold them together and smell them, before adding to the carrier. Consult your client and let them smell your choice.

Aromatherapy record card

Treatment needs	1	2	3
Carrier	Essential oil 1	Essential oil 2	Essential oil 3

Tip

The amount of essential oil in your blend will vary from 0.5–3 per cent depending on a person's condition and size. The average is:

2–2.5 per cent for an adult, or small areas

1 per cent for face, children, elderly, very slim or pregnant clients

3 per cent for obese clients.

Tip

Working out quantities

Face treatment = 5 ml carrier oil + 1 drop (1% blend)

Back treatment = 10 ml 2–2.5% blend

Full body treatment = 25 ml 2–2.5% blend

Very large client = 50 ml 2.5%–3% blend

When working out quantities a quick guide is to divide the total of carrier by 2 for a 2.5 per cent blend.

Interesting fact

Calculating blends
When calculating blends:
1 ml = 20 drops essential oil.

- Drop half the required amount into the carrier; mix the oils into the carrier and smell.
- Ask the client for approval.
- Make up to the required percentage or adjust the blend and make note of any changes.
- Record the quantities of each oil used in a table like that shown above.

Blending

Before starting the treatment, apply a little of the blend to the client's skin and ask the client to smell. Remember that the chemicals on the surface of our skin will alter the aroma. Like perfume, a blend that smells great on one person may not be so great on someone else!

When treating male clients, try to use aromas that will be more masculine. If you really need to use a 'feminine' oil, blend it with woods, spices or citrus aromas.

Quantities of essential oil

Essential oils usually form between 0.5 and 3 per cent of the total blend. It is not practical to measure essential oils in millilitres; essential oils are therefore measured in drops.

Working out percentages: a quick guide

0.5% = 1 drop essential oil per 10 ml
1% = 2 drops essential oil per 10 ml
1.5% = 3 drops essential oil per 10 ml
2% = 4 drops essential oil per 10 ml
2.5% = 5 drops essential oil per 10 ml
3% = 6 drops essential oil per 10 ml

The rule of thumb is *1 drop per every 10 ml*.

Blending with skin and hair care products

In the salon blending is typically an oil carrier and essential oils. However, other products can be enhanced with the use of essential oils. Use products that have been formulated for this purpose to avoid any possible conflict between ingredients. Suggestions are:

- cleanser base
- flower waters as skin tonics and toners
- clay masks – add to flower water and then mix to a creamy paste before applying
- eye compresses – flower waters
- shampoos and conditioners
- bath products.

The aromatherapy treatment

The aromatherapy treatment may take many forms. It may be a modification of a Swedish massage omitting most tapotement/percussion movements (common when using pre-blended oils) or a more specialized treatment incorporating pressure points and lymphatic massage. The treatment is generally more passive and less physical for the therapist to perform than Swedish massage.

Suggested routine

Tip

Aromatherapy treatment is unique depending on the views of the trainer. Do not be put off by this; this just demonstrates the flexibility of the treatment. The routine given is for guidance and to give you ideas to work with. Use the routines you are given as you train and learn these. If the ideas are different in this book use these to develop your skill.

A typical aromatherapy treatment routine (whether using pre-blended or blended oils) is as follows:

- back (using diagnostic techniques)
- back of legs
- front of legs
- abdomen
- arms (if included)
- chest
- face and scalp.

The aromatherapy sequence

Back

Why begin with the back?

The routine begins on the back for several reasons.

Tip

An aromatherapy massage should take you approximately 1 hour plus about 15 minutes for an initial consultation. The following is an outline of how the time should pan out:

- the back should take you a good 20 minutes
- back of legs, 5 minutes each
- front of legs and feet, 5 minutes each
- abdomen, 5 minutes
- arms, 5 minutes for both
- the face and scalp, 10 minutes.

You should be aiming for between four and six repetitions of each movement or to ensure an area has been totally covered with a movement. Slow down the pace of the movements rather than increase the number of repetitions if you are too quick.

- The back can be a useful diagnostic tool. The type of skin reaction obtained when working down either side of the spine using neuromuscular techniques can be seen to indicate weaknesses in the body. The fascia over the muscles on the back lies diagonally out from the vertebrae. Tension within the muscle can be detected easily. There is a strong relationship between the tension in the fascia and the organs directly related to the nerve supply running from the vertebrae. Patchy skin reactions (rather than a definite erythema) may be an indicator of problems in the corresponding area.

- Many clients view the back as the most relaxing part of the treatment. By beginning with this area the client can begin to relax more easily from the start of the treatment.

- The client will finder it harder to chat lying prone and so can be encouraged to rest. When the client turns over they are ready to go into a deeper state of relaxation, for most relaxation is easier to achieve while lying on the back. On completion of the treatment it is also easier to sit the client up, to allow them to rest and adjust before helping them off the couch.

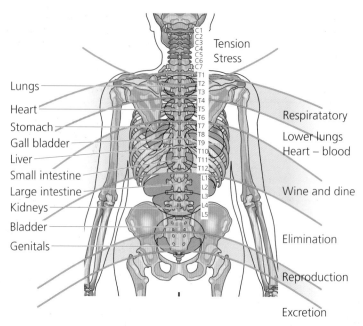

Lungs
Heart
Stomach
Gall bladder
Liver
Small intestine
Large intestine
Kidneys
Bladder
Genitals

Tension
Stress

Respiratatory
Lower lungs
Heart – blood

Wine and dine

Elimination

Reproduction

Excretion

Seven sections of the back

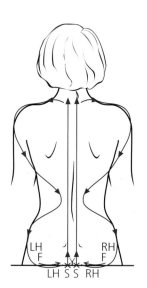

Back 1 Figure of 8

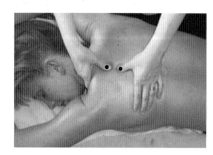

Back 1 Thumb pressures

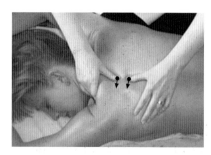

Back 2 Neuromuscular release

Back procedure

Expose the back so that the sacrum and middle of the gluteals can be seen. Don't skimp! You need to be able to work the whole back.

There are seven sections to the back. Patchy reactions in the area will guide you to imbalances. The length of these will vary according to the length of the back.

1   tension – stress

2   respiration

3   bottom of lungs, heart, spleen (blood)

4   wine and dine – liver, gall bladder

5   elimination – colon, kidneys, bladder

6   reproduction

7   coccyx – excretion (bowels).

1   *Figure of eight*
    Using middle and index finger with pressure, glide up the spinal tracks from coccyx to top of the cervical vertebrae. Feel for tightness, texture, pockets of resistance and thickenings. Hands return moulded to the sides of the body, crossing over the waistline and back out over the gluteals. Repeat ×6.

2   *Thumb pressure*
    With thumbs flat and parallel to each other, press and release, working down the spine feeling for the spinal tracks (approx. 1 inch). Start from T1 (first thoracic vertebra) and work down to the sacrum. Thumbs should stay in continual contact, i.e. one thumb moves to next position; when in place the second thumb repositions. Repeat twice on each side of the spine.

3   *Neuromuscular release*
    Starting at T1 work down one side of the spine, again with thumbs. Feel for the ripples or dips between each vertebrae. Slowly press in

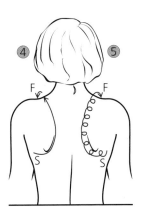

Back 4/5

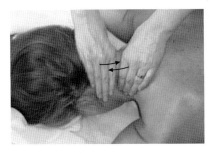

Back 7 Pull and push kneading to neck

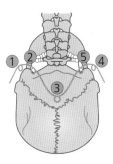

Back 10 Cranium points

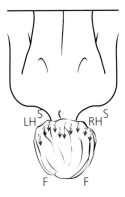

Back 11 Press and release to scalp

between the vertebrae with the thumbs then lift muscle to push away from the spine. Move down to the next vertebra, position thumbs and apply technique. Work down to L5 (fifth lumbar). Repeat twice on each side of the spine.

Observe skin reaction.

4   With the index finger reinforced (middle finger on top of the index finger), drain around scapula from axillary region to the clavicle bone at the front of the body.

5   Using middle and index fingers work around scapula to clavicle with circular movements.

6   Reinforced effleurage figure of eight.
    Work with hands flat tips of fingers pointing towards the client's head to make a figure of eight over the scapula and tops of shoulders. Repeat ×6.

Client to place forehead on hands if no face hole.

7   Picking up of neck with a pull and push action creating a localized figure of eight.

Stand at head of client.

8   Working each side separately, knead with deep circles around scapula in anticlockwise direction from the top to the axillary nodes.

9   Circle up neck using fingers with a press and release.

10 Pressure points at base of the skull along occipital bone. Check for sensitivity (tender or bruised feeling). If sensitive use a gentle pumping action.

> ✎ **Tip**
>
> **Cranial points**
> The points of the cranium are as follows:
>
> 1 + 5 outside of face, sinus, throat, ears, back teeth, recent ear piercing
>
> 2 + 4 sinus, dry sinus, neuralgia, high teeth
>
> 3 high point; instability, emotional, addictions

---

11 Press and release over back of scalp.
    With fingers open, gently work over the back of the skull with a press and release pumping action. Work from the base of the cranium over the head until the fingers lose contact (the front will be treated later).

12 Run fingers over the scalp in a zigzag action.

13 Knead over scalp with the fingers (shampooing). Rotate fingers out so that the hands fit the side of the head and then pump with the fingertips down to base of cranium. Work down the sides of the neck onto trapezius. Turn the hands around so that you can continue to pump and drain to the clavicle and the deep cervical nodes.

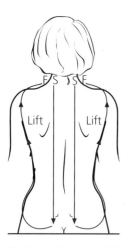

Back 14 Reverse effleurage

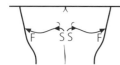

Back 15 Thumb drain pelvis

14   Reverse effleurage.
Work down the spine to sacrum, divide hands. Apply pressure as you come back up the sides of the body, firmly pull scapula, then continue around shoulders. Repeat ×6.

15   Thumb drain over pelvis.

Move to side of body

16   Hands flat, side by side, one side of the back fingers pointing away from the body. Lift tissue between the index fingers, squeeze and release (do not pinch). Work down the back to the gluteals and repeat for other side.

17   Transverse effleurage.

18   Fanning.
Drain each side of the back using both hands with fingers open. Start at the bottom and drain towards axillary nodes using swift movements (four movements with alternating hands to cover area). Repeat ×6. Repeat for other side.

19   Repeat but just drain over gluteal muscles to abdominal nodes. Repeat for other side.
Place hands parallel and flat on back just below scapula (over solar plexus). Stretch hands way from each other (one goes to head, one to bottom) to ease erector spinae. Repeat ×6 (you can use the palm, full hand or forearms depending on the depth required).

20   Effleurage, stroking to finish.

21   Rest hands over solar plexus and pause.

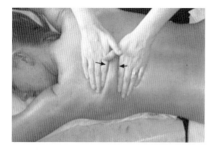

Back 16 Chopping

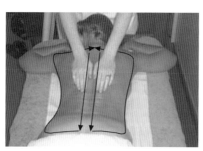

Back 17 Transverse effleurage

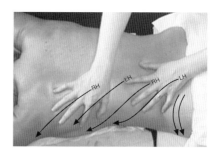

Back 19 Fan drain

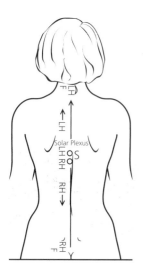

Back 20 Spine stretch

Back of legs

Start with client's left leg.

1   Left leg, left hand, one stroke, firm effleurage ankle to thigh. Right hand, firm effleurage ankle to knee, creating a ripple only. Repeat ×6. (Reverse hands when working on other leg.)

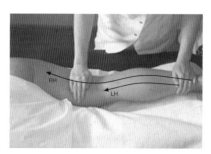
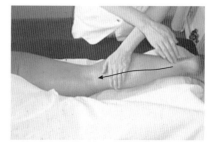

Back of leg effleurage

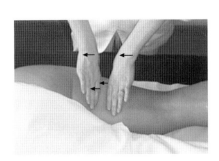

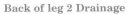

Back of leg 2 Drainage

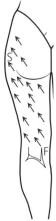

Back of leg 3 Thumb knead

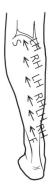

Back of leg 5 Drainage to gastrocnemius

2 Drainage
Work from top of thigh to knee. With a slow drainage movement push with alternate hands, index fingers turned into flesh and hands tilted in towards each other.

3 Thumb knead
Using large sweeping thumb movements, knead thigh. Work from the gluteals down the thigh until the area is covered.

4 Transverse effleurage across thigh.

5 Drainage to gastrocnemius.

6 Palm stroke
Support foot, lift ankle to raise leg. Stroke with palm of hand (thumb tucked in) from ankle to knee running along centre of gastrocnemius (Should not be uncomfortable.) Repeat ×6.

7 Thumb slide
Start with thumbs side by side pointing up to knee. Slide up gastronomies from the ankle to back of knee. Slide hands back down sides to ankle. Repeat ×6.

8 Palm effleurage to sole of foot.

9 $1^1/_2$ drain.

Repeat step 1 but with fingers splayed ankle to thigh, ankle to knee.

Repeat for right leg.

Cover client and turn client over.

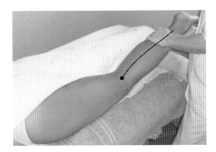

Back of leg 6 Palm stroke

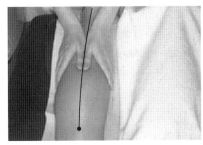

Back of leg 7 Thumb slide

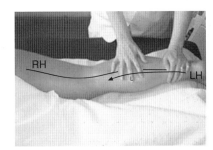

Back of leg 9 Drain fingers open

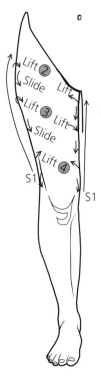

Front of leg finger lift

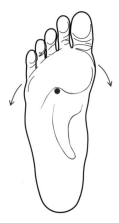

Foot 5 Solar plexus and open chest

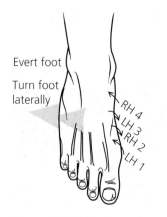

**Foot 11 Medial twist to foot.
Turn foot out laterally**

Front of legs

Place support under knees.

Start with left leg.

1    $1\frac{1}{2}$ hand effleurage.
     Ankle to thigh, ankle to knee. (Do not apply pressure over patella.)

2   Thumb knead thigh working from the top down until the area has been sufficiently covered.

3   Finger lift and slide to hamstrings.
     Slide fingers under thigh and up the back of thigh, thumbs on the front of thigh. At the top of thigh lift the muscle up using the fingers, so that thumbs cross over on the front of the thigh. Slide fingers back a few centimetres and repeat until the thigh area has been covered. Finish at the knee.

4   Transverse effleurage across thigh.

5   Fingers knead around patella.

6   Fingers knead popliteal space behind knee.

7   Thumb knead tibialis anterior.

(For steps 5–7 see Chapter 9, p.203.)

8    $1\frac{1}{2}$ effleurage with fingers splayed up front of leg.

Cover leg.

Foot

1   Thumb stroking front of foot around ankle.

2   Extend ankle and pull leg gently.

3   Knead down Achilles tendon.

4   Using the fingertips pump around ankles.

5   Thumbs on solar plexus, finger across top touching, slide fingers out to stretch foot (open chest).

6   Thumb knead with little circles on ball of foot.

7   Knead sole of foot with knuckles and thumb frictions.

8   Finger slide between metatarsals on top of foot.

9   Apply tiny finger frictions between metatarsals.

10   Rotate each toe clockwise and anticlockwise.

11   Hands clasp inner foot (arch), gently twist between hands (wringing).

12   Support foot and rotate ankle clockwise and anticlockwise.

Repeat for left leg and foot.

Arms

Place support under the arm.

1   Effleurage arm.

2   Drainage movement to arm starting at top. Work down. Form rings with thumb and finger and push upwards using alternate hands.

3   Thumb knead biceps and deltoid.

4   Rest forearm across chest and continue to thumb knead triceps.

5   Effleurage arm.

6   Thumb knead radialis lower arm.

7   Using fingers and thumb grip around wrist and scoop up arm elbow. Repeat ×6.

8   Using light finger movements feather down arm to hand.

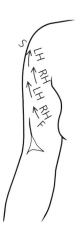

Arms 2 Drainage

Hand

1 Thumb stroking back of hand.
2 Finger slide between metacarpals on back of hand.
3 Tiny finger frictions between metacarpals.
4 Knead down each finger and rotate clockwise and anticlockwise.
5 Thumbs on solar plexus point, fingers across top touching. Slide fingers out keeping thumbs pressing into solar plexus to stretch hand (open chest).
6 Thumb knead with little circles the palm of hand.
7 Using the thumbs apply frictions to palm of hand.
8 Frictions up carpals and forearm.
9 Rotate wrist clockwise and anticlockwise.

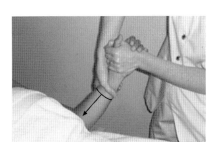

Lower arm scoup

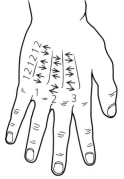

Hand 3 Finger frictions to metacarpals

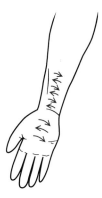

Hand 8 Frictions up carpals and forearm

Tip

Male clients
When treating the abdomen on male clients:

- avoid contact below the navel
- work higher onto the chest with effleurage.

Abdomen

Place support under knees to relax the pelvis.

1 Transverse effleurage across abdomen.
2 Thumbs on base of sternum, draw thumbs down in a line to umbilicus. Repeat ×4.
3 Repeat with a pumping action ×4.
4 Repeat drawing the thumbs down alternately in quick succession to drain.
5 Reinforce hands, using fingers, work from centre outwards along the bottom of the rib cage with a pumping action.

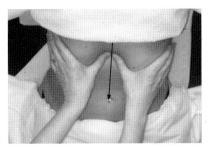

Abdomen thumb drain from sternum

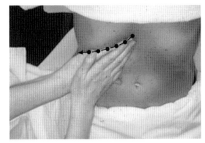

Abdomen pumping along base of rib cage

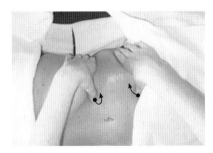

Abdomen colon elimination

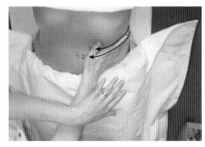

Fan drain sides of abdomen

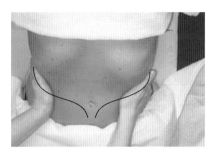

Effleurage to abdomen

6 **OPTIONAL**: 'colon elimination' movement. Use where there is sluggish digestion or constipation – this really does the trick. Ask the client to raise the knees for comfort. Mark transverse colon (sternum to umbilicus and out to approx. mid-line). Fingers lift side of abdomen to ensure position of the end of the colon. Walk to pelvic bone and move in two finger widths. Rock the thumbs back and forth on the two points in a pedalling action to empty the colon.

7 Using deep effleurage drain ascending, descending and colon with deep effleurage. Maintain contact over lower abdomen but apply no pressure.

8 Drain from the back around the waist to the pelvis using alternate hands, with a brisk effleurage, fingers open. Repeat for other side.

9 Effleurage both sides of the abdomen, one hand to each side. Lift and drain slowly back to front.

10 Symbolic drain from base of sternum. Run thumbs along line of the rib cage to finish.

Head, face, neck and chest

The head, face, neck and chest complete the treatment. A simple routine would incorporate the following:

- lymphatic drainage and pressure point to face
- drain into thoracic duct
- massage back of neck
- complete with head and scalp massage.

For further guidance go to Chapter 12, p.294 and Chapter 13, p.307.

After care

Tip

Review your blend every time you see the client, even if it has been effective previously. Remember that the person we are today is not the same person we will be next week. Always monitor the client and update the consultation *each* time you see them.

Sit the client up slowly and give them a glass of water to drink. Allow the client to rest for several minutes after treatment. Advise them of the after care that they should follow, reminding them at the end of each treatment.

To ensure you are familiar with after care and contra actions, go to Chapter 5, p.137.

Future treatments

The client should be encouraged to have regular treatments; once a month is ideal to maintain the body's equilibrium. If there are specific areas of concern or weaknesses then a course of weekly treatments for about six weeks will be beneficial.

Home treatment and other uses for essential oils

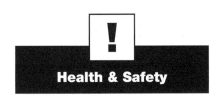
Clients should be encouraged to follow up their treatment at home and this can be achieved in a variety of ways depending on the client's needs. This will also give you an opportunity to retail suitable products to your client. Products can be pre-blended for retail or blended specifically for the client.

Massage

An excellent way to supplement treatment with essential oils. This can be carried out daily or as required.

Vaporizer/burner

Place 5 drops (approx.) of the oil into a burner or vaporizer depending on the size of room. This procedure is beneficial for a variety of reasons: as a room deodorizer and as a mood enhancer.

Direct application

As a general rule don't encourage clients to use oils neat. Be aware that the client could misuse the oils. Only suggest using of oils which can be used safely, to avoid possible skin sensitivity. Give clear guidance to the client on use and write it down. Tea tree and lavender are the usual oils recommended for neat applications.

Method of application: soak a cotton bud with water and add 2 drops essential oil.

Specific application: e.g. spot, verrucae; daily until cleared.

Inhalation

Add a few drops to a hankie/tissue of an appropriate oil. Useful method for travel sickness, nausea, to keep alert, on pillow for insomnia, for restlessness and a stuffy nose. Alternatively, for ladies, a small piece of cotton wool with a couple of drops can be placed in the bra at the front of the chest. The warmth of the body will release a gentle aroma.

Recommended use: twice a day for a maximum of four days.

Steam inhalation

Excellent for upper respiratory infections.

Add a maximum of 6 drops of an appropriate essential oil(s) into very hot water in a bowl or sink (boiling water will scold). Cover the head with a towel to prevent the steam escaping and keep eyes closed. Inhale slowly and breathe deeply. Duration is for between 2 and 10 minutes maximum. (Use extreme caution if asthmatic.)

Sauna or steam room

Add to water, *never* to the stove.

Bath (or douche)

This is an easy way to benefit from the properties of essential oils and can be undertaken daily if required.

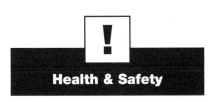

Mix drops into a teaspoon of a milk, vodka or carrier oil before adding to the bath and agitate the water ensure oils are dispersed. Add no more than 8 drops. Advise the client on the temperature of the bath.

Footbath: use a maximum of 6 drops for a 10-minute soak.

Douche: as above but use about 4 drops.

Compresses

Compresses can be used hot or cold depending on their purpose and are an effective way of using essential oils to relieve pain and reduce inflammations.

Method of application: add 4–5 drops essential oil to water (hot/cold), soak a cloth, towel and cotton wool. Remove excess water and apply to the area to be treated.

Specific application: cold compresses reduce body temperature, inflammation, sunburn, headaches, varicose veins and bruises; hot compresses ease rheumatism, menstrual pain, back pain, abscesses, earache and toothache.

Knowledge review

1 List the main methods of extracting essential oils and briefly describe the process(es) used. How many oils can you associate with each method of extraction?

2 Explain why mineral oils should not be used.

3 What would you look for when buying essential oils?

4 How would you store essential oils?

5 What legislation covers the storage of essential oils and what guidelines does this give?

6 What is the purpose of a carrier oil?

7 What options are there for applying essential oils other than using a carrier oil?

8 What percentage is a 12.5 drop of essential oil in 25 ml carrier oil?

9 Design an after care leaflet for aromatherapy including methods the client can use to practice aromatherapy at home.

10 List the contra actions a client could potentially experience. Think about each one and give a reason why it occurs.

11

Chemistry and essential oils directory

Learning objectives

This chapter covers the following

- **classification of essential oils**
- **chemotypes**
- **categories of essential oils**
- **synergy**
- **harmony**
- **directory of essential oils**

This chapter explores the underpinning knowledge of the essential oils. It is important to have a good understanding of the information contained in Chapter 2, Foundations of chemistry, before you work through this directory as this is essential to your understanding of the classification of essential oils.

The chapter is laid out so it can be used as a reference guide to develop your blending skills. It lists the properties of each oil, its uses and other information essential for safe use.

Classification of essential oils

When an essential oil is analysed it will reveal that the following.

- It has only a few chemical constituents that can be classified as *major*, e.g. limonene in lemon oil.
- There are a large number of *minor* constituents, which give the character to the essential oil odour.
- There are hundreds of *trace* constituents giving individual qualities to each oil.

There is no simple link between the chemical constituents and the therapeutic value or hazards of an essential oil. However, having an awareness of the chemical composition of an oil will help give guidance.

Every essential oil can be classified in several ways. Each essential oil has a basic building block made of the compounds hydrogen, carbon and oxygen. Different combinations of these three molecules create different compounds.

These compounds can also be divided into two groups

1   *Hydrocarbons* comprise carbon and hydrogen only and mainly consist of terpenes (monoterpenes, sesquiterpenes, diterpenes).
2   *Oxygenated compounds* are hydrocarbons which have been oxidized, i.e. oxygen has been added. Oxygenated compounds consist mainly of alcohols, aldehydes, esters, ketones and phenols.

Oxygen atoms can replace hydrogen atoms in different ways. These make up what is known as a *functional group*, e.g. ester, alcohol.

Some building blocks are not in straight lines and form circles of 6 carbon atoms. These are known as *benzene rings* (or aromatic rings). The rings can also attach themselves to chains, creating new molecules, including phenols, aldehydes and organic acids.

a. Terpenes

Terpenes are present in virtually all essential oils. Their therapeutic effect is somewhat weak but their value is still significant. Terpenes are hydrocarbons, i.e. they are made up of carbon and hydrogen atoms in a chain. They are termed aliphatic because the hydrocarbons form chains. Specific groups of atoms are attracted to these chains forming new compounds of alcohols, aldehydes and organic acids. Each of these has a different molecular structure and different therapeutic properties.

● Terpenes absorb oxygen easily and are easily oxidized by the air; this process results in hydrogen peroxide. Their effect on the skin is antiseptic.
● Terpene may be partially or completely removed, creating fractionated oil. This results in the therapeutic value of the oil being affected.
● Some terpenes may be slightly irritating to the skin; indeed all citrus oils (except bergamot) have a high proportion of terpenes.

Monoterpenes

These comprise 2 isoprene units. Each unit comprises 5 carbon atoms in a branched chain. They occur in practically all essential oils but their effect is weak. Examples are limonene, pinene and terpinene.

Properties – stimulating
Antiseptic in the air, bactericidal, expectorant, decongestant and mildly analgesic. A few are anti-viral.

Sesquiterpenes

These comprise 3 isoprene units.

A high proportion of essential oils contain sesquiterpenes. Examples include caryophyllene, cadinene and germacrene.

Properties – balancing
Slightly antiseptic, bactericidal, slightly hypotensive, astringent, calming and anti-inflammatory. A few are analgesic and anti-spasmodic.

Diterpenes

These have 4 isoprene units. Few oils can be classified with diterpenes; because of their size they tend not to transfer during distillation.

Properties – clearing
Slightly bactericidal, expectorant and purgative. A few are anti-fungal and anti-viral. Some may have a balancing effect on the hormonal system.

b. Alcohols

Alcohols are formed from 1 hydrogen atom bonded to 1 oxygen atom. This is called a hydroxyl group. When this attaches itself to a carbon in an aliphatic terpene chain it becomes an alcohol. Examples include citronellol, linalool, geraniol and terpineol.

General properties
Stimulating, antiseptic, anti-viral, bactericidal, balancing, hormone-like, warming, diuretic.

Monoterpenols

Monoterpenol = monoterpene compound + hydroxyl group.

Properties
Anti-fungal, anti-infectious, anti-viral, bactericidal, immune system balancer, hepatic, stimulating, warming, vasoconstrictor, general tonic.

Non-toxic, non-hazardous, usually non-irritant.

Sesquiterpenols

Sesquiterpenes = hydrogen and oxygen (–OH) + sesquiterpene.

Properties
Decongestant, hepatic, hypotensor, temperature-reducing, nervine, uplifting, tonic. Some aphrodisiac properties. Particularly calming.

Non-irritant.

Diterpenols

Diterpenols = hydrogen and oxygen –OH + diterpene molecule.

Not very volatile and do not generally come through to the essential oil during distillation. Their structure is similar to that of human hormones (steroids).

Properties
Hormone-balancing, e.g. sclareol in clary sage.

c. Phenols

Phenols are stronger than alcohols. Phenol = hydrogen + oxygen (–OH) attached to a carbon in a phenol ring. Examples include carvacol, eugenol, thymol, *trans*-anethole, methyl chavicol.

Properties
Analgesic, powerful antiseptic, bactericidal, anti-viral, stimulant for the nervous and immune systems, sedative, digestive, diuretic, expectorant, emmenagogue, hypertensive. Can causes skin irritation and should be used with discretion.

d. Aliphatic aldehydes

Carbonyl group + hydrogen atoms attached to a carbon atom in a chain or ring molecule. Often have a powerful aroma.

May be a sensitizer (some only when isolated from the oil as some constituents act as a quencher to counteract these sorts of effects). Examples include citral, citronellal, neral and geranial.

Properties – relaxing
Antiseptic, anti-fungal, anti-infectious, anti-viral, hypotensive, calming, nervine. May reduce temperature.

e. Ketones

Ketone = carbonyl O attached to a carbon in a chain or ring molecule.

Not pleasant therapeutically; some are neuro-toxic, some are harmless. Aniseed, caraway, hyssop, pennyroyal and sage are all high in ketones. Essential oils with high ketones should be used at a maximum 2 per cent and should ideally be well diluted. Examples include camphor, carvone, menthone and thujene.

Properties – relaxing
Abortifacient, cicatrisant, expectorant, lipolytic, mucolytic, calming, sedative; some are analgesic, digestive, anti-coagulant, anti-inflammatory, anti-fungal. Parasiticidal. Emmenagogue.

f. Acids and esters

Based on the carboxyl group. Organic acids are not like inorganic acids, which have the potential to be hazardous.

Acids

Organic acids react with alcohol to form esters + water.

Acids in their free state are rare in essential oils and occur only in minute quantities. Examples include benzoic acid and phenylacetic acids.

Properties – stimulating
Anti-inflammatory, deodorant.

Ester

Ester is produced as a result of the reaction between an organic acid (carboxylic acid) and an alcohol = ester + H_2O.

Properties – relaxing
Anti-fungal, anti-inflammatory, anti-infectious, balancing, cicatrisant, relaxing, uplifting, tonic. Good for skin rashes and skin problems.

g. Oxides

These are linked with phenols or phenolic ethers and are rare, e.g. 1,8 cineole.

Properties – stimulating
Expectorant, mucolytic, warming, anti-coagulant, decongestant. Can be an irritant.

h. Lactones

Occur mainly in expressed oils and may also be found in jasmine absolute.

Properties
Mucolytic, temperature-reducing. Responsible for photosensitivity.

i. Coumarins and furocoumarins

Properties
Anti-coagulant, hypotensive, phototoxic, calming, uplifting, sedating, tonic. Furocoumarins are photosenitizers, e.g. bergaptene in bergamot oil.

Chemotypes

Chemotypes are variations in the chemical constituents of essential oils. There are many groups of essential oils which contain different species under the same name, e.g. lavender, chamomile, eucalyptus. The odour and value of each species varies and this is why it is important to be familiar with the Latin names.

It is also important to be aware of the impact of different growing conditions as well as growth stages. Some plants show great variation in chemicals between night and day, hence why there are specified harvesting times.

Categories of essential oils

There are differing opinions as to which oils fall into which category. Oils are classified for simplicity and are described by their volatility, i.e. how quickly their odour evaporates. The most volatile oils are known as *top notes* (T.♪), e.g. eucalyptus. Oils which evaporate at a medium rate are known as *middle notes* (M.♪), e.g. lavender. A *base note* (B.♪) has a low volatility rate and evaporates slowly, e.g. rose. It is the last scent left on the skin in a blend. Each of these notes has specific characteristics. Please go to www.thomsonlearning.co.uk/hairandbeauty/beckmann for more detailed information on the categories of oils.

Synergy

Some oils when blended work together to enhance each other's properties. Others clash however and inhibit the blend's potential. Here are a few guidelines for achieving a synergistic blend.

- The holistic approach is important here in that the blend should work to balance all the body's needs. It should take into account, physical, emotional and psychological well-being.
- Oils from the same botanical family blend well.
- Oils which share common constituents blend well.
- Oils from within the same group generally blend well, e.g., spices, florals, etc.
- Lavender, jasmine and rose enhance any blend.
- The aroma must be pleasing to the user.
- Your intuition will be important as you make your choice.

Harmony

Some aromatherapists believe that a good blend is created from a balance of oils from each category, i.e. top, middle and base. These notes create harmony in the blend and give the aroma lasting power. Creating a harmonious blend is not always possible and does not really affect the therapeutic value of a blend. Odours are subjective and will be described differently by different individuals.

Directory of essential oils

Basil *Ocimum basilicum* (family: labiatae/lamiaceae)

Origin Delicate herb with mid-dark green, hairy, oval leaves. Produces a white flower.

Extraction Steam distillation of the leaves.

Appearance Colourless → yellowish, mobile liquid.

Odour T.♪ sweet, herbaceous, spicy, rich, camphorous, with distinct aniseed tones.

Precautions May cause skin sensitivity in some individuals. Recommended use is in lower concentrations. Do not use during pregnancy. Has been found to cause depression.

Main constituents

Alcohols	Linalool, α-terpineol, citronellol
Esters	Linalyl acetate, fenchyl acetate, *methyl cinnamate
Ketones	Camphor octanane
Oxides	1,8-cineole, *trans*-ocimene
Phenols	**Methyl chavicol (40–80%), methyl eugenol, eugenol
Monoterpenes	α-pinene, β-pinene
Sesquitperpenes	†β-caryophyllene

†Sweet – linalool type *alcohol*. 50%
*methyl cinnamate – *ether* 90% (type 2)
**Exotic – estrogole type (type 1)

Geographical source
Mediterranean, France, Italy, Reunion, Spain, USA, India, Egypt.

Blends well with
Top: Clary sage, bergamot
Middle: Geranium
Base: Frankincense, neroli

Home use
Burner – whilst studying to improve mental awareness

Properties – clearing	Use – tonic, stimulating
Adrenal cortex stimulator	Stress
Anti-depressant	Depression, uplifting, anxiety
Antiseptic	Intestinal
Anti-spasmodic	Gastro-intestinal, muscular aches and pains, tired overworked muscles, cramp
Cephalic	Excellent cephalic, headaches, migraines, mental fatigue, clears the head, sharpens functions
Digestive	Colic, indigestion, nausea, to stimulate digestion
Emmenagogue	Amenorrhoea and dysmenorrhoea
Expectorant	Clarifying, sinus and chest congestion, colds, flu, etc.
Febrifugal	Reducing a fever or flu
Hypertensor	Hypotension, palpations
Nervine	Nervous disorders, insomnia, weakness, fatigue, epilepsy
Muscular	Flaccid muscles, warming
Stomachic	Digestive problems, jaundice
Skin	To improve general tone and appearance

Benzoin *Styrax benzoin* (family: styracaceae)

Origin Tropical tree. The crude resin (gum) is collected from trees by making deep incisions into the tree trunk.

Extraction Solvent extraction of the resin/gum. It is dissolved in a solvent to make it easier to use.

Appearance Dark golden brown, very viscous.

Odour B.♪ heavy, sweet, with distinct vanilla aroma.

Precautions Possible sensitizer.

Geographical source
Tropical Asia.

Blends well with
Top: Coriander, lemon
Middle: Cypress, juniper
Base: Frankincense, jasmine, myrrh, rose, sandalwood

Home use Inhalation, sore throats and laryngitis

Main constituents – esters (approx. 70%)

Acids	Benzoic acid, cinnamic acid, sumaresinolic acid
Aliphatic aldehydes	Benzaldehyde, vanillin
Esters	Coniferyl benzoate, coniferyl cinnamate

Properties – expectorant	Use – warming
Anti-inflammatory	Inflamed or irritated skin, rheumatism, arthritis, coughs
Antiseptic	Laryngitis
Astringent	Urinary, pulmonary
Carminative	Flatulence, heartburn
Cordial	Colic, flatulence
Deodorant	Warms and tones the heart and circulation
Diuretic	Cystitis, diuretic, fluid retention
Expectorant	Asthma, bronchitis, coughs, flu
Genito-urinary	Leucorrhoea, antiseptic

Properties – expectorant	Use – warming
Sedative	Stress, nervous tension, anxiety
Vulnerary	Cuts, chapped skin
Skin	Chapped, inflamed and irritated skins, mature skin, chilblains

Bergamot *Citrus bergamia* (family: rutaceae)

Origin Small tree with oval leaves producing fruits which resemble miniature oranges. Do not confuse with the herb bergamot.

Extraction Cold expression of the rind of the almost ripe, freshly picked fruit.

Appearance Green or yellowish-green mobile liquid. Natural bergamot oil. Yields a white deposit of furocoumarins on standing in a cool place for some time.

Odour T.♪ sweet, fresh and lemony in the top note, followed by a sweet, rich, herbaceousm floral and delicately peppery body.

Precautions Do not use for epileptics. Bergamot is phototoxic due to furocoumarin (bergapten) content; bergapten free oil is available.

Geographical source Southern Calabria, in Italy (famous for bergamot oil of high quality), Sicily, Ivory Coast.

Blends well with
Top: Other citrus oils, basil, coriander
Middle: Geranium, tea tree, lavender, chamomile, juniper, cypress
Base: Sandalwood, rose, neroli, jasmine

Home use
Baths – deodorant, cystitis
Burner – insect repellent

Main constituents – esters (40%)

Aliphatic aldehydes	Citral
Alcohols	Linalool (up to 22%), geraniol
Esters	Linalyl acetate (up to 45%)
Lactones and coumarins	Bergaptenes
Monoterpenes	Limonene (19–38%), β-pinene (up to 13%), γ-terpinene, α-terpinene (up to 13%)
Sesquiterpenes	β-bisabolene

Known to have about 300 compounds in expressed oil

Properties – uplifting	Use – cooling
Anti-depressant	Depression, anxiety, PMS, agitation, insomnia
Antiseptic	Pulmonary (colds, flu), genito-urinary, thrush, cystitis, leucorrhoea
Anti-spasmodic	Gastric, muscular aches
Carminative	Balancing, indigestion
Febrifugal	Reduces fever
Laxative	Constipation
Parasiticidal	Intestinal, skin infestations
Stimulant	Stimulates bile and gastric secretions
Stomachic	Colic, anorexia nervosa, eating problems, loss of appetite
Tonic	Nerves, stress, promotes restful sleep
Vermifugal	Intestinal, parasites and infection
Vulnerary	Stimulates the circulation, muscular aches
Skin	*Psoriasis eczema*, acne, oily skin, skin infestations, infections, rashes

Black pepper *Piper nigrum* (family: piperaceae)

Origin Sun-dried red berries of the woody, perennial, climbing vine.

Extraction Steam distillation of the fruit (ripe black peppercorns).

Appearance Mobile, colourless → light amber.

Odour M.♪ sharp, warm and spicy.

Precautions May cause irritation if used in high quantities due to rubefacient effect. Use with caution on anyone with a history of kidney problems.

Geographical source India, Indonesia, Malaysia, China.

Blends well with Spices and florals
Top: Lemon, coriander
Middle: Lavender, rosemary, marjoram, fennel, pine
Base: Frankincense, sandalwood, benzoin, patchouli, rose, vetiver

Home use
Burner – fevers, colds, to combat mental fatigue, stomach upsets

Main constituents – terpenes

Aromatic aldehydes	Piperonal
Ketones	Piperitone
Oxides	Caryophyllene, 1,8-cineaole
Monoterpenes (60%)	Limonene, α-pinene, β-pinene, sabinene, terpenes, phellandrene, myrcene, camphene
Sesquiterpenes (30%)	β-caryophyllene

Properties – warming	Use – stimulating
Analgesic	Muscular aches, rheumatic pain
Anti-rheumatic	Rheumatic pain
Anti-spasmodic	Digestive, colic
Aphrodisiac	Mild
Carminative	Flatulence, heartburn
Cephalic	Headache, vertigo, mental fatigue, stimulates the mind
Detoxifying	Diuretic, cellulite
Digestive	Sluggish digestion, stimulating, colic, colitis, nausea, vomiting
Diuretic	Cellulite
Expectorant	Colds, flu, sinusitis, respiratory disorders
Febrifugal	Induces sweating (brings out colds, etc.)
Genito-urinary	Cystitis, diuretic, fluid retention, urinary infections
Laxative	Constipation
Rubefacient	Stimulate the superficial circulation (cold limbs)
Stimulant	Circulation, nervous and digestive systems, kidneys
Stomachic	Loss of appetite, nausea
Sudorific	Increases sweating
Skin	Lack of skin of tone (body)

Cajeput *Melaleuca leucadendron* (family: myrtaceae)

Origin Tall evergreen tree with white wood. The bark is loose and fibrous.

Extraction Steam distillation of the twigs, leaves and buds.

Appearance Pale liquid with a hint of yellowy green.

Odour T.♪ penetrating aroma with camphorous peppery tones. Leaves a cool clearing feeling.

Precautions Odoriferous oil. Use in low concentrations to avoid skin irritation. Be aware of adulterated oils.

Geographical source Native to Australasia, Malaysia, Indonesia, Australia, South Eastern Asia, Philippines.

Blends well with
Top: Bergamot, lemon, eucalyptus
Middle: Pine, rosemary, cypress, juniper, lavender
Base: Cedarwood

Home use
Inhalations – sore throats, colds (not before sleep)
Direct – earache on cotton bud

Main constituents – oxides

Alcohols	Linalool, terpineal
Ester	Terpinyl acetate
Oxides	1,8-cineole (up to 70%)
Monoterpenes	α-pinene, β-pinene, limonene

Properties – pulmonary	Use – pulmonary
Analgesic	Muscular aches and pains, neuralgia, arthritis
Anti-microbial	Resists and destroys micro-organisms
Anti-spasmodic	Muscular pain, coughs, asthma, colitis
Antiseptic	Upper respiratory
Expectorant	Coughs, colds, catarrh
Febrifugal	To reduce a fever
Genito-urinary	Cystitis, urinary infections
Insecticidal	Insect repellent
Pulmonary	Asthma, respiratory infections
Rubefacient	Mild effect, for poor circulation
Sudorific	To promote sweating
Tonic	Pulmonary
Skin	Skin diseases (psoriasis, acne), insect bites

Cedarwood *Cedrus atlantica* (Cedarwood atlas) (family: pinaceae)

Origin Evergreen conifer tree.

Extraction Steam distillation of the wood (including sawdust).

Appearance Dark yellow → dark amber viscous liquid.

Odour B.♪ sweet, rich, woody aroma with musky undertones. Improves with age.

Main constituents – sesquiterpenes (approx. 50%)

Alcohols	Atlantol, cedrol
Ketones	α-altantone
Sesquiterpenes	α-cedrene, β-cedrene, caryophyllene, thujopsene, cadinene

Precautions Do not use
during pregnancy. Do not
use in conjunction with
chemotherapy treatments.
A possible skin irritant on
sensitive skins. There are
several trees that yield
essential oils sold as
cedarwood. Ensure that you
are using *Cedrus atlantica*.

Geographical source Atlas
Mountains of Algeria, but
oil is mainly produced in
Morocco.

Blends well with
Top: Clary sage, bergamot
Middle: Cypress, juniper,
rosemary
Base: Benzoin, frankincense,
neroli, patchouli, rose,
sandalwood, vetiver

Home use
Burner – insect repellent

Properties – mucolytic	Use – masculine
Antiseptic	Pulmonary, urinary, skin eruptions
Astringent	Greasy skin
Diuretic	Cystitis, cellulite
Expectorant	Bronchitis, catarrh, congestion, coughs, TB
Fungicidal	Fungal infections
Genito-urinary	Cystitis, leucorrhoea, PMT
Mucolytic	Dissolves and breaks down catarrh
Sedative	Stress and nervous tension, anxiety, panic
Stimulant	Circulatory, decongests and clears arteries, stimulates lymph
Tonic	Circulatory, kidney
Skin	Balances sebum (greasy skin, dandruff, eczema, dermatitis, fungal infections)

Chamomile
German (true chamomile) – *Matricaria recutica, Matricaria chamimilla*
Roman (lawn chamomile) – *Anthemis nobilis, Chamaemelum nobile*
Moroccan – *Ormenis multicaulis, Ormenis mixta*
(family: asteraceae (compositae))

Origin Aromatic herb.
German: low-growing annual
herb with sparse fine
leaves and white daisy-like
flowers.
Roman: low-trailing perennial
herb with delicate feathery
leaves and daisy-like
flowers.
Moroccan: wild chamomile.

Extraction Steam distillation
of the dried florets.

Main constituents

Alcohols	α-bisabolol, **farnesol, α-terpineol, ***santolina alcohol, ***transpino-carveol, ***yomogi alcohols, ***artemisia alcohol
Esters	**methyl angelates, **tiglates, **methylpenty-lisobuterate, ***bornyl acetate, ***bornyl buterate
Oxides	*α-bisabolol A/B, ***1,8-cineole
Phenols	***eugenol
Monoterpenes	***α-pinene, ***myrcene
Sesquiterpenes	*/**chamazulene, *farnesene, ***germacrene, ***β-carophyllene, ***bisabolene

*German – *sesquitperene/oxides* (35/35%)
**Roman – *esters* (75%)
***Maroc – *alcohols* (40%)

Appearance
German: deep, inky blue (due to high azuelene content); viscous liquid.
Roman: pale blue, mobile liquid which turns very pale blue or becomes colourless with age.
Moroccan: pale yellow.

Odour M.♩♪
German: pungent, intense, warm, rich, herbaceous and hay-like.
Roman: less pungent with a fruity undertone (overripe apples).
Moroccan: sweet, fresh, herbaceous.

Precautions
May cause dermatitis. Moroccan is not as safe as the other two.

Geographical
German: Hungary, Egypt.
Roman: Europe (Belgium, England, France and Italy), S. America.
Moroccan: North-west Africa (Morocco), Spain, Israel.

Blends well with
Top: Citrus, bergamot, clary sage
Middle: Lavender, juniper, marjoram, geranium
Base: Rose, benzoin, jasmine, neroli, patchouli, sandalwood, cedarwood, myrrh

Home use
Burner – calming
Bath – soothes skin, calming, general tonic, aches and pains

Properties – soothing	Use – anti-inflammatory
Analgesic	Lumbar backache, general aches and pains, migraine, neuralgia sciatica (r/m)
Anti-allergenic	Dry skin, eczema (anti-allergenic) (r)
Anti-inflammatory	Inflamed joints, skin
Anti-rheumatic	Rheumatic pains (r/g)
Antiseptic	Conjunctivitis (r)
Anti-spasmodic	Muscular, digestive (colic) (g/r)
Bactericide	Skin conditions (g/r)
Carminative	Upset stomachs, colic (g/r)
Cicatrisant	Wounds (g/r)
Choloagogue	To stimulate production of bile (g/r)
Cytophylactic	To fight infection, increase production of white blood cells (g/r)
Digestive	Ulcers, heartburn, colic, nausea (r/m)
Diuretic	Cystitis, fluid retention (r)
Emmenagogue	All menstruation problems, PMS, menopausal (g/r/m)
Genito-urinary	Menopausal (m), fluid retention, cystitis (g/r)
Hepatic	AIDS, liver and spleen congestion (g/r/m)
Immuno-stimulant	Stimulates production of leucocytes (g/r)
Nervine	Sedating, insomnia, stress (g/r/m)
Pulmonary	Tickly coughs (g/r/m)
Sedative	Nervous irritability, anger, agitation, insomnia (g/r/m)
Stomachic	Loss of appetite (r/g)
Sudorific	To induce sweating (g/r)
Tonic	General (g/r/m)
Vasoconstriction	Local constrictions of small blood vessels, thread veins (g/r)
Vulnerary	General skin healing, boils, burns (g/r)
Skin	Eczema, sensitive skin, dry flaky skin (r/g)

'Clary' sage *Salvia sclarea* (family: labiatae)

Origin Small shrub with broad, purplish, wrinkled leaves and small blue flowers.

Extraction Steam distillation of the dried leaves of wild-growing plants.

Appearance Pale yellow, mobile liquid.

Odour M.♪ strong, fresh, with a floral, nutty and musty scent.

Precautions Do not use during pregnancy and do not drink alcohol as it may induce nightmares and nausea (as with all applications). Avoid if driving due to sedative effect. Use with restraint as large doses can cause headaches.

Geographical source Mediterranean (France), Russia, USA.

Blends well with
Top: Citrus, coriander
Middle: Geranium, lavender, juniper, pine, marjoram, melissa
Base: Rose, frankincense, jasmine, cedarwood, sandalwood, benzoin, vetiver

Main constituents – esters

Alcohols	Linalool, sclareol, α-terpineol
Esters	Linalyl, acetate (up to 75%)
Oxides	1,8-cineole, caryophyllene
Monoterpenes	α-pinene, β-pinene myrcene, limonene, phellandrene, camphene
Sesquiterpenes	Caryphyllene, germacrene

Properties – euphoric | **Use – female hormones**

Property	Use
Anti-convulsive	Epilepsy
Anti-spasmodic	Powerful action, nervous tension and stress, post-natal depression
Antiseptic	Asthma, coughs, anxiety
Bactericidal	Skin
Carminative	Colic, digestive cramps
Cicatrisant	To promote healing of the skin
Deodorant	To combat odour and prevent excessive sweating
Digestive	Flatulence, indigestion
Emmenagogue	Menopausal, tensions and hot flushes, dysmenorrhoea, PMS
Euphoric	To uplift spirits (may heighten dreaming)
Hypotensor	Hypertension
Sedative	Powerful relaxant, muscular tension, emotional, mental stress, insomnia
Stomachic	Calming, flatulence, colic
Vasoconstrictor	Local vasoconstrictor, varicose veins
Skin	Controls sebum production (acne, oily skin)

Coriander *Coriandrum sativum* (family: umbilliferae)

Origin A small, bright green herb with very pale pink flowers.

Extraction Steam distillation of ripe crushed seeds.

Appearance Colourless → pale yellow.

Odour T.♪ sweet, woody-spicy aroma with a hint of musk.

Precautions Stupefying if used in large doses.

Geographical source Far East, Spain, North Africa, Russia.

Blends well with
Top: Citrus, petitgrain
Middle: Cypress, juniper, pine
Base: Sandalwood, jasmine, frankincense, neroli

Main constituents – alcohols (70%)

Aliphatic aldehydes	Decyl aldehyde
Alcohols	Linalool (up to 75%), α-terpineol, geraniol, borneal
Esters	Geranyl acetate, linalyl acetate
Ketones	Camphor, carvone
Lactones and coumarins	Bergaptene, umbelliferone
Monoterpenes	γ-terpinene, ρ-cymene, α-pinene, limonene

Various chemotypes

Properties – digestive	Use – digestive tonic
Analgesic	Neuralgia, rheumatism, arthritis, general aches and pains
Anti-rheumatic	Rheumatism
Anti-spasmodic	Muscle spasms, colic
Aperitive	To stimulate appetite, anorexia
Carminative	Flatulence, colic, indigestion
Depurative	To detoxify impurities
Digestive	Flatulence, colic, indigestion, loss of appetite
Stimulant	Digestive system
Stomachic	To stimulate digestion

Cypress *Cypressus sempervirens* (family: cupressaceae)

Origin A tall, conical-shaped, evergreen tree with small flowers and round cones or nuts.

Extraction Steam distillation of the green leaves and sometimes flowers, cones and or the twigs.

Appearance Very pale yellow, mobile liquid.

Odour M.♪ sweet, refreshing, smoky balsamic aroma, with a woody, nutty tone.

Main constituents – terpenes (75%)

Alcohols	Cedrol, α-terpineol, sabinol
Esters	α-terpinyl acetate
Oxides	1,8-cineole
Monoterpenes	α-pinene β-pinene, ρ-camphene ?3-carene limonene
Sesquiterpenes	Cadrene, cadinene

Precautions Beware of prolonged use on sufferers of high blood pressure.

Geographical source Southern Europe, North Africa, southern France.

Blends well with
Top: Citrus notes
Middle: Juniper, lavender, chamomile
Base: Sandalwood

Home use
Burner – insect repellent; to ease coughs
Bath – haemorrhoids, deodorant, varicose veins
Foot bath – sweaty feet

Properties – astringent	Use – vascular
Anti-rheumatic	Rheumatism
Anti-spasmodic	Period pains, coughs
Astringent	Oily skin
Bactericide	Pulmonary
Genito-urinary	Menstrual, menopausal problems, regulates ovaries, diuretic, fluid retention
Hepatic	Stimulates the secretions of the liver
Nervine	Balances nerves, reduces stress, nervous tension
Sudorific	Excessive perspiration
Tonic	Circulatory
Vasoconstriction	Poor circulation, varicose veins
Skin	Oily skin, sweating, thread veins

Eucalyptus *Eucalyptus globulus*

Other eucalyptus species include *Eucalyptus radiata, Eucalptus citriodora* (lemon eucalyptus)
(family: myrtaceae)

Origin Tall evergreen tree with sword-shaped bluish leaves. Also known as blue gum tree.

Extraction Steam distillation of the partially dried leaves.

Appearance Colourless, mobile liquid.

Odour T. ♪ crisp, camphorous, distinctive and refreshing.

Main constituents – these are quite different for the three species

Aliphatic aldehydes	*Citronellal (80%)
Alcohols	Globulol, *citronellol, *geraniol
Ketones	*Methone
Oxides	1,8-cineole (up to 90%), α-pinene epoxide
Monoterpenes	α-pinene, limonene, ρ-cymene, phellandrene

There are over 300 chemotypes
Eucalyptus blue gum – eucalyptus globules – *oxides* (approx. 80%)
*Eucalyptus citriodora (lemon-scented) – aliphatic aldehydes (approx. 80%)

Precautions Toxic if
ingested. Do not use with
homeopathic remedies or
in cases of high blood
pressure or epilepsy. Patch
testing may be advisable on
allergic skins.

Geographical source The
tree grows in almost all
tropical and semi-tropical
regions, Algeria, South
Africa, India, China,
California.

Blends well with Spices
Top: Thyme, lemon, basil
Middle: Lavender, marjoram,
pine, rosemary, chamomile
Base: Cedarwood, benzoin

Home use
Burner – insect repellent,
air antiseptic, colds, flu
Infusion – decongestant
In conditioner for treatment
of head lice (adults)

Properties – see oxides (g) and aliphatic aldehydes (c/r)	Use – lungs
Analgesic	Muscular aches and pains
Anti-rheumatic	Rheumatism
Antiseptic	Pulmonary, urinary, candida
Anti-spasmodic	Muscular pain, asthma
Anti-viral	Preventative against measles and other viruses
Cicatrisant	Skin healing and scar tissue
Decongestant	Congested head, hay fever, cold, flu
Depurative	To detoxify and remove toxins
Diuretic	To detoxify
Expectorant	Bronchitis, influenza, TB, any chest infection with mucus
Febrifugal	Fever
Hypertensive	Hypotension, increase circulation
Parasiticidal	Insect repellent
Prophylactic	To prevent disease
Rubefacient	Increase superficial circulation, muscular aches
Stimulant	Poor circulation, stimulate pancreas (diabetes)
Vulnerary	Skin healing
Skin	Skin eruptions, skin infections, helps to remove toxins

Fennel – sweet *Foeniculum vulgare* (family: apiaceae)

Origin Perennial or biennial
herb with feathery leaves.
Bears golden-yellow
flowers. Prefers cultivation
near the sea.

Extraction Steam distillation
of the crushed seeds.

Appearance Colourless →
pale yellow liquid.

Odour M.♪ Aniseed-like,
sweet and warm with
liquorice undertones.

Main constituents – phenols (approx. 60%)

Acids	Anisic acid
Alcohols	Fenchol
Aromatic aldehydes	Anisaldehyde
Ketones	Fenchone
Oxides	1,8-cineole
Phenols	*Trans*-anteole, methyl chavicol (estragole)
Monoterpenes	α-pinene, α-thujene, γ-terpinene, limonene, myrcene, phellandrene

Geographical source
Mediterranean (Italy, France, Greece).

Blends well with
Middle: Lavender, geranium
Base: Rose, sandalwood

Properties – carminative	Use – poor digestion
Anti-inflammatory	Rheumatism, joints
Anti-microbial	Resists and destroys micro-organisms
Antiseptic	Destroy and prevents the growth of micro-organisms
Anti-spasmodic	Asthma, coughs, hiccoughs, menstruation
Aperitive	Anorexia
Carminative	Flatulence, dyspepsia, colic, nausea, indigestion
Depurative	Detoxifying, combats impurities in the blood and organs
Diuretic	Cellulite, obesity, oedema, fluid retention
Emmenagogue	Amenorrhoea, menopausal problems (increases production of breast milk)
Expectorant	Chest infections, coughs
Genito-urinary	Amenorrhoea, menopausal problems, PMT
Stimulant	Circulatory
Stomachic	Flatulence, dyspepsia, colic, nausea, constipation
Tonic	Digestive, kidney
Skin	Bruises, dull oily skin, mature complexions; good for maintaining muscle tone, skin elasticity and connective tissue; cellulite

Frankincense *Boswellia carteri* (family: burseraceae)

Origin Small tree or shrub with pinnate leaves. Flowers are white or pale pink. Produces abundant oleo gum resin, at first a milky-white colour. This hardens into 'tears' (amber to orange-brown lumps), which are collected for extraction.

Extraction Steam distillation of the gum resin.

Main constituents – terpenes

Alcohols	Octanol, farnesol, linalool
Esters	Octyl actetate
Monoterpenes	α-pinene, β-pinene, α-terpinene, diterpene, ρ-ctmene, thujene, myrcene, phellandrene, limonene
Sesquiterpenes	*Trans*-carophyllene

There are profound differences in the chemotypes from different regions.

Appearance Colourless →
pale yellow or greenish,
mobile liquid.

Odour B.♪ warm, spicy,
woody, with a sweet fresh
balsamic undertones.

Precautions Avoid during
pregnancy – stimulates
bleeding.

Geographical source
Somalia, Ethiopia, Saudi
Arabia, the Red Sea region,
China.

Blends well with
Top: Citrus, bergamot, basil
Middle: Lavender, black
pepper, geranium, pine
Base: Benzoin, neroli,
sandalwood, rose, vetiver

Home use
Inhalations – respiratory
problems
Bath – skin conditioning
Burner – to aid mediation/
relaxation and respiratory
conditions

Properties – see terpenes	Use – meditation
Anti-inflammatory	Pulmonary
Antiseptic	Cystitis, pulmonary
Carminative	Calming
Cicatrisant	Scar tissue, wounds
Cytophylactic	Immuno-stimulant (colds, flu)
Digestive	Indigestion
Diuretic	Cystitis
Emmenagogue	Amenorrhoea, dysmenorrhoea
Expectorant	Respiratory ailments, coughs
Genito-urinary	Cystitis, leucorrhoea, dysmenorrhoea
Sedative	Stress, calms emotions, PMS, slows and calms breathing (produces heightened awareness), asthma, nervous tension
Tonic	Emotional and skin
Uterine	General tonic
Vulnerary	To assist the healing of scars and wounds
Skin	Mature skins, wrinkles, rejuvenating, skin tonic, slack skin

Geranium oil *Pelargonium graveolens* (family: geraniaceae)

Origin Aromatic shrub with
serrated, pointed leaves
bearing small pink flowers.

Extraction Steam distillation
of the leaves, stalks and
flowers.

Appearance Pale green, or
greenish-yellow, mobile
liquid.

Odour M.♪ powerfully mint-
green and rose-like, with a
'cabbage like' top note,
sweet and heavy.

Precautions May
cause dermatitis in
hypersensitive skins.
May cause restlessness if
used in large quantities
late on in the day.

Main constituents – alcohols (approx. 70%)	
Aliphatic aldehydes	Citral
Alcohols	Geraniol, citronellol, linalool
Esters	Methone
Ketones	Menthone
Oxides	*Cis*-rose
Monoterpenes	Phellandrene, limonene, α-pinene
Sesquiterpenes	β-caryophyllene

Geographical Reunion,
China, Egypt.

Blends well with
Top: Bergamot (citrus), basil,
coriander
Middle: Lavender, juniper,
rosemary
Base: Rose, sandalwood, clove,
jasmine, neroli, vetiver

Home use Burner and bath
for balancing

Properties – balancing	Use – hormones
Adrenal cortex stimulant	To balance, stress
Analgesic	Mild pain relief
Anti-depressant	Depression, mood adjuster/balancer
Anti-inflammatory	Soothing, eczema
Antiseptic	Cystitis, upper respiratory infections
Astringent	Oily skin
Balancing	Fluctuating hormones (menopausal, PMS), diabetes
Cicatrisant	Scar tissue, wounds
Diuretic	Fluid retention, oedema, cellulite
Fungicidal	Athlete's foot
Haemostatic	Slows bleeding
Nervine	Mood balancer, uplifting, stress, nervous tension
Parasiticidal	Insects, head lice
Stimulant	Poor circulation, lymphatic system, liver, gall bladder
Stomachic	Gastric problems, ulcers, balancing
Tonic	Kidneys, reproductive system, skin
Vulnerary	Burns, wounds, eczema
Skin	Balancing, antiseptic, good astringent, thread veins

Ginger *Zingiber officinale* (family: zingineraceae)

Origin Spice. Perennial herb
with long narrow leaves,
growing up to 1m. Has a
thick, spreading, tuberous,
rhizome root.

Extraction Steam distillation
of the dried rhizomes
(roots).

Appearance Greenish yellow
or pale amber liquid.

Odour B.♪ warm, sweet,
fresh and woody.

Precautions Slightly
phototoxic if used neat.
Use in low concentrations
as may cause irritation.

Main constituents – sesquiterpenes (approx. 55%)

Aliphatic aldehydes	Geranial, citronellal
Alcohols	Citronellol, linalool, borneaol, gingerol
Ketones	Gingerone
Oxides	1,8-cineole
Monoterpenes	α-pinene, β-pinene, camphene, limonene, phellandrene
Sesquiterpenes	β-sesquiphellandrene, α β-zingiberen ($\rightarrow$ 51%), *ar*-cumcumene ($\rightarrow$ 33%)

Geographical source West Indies, Nigeria, China, Jamaica, Japan.

Blends well with
Top: Coriander, orange (citrus), petitgrain
Middle: Rosemary, lavender, fennel, chamomile
Base: Cedarwood, frankincence, neroli, patchouli, rose, sandalwood, vetiver

Home use
Compress – rheumatic pains, muscular aches and pains
Inhalation – nausea, travel sickness

Properties – see sesquiterpenes	Use – warming
Analgesic	Arthritis, muscular aches and pains, rheumatism
Anti-rheumatic	Rheumatism
Antiseptic	Air antiseptic
Anti-spasmodic	Arthritis, muscular aches and pains, rheumatism
Aperitive	Loss of appetite
Aphrodisiac	Mild, impotence
Bactericidal	Air antiseptic
Carminative	Diarrhoea, colic, flatulence, travel sickness, indigestion
Cephalic	Mental fatigue, nervous exhaustion, sharpens the senses, aids memory
Expectorant	Coughs, colds, sore throats, sinusitis, warming chills and shivering
Febrifugal	Reduces fever
Rubefacient	Poor circulation, muscular aches
Stimulant	Mental fatigue
Stomachic	Indigestion
Sudorific	Increases sweating
Skin	Bruises

Grapefruit *Citrus paradisi* (family: rutaceae)

Origin Evergreen tree with shiny leaves producing white flowers and large yellow fruits.

Extraction Cold expression of the fresh fruit peel.

Appearance Pale yellow or greenish, mobile liquid.

Odour T. fresh, citrus, tangy with sweet undertones.

Precautions Phototoxic. Oxidizes quickly and therefore has a short shelf life.

Main constituents – terpenes (approx. 90%)

Aliphatic aldehydes	Citronellal, citral, sinensal
Alcohols	Paradisiol, geraniol
Esters	Geranyl acetate
Lactones and coumarins	Auraptene, limettin
Monoterpenes	Limonene
Sesquiterpenes	Cadinene

Geographical source Brazil, California, Florida.

Blends well with
Top: Clary sage, bergamot
Middle: Juniper, lavender, geranium
Base: Sandalwood, neroli, ylang ylang

Home use
Bath – detox

Properties – detoxifying	Use – detox
Antiseptic	Destroys and prevents the development of micro-organisms
Anti-toxic	To prevent or treat the build up of toxins
Astringent	Congested skins
Bactericidal	Congested skin
Depurative	Detoxifying, obesity
Digestive	Stimulates the appetite
Diuretic	Cellulite, fluid retention
Tonic	Depression, nervous exhaustion, chills, kidneys, stomach, liver
Other	Preparation for exercise, balancing effect on emotions
Skin	Oily, acne, congested skins, cellulite

Jasmine absolute

Jasminum offininale (common jasmine)
Jasminum grandiflorum
Other varieties include *Jasminum paniculatum*, *Jasminum auriculatum*, *Jasminum sambac*
(family: jasminacea)

Origin Evergreen shrub or vine, which grows up to 10m. Has delicate leaves and white or star-shaped highly fragrant flowers.

Extraction Solvent extraction of the flowers (picked after dusk when at their most fragrant due to changes in the plant's chemistry) producing a concrete. This is then steam distilled to produce the absolute.

Appearance Orangey-brown viscous liquid.

Odour B.♪ rich, intense, floral, heady aroma with musky undertones.

Main constituents – esters (approx. 55%)	
Alcohols	Linalool, nerol, geraniol, benzyl alcohol, farnesol, terpineol, phytols
Esters	Benzyl acetate, linalyl acetate, benzyl benzoate, methyl jasmonate, methyl anthranilate
Ketones	*Cis*-jasmone
Phenols	Eugenol
Others	Indole

Precaution An allergic reaction is possible in some; patch testing advisable in those prone to allergies. Avoid during the first four months of pregnancy

Geographical source Egypt, India, Morocco, France, China, Japan, Algeria, Turkey.

Blends well with florals
Top: Bergamot, clary sage, citrus
Middle: Geranium, melissa
Base: Neroli, rose, sandalwood

Home use
Burner – aphrodisiac qualities
Bath – during labour, for those who lack confidence, or suffer from lethargy, depression

Properties – tonic	Use – uterine
Analgesic	Mild, muscular aches and pains, easing tension in tight muscles, dysmenorrhoea
Anti-depressant	Depression, stress, creates feeling of optimism
Anti-inflammatory	Upper respiratory infections, loss of voice
Antiseptic	Air antiseptic
Anti-spasmodic	Coughs, labour pains
Aphrodisiac	Impotence
Cicatrisant	Irritated skin
Expectorant	Catarrh, coughs, upper respiratory infections (laryngitis)
Parturient	To ease labour pains
Sedative	Stress, feeling of euphoria
Tonic	Uterine, male reproductive organs
Skin	Dry irritated skin, to improve elasticity, warms the skin but does not have rubefacient qualities

Juniper berry oil *Juniperus communis* (family: cupressaceae)

Origin Small evergreen bush/tree with short spiny needles and blue-black berries.

Extraction Steam distillation of the crushed, partially dried, ripe berries (fruit).

Appearance Colourless to pale green-yellow tinge, mobile liquid.

Odour M.♩ fresh, pine-like, woody, warm, rich and balsamic.

Precautions Do not use during pregnancy or if there is kidney disease.

Geographical source Widely distributed throughout Europe, Canada.

Main constituents – terpenes (approx. 80%)

Alcohols	Terpinene-4-ol α-terpineol
Esters	Bornyl acetate, terpinyl acetate
Monoterpenes	α-pinene ($\rightarrow$ 70%), β-pinene, γ-terpinene, ρ-cymene, limonene, sabinene ($\rightarrow$ 27%), thujene, mycrene, camphene
Sesquiterpenes	Caryophyllene, cadinene, humulene, germacrene

Properties – anti-toxic	Use – purify
Anti-rheumatic	Rheumatism and arthritis, gout
Antiseptic	Urinary, air antiseptic
Anti-spasmodic	Muscular aches and pains, dysmenorrhoea
Anti-toxic	Counter effects of toxic build up
Carminative	Colic, diarrhoea
Cicatrisant	Skin disease and disorders, scar tissue, wounds
Depurative	To detoxify, purify the blood, cellulite, obesity
Diuretic	Cystitis, kidney stones, fluid retention
Emmenagogue	Amenorrhoea, dysmenorrhoea, leucorrhoea, PMS

Blends well with
Top: Bergamot, cypress, clary
  sage, citrus, petitgrain
Middle: Chamomile,
  geranium, lavender, pine,
  rosemary
Base: Sandalwood, benzoin,
  cedarwood, vetiver,
  frankincense, benzoin

Home use
Burner – to give protection
  from infections
Bath – menstrual problems,
  diuretic and to detox

Properties – anti-toxic	Use – purify
Nervine	Stress, nervous tension, anxiety, insomnia, epilepsy
Parasiticidal	Skin infestations
Rubefacient	Stimulates the superficial circulation, muscular aches and pains
Sedative	Calms the nervous system
Stomachic	Loss of appetite
Sudorific	Increases perspiration
Tonic	Digestive (incl. liver), kidney, spleen
Vulnerary	Skin diseases and disorders
Other	Diabetes
Skin	Acne, dermatitis, eczema, oily skin and hair, lack of skin tone, psoriasis

Lavender oil
Lavendula agustfolia (true lavender)
Lavendula officinalis (common lavender)
Lavendula lactifolia (spike lavender)
(family: labiatae/lamiaceae)

Origin Aromatic, woody
  shrub with grey-green,
  small, pointed leaves and
  delicate violet-blue flowers.
  Spike lavender has broader
  leaves with grey-blue
  flowers.

Extraction Steam distillation
  of the freshly cut entire
  aerial parts.

Appearance Colourless →
  pale yellow, mobile liquid.

Odour M.♪ fresh, sweet,
  floral and herbaceous, with
  woody undertones. Spike
  lavender has a hint of
  rosemary.

Geographical source
  Southern France, UK,
  Italy.

Main constituents –

Aromatic aldehydes	†Cuminaldehyde, †benzaldehyde
Alcohols	Borneol, linalool ($\to$ 50%), lavandulol, †terpinene-4-ol, †α-terpinene, †geraniol
Esters	Linalyl acetate (†$\to$ 55%), geranyl acetate, lavandulyl acetate
Oxides	1,8-cineole (*$\to$ 37%)
Ketones	Camphor (*$\to$ 60%), †octane
Monoterpenes	†Ocimene, camphene, limonene
Sesquiterpenes	*Caryophyllene, †β-caryopyllene

†True lavender – *esters* (approx. 50%)
*Spike lavender – *oxides* (approx. 34%)/ketones

Properties – see esters (t) and oxides (s)	Use – universal
Analgesic	Muscular aches and pains, rheumatism, dysmenorrhoea, sciatica, migraine, headache
Anti-depressant	Depression, nervous tension, stress
Anti-microbial	Resists and destroys micro-organisms
Anti-rheumatic	Rheumatism and arthritis
Antiseptic	Destroys and prevents growth of micro-organisms

Blends well with Floral oils,
   spices
Top: Citrus, clary sage,
   coriander, petitgrain
Middle: Geranium, pine,
   chamomile, juniper
Base: Cedarwood, clove,
   patchouli, vetiver, rose,
   neroli, frankincense, ylang
   ylang, benzoin

Home use
Burner – insect repellent,
   air antiseptic, headaches
Neat – burns, bites, a little to
   temples to help headaches
Compress – muscular aches,
   sprains, bruises

Properties – see esters (t) and oxides (s)	Use – universal
Anti-spasmodic	Muscular, colic, dysmenorrhoea, asthma, coughs
Anti-toxic	Counters the effect of toxins
Carminative	Colic, flatulence, nausea
Cholagogue	Stimulates gall bladder and bile secretions
Cicatrisant	Scars, skin disorders and disease
Cordial	Stimulant and tonic
Cytophylactic	Increases the productions of white blood cells
Deodorant	Masks unpleasant odours
Diuretic	Cystitis
Expectorant	Asthma, upper respiratory infections
Emmenagogue	Dysmenorrhoea, leucorrhoea, candida
Hypotensive	Hypertension, palpitations
Insecticidal	Insect repellent
Nervine	Nervous tension, stress, insomnia, PMT, shock, epilepsy
Parasiticidal	Infestations
Rubefacient	Varicose veins, poor circulation, bruises
Sedative	Insomnia, stress, palpitations
Stimulant	Immune system, circulation
Sudorific	Induces perspiration
Tonic	Heart, nerve, emotional
Vulnerary	Healing wounds, skin diseases and disorders
Skin	Skin diseases and disorders, infections, bites, deodorant, bruises, skin rejuvenator, stretch marks, burns

Lemon *Citrus limonum* (family: rutaceae)

Origin Evergreen tree with
   shiny oval leaves, bearing
   very pale-pink flowers and
   yellow fruit. (3000 lemons
   = 1 kilo essential oil.)

Extraction Expression of the
   outer rind of the fruit.

Appearance Yellow mobile
   liquid.

Main constituents – terpenes (approx. 85%)

Aliphatic aldehydes	Citral, citronellal, octanol
Alcohols	Linalool, geraniol, octanol, α-terpineol, nonanol
Esters	Neryl acetate, geranyl acetate, terpinyl acetate
Lactones and coumarines	Bergaptene
Monoterpenes	Limonene (→80%), α-pinene, β-pinene, γ-pinene, camphene, phellandrene, ρ-cymene, sabinene, myrcene
Sesquiterpenes	α-bergamotene

Odour **T.**♪ sharp, crisp, fresh, citrus smell.

Precautions Lemon is a fairly strong astringent and the oil may cause skin irritation and sensitization. Phototoxic.

Geographical source Mediterranean, California, Florida, Israel, Italy, Spain.

Blends well with
Top: Bergamot, orange, eucalyptus
Middle: Lavender, juniper, chamomile, fennel, geranium
Base: Neroli, ylang ylang, benzoin, rose, sandalwood, myrrh

Home use
Infusion – head colds, sinusitis
Neat application to

- warts and verrucae twice a day until cleared
- cuts or infected wounds (insect bites)
- brittle nails

Burner – head colds, air antiseptic, insect repellent

Properties – see terpenes	Use – cooling
Anti-microbial	Resists and destroys micro-organisms
Anti-rheumatic	Rheumatism, arthritis, gout
Antiseptic	Destroys and prevents growth of micro-organisms
Anti-spasmodic	Rheumatism
Anti-toxic	Counteracts the effect of toxins
Astringent	Oily skin, hair
Bactericidal	General
Carminative	Indigestion, vomiting, counteracts acidic conditions
Cicatrisant	Prevents hardening of scar tissue
Cytophylactic	Stimulates the production of white blood cells
Depurative	Cleanses the body of toxins
Diuretic	Kidney stones
Febrifugal	Reduces fever, colds, flu
Haemostatic	Arrests bleeding
Hypotensive	Hypertension, regulates blood pressure, poor circulation, arteriolosclerosis
Insecticidal	Insect repellent
Rubefacient	Poor circulation, chilblains, varicose veins
Sudorific	Increases perspiration
Tonic	Digestive (stomach, liver), heart, kidney, nervous system
Skin	Oily skin, skin infections (warts, herpes, pustules), brightens pale and dull complexions

Lemongrass *Cymbopogon citrates* (West Indian)
Cymbopogon flesuosus (East Indian)
(family: poaceae (gramineae))

Origin Fragrant, fast-growing, tall, perennial grass.

Extraction Steam distillation of fresh, partially dried, grass.

Appearance Yellow → reddish-brown mobile liquid.

Main constituents – aliphatic aldehydes (approx. 80%)

Aliphatic aldehydes	Citral (approx. 80%) (neral, geranial)
Ketones	Methyl heptenone
Monoterpenes	Limonene, dipentene, myrcene (approx. 12–25%)
Sesquiterpenes	Borneal, geraniol, nerol

Many chemotypes

***Odour* T.♪** highly odiferous, strong lemony aroma with sweet, earthy undertones. East Indian lemongrass a little lighter.

Precautions May cause dermal irritation.

Geographical source Madagascar, native to India, Tropical Asia (Sri Lanka, Indonesia), Brazil, Guatemala, Central Africa.

Blends well with
Top: Basil, bergamot, coriander, palmarosa, tea tree, ginger, eucalyptus
Middle: Geranium, lavender, rosemary
Base: Jasmine, neroli, cedarwood, clove, patchouli, sandalwood

Home use
Bath – general antiseptic, deodorant; low dilution (no more than 3 drops due to possible skin irritation)
Foot bath – fungal infections, sweaty feet
Burner – insect repellent and to lift mood

Properties – see aliphatic aldehydes	Use – various
Anti-depressant	Depression, uplifting, stress
Anti-microbial	Resists and destroys micro-organisms
Anti-oxidant	Prevents deterioration of a substance
Antiseptic	General, upper respiratory infections
Bactericidal	Destroy bacteria
Cephalic	Headaches, clears the head
Digestive	To stimulate digestion, combat flatulence, liver tonic, colitis
Diuretic	Fluid retention, cellulite, eliminates lactic acid
Fungicidal	Athlete's foot
Insecticidal/parasiticidal	Insect repellent
Sedative	Nervous tension
Tonic	Digestive system
Vasodilatation	Stimulates circulation
Skin	To improve skin tone (body)

Mandarin *Citrus reticulata* (family: rutaceae)

Origin A small evergreen tree with glossy leaves, growing to a height of approx. 6 m. Bears fragrant white flowers followed by small, loose-skinned, orange fruits.

Extraction Cold expression of the outer peel of the fruit.

Appearance Golden-yellow, mobile liquid.

***Odour* T.♪** intensely sweet, delicate citrus aroma with a hint of floral.

Precautions Avoid exposure to sunlight/ultra violet; possibly phototoxic.

Main constituents – terpenes (approx. 90%)

Aliphatic aldehydes	Decanal, sinensal, citral, citronellal
Alcohols	Linalool, citronellol, octanol, geraniol
Esters	Methyl anthranilate
Phenols	Thymol
Monoterpenes	γ-terpinene, limonene, pinenes, myrcene, ρ-cymene

Properties – see terpenes	Use – pregnancy
Antiseptic	Destroys and prevents growth of micro-organisms
Anti-spasmodic	Colic, hiccoughs
Carminative	Indigestion, flatulence, colic, nausea, breaks down fats
Diuretic	Very mild, fluid retention, obesity
Laxative	Mild

Geographical source
Algeria, Brazil, Cyprus, Greece, Italy, Spain; as a tangerine: Texas, California, Florida.

Blends well with
Top: Citrus, petitgrain, coriander, lemongrass
Middle: Chamomile (g), geranium
Base: Clove, cinnamon, neroli

Properties – see terpenes	Use – pregnancy
Sedative	Insomnia, nervous tension, stress
Stimulant	Digestive, lymphatic
Tonic	Digestive (incl. liver), balances the metabolic rate, emotionally strengthening
Other	Good to use during pregnancy, for children and the elderly for restlessness
Skin	Oily, congested, acned skins, scars, to prevent stretch marks during pregnancy, regenerative

Marjoram – sweet *Origanum marjorana* (family: labiatae/lamiaceae)

Origin Tender, perennial, aromatic bush with hairy stems, small soft leaves and pinkish flowers.

Extraction Steam distillation of the leaves.

Appearance Pale amber-coloured mobile liquid.

Odour M.♪ warm, woody, camphorous aroma.

Precautions Do not use during pregnancy. Do not confuse with Spanish marjoram – (*Thymus mastichina*) which has chiefly oxide constituents and has a different botanical classification and therapeutic properties to sweet marjoram.

Geographical source
France, Tunisia, Morocco, Egypt, Bulgaria, Hungary, Germany.

Blends well with
Top: Bergamot, tea tree, eucalyptus
Middle: Lavender, rosemary, chamomile, cypress
Base: Rose, cedarwood

Main constituents – alcohols (approx. 50%)

Aliphatic aldehydes	Citral
Alcohols	Linalool, borneol, α-terpineol, terpinene-4-ol
Esters	Linalyl acetate, terpinyl acetate, geranyl acetate
Monoterpenes	β-pinene, α-terpinene, γ-terpinene, ρ-cymene myrcene, limonene, ocimene, sabinene
Phenols	Carvacrol, eugenol
Sesquiterpenes	β-caryophyllene, cadinene

Properties – see alcohols	Use – warming
Analgesic	Neuralgia, muscular aches and pains, rheumatism, arthritis, strains
Anaphrodisiac	Reduces sexual responses and physical sensation
Anti-oxidant	Prevents or delays oxidation on exposure to the air
Anti-spasmodic	Rheumatism arthritis, muscular aches and pains, cramp, tickly coughs, asthma,
Anti-viral	Colds, bronchitis, respiratory viruses
Carminative	Colic, flatulence, indigestion
Cephalic	Headache, migraine
Cordial	Heart tonic
Digestive	Stimulates digestion
Emmenagogue	Amenorrhoea, dysmenorrhoea, leucorrhoea, PMT
Expectorant	Coughs, colds, flu
Hypotensive	Hypertension, low body temperature, poor circulation
Nervine	Anxiety, insomnia, exhaustion, stress, vertigo, epilepsy

Home use
Bath – colds; with lavender
for insomnia
Steam inhalation – to clear
chest and respiratory
problems

Properties – see alcohols	Use – warming
Sedative	Insomnia
Stomachic	Stimulates digestion
Tonic	Nervous, heart
Vasodilative	Relaxes blood vessels, poor circulation, warms muscles
Vulnerary	Aid to healing wounds, chilblains, bruises

Melissa *Melissa officianalis* (family: labiatae/lamiaceae)

Origin Perennial herb with
small, bright-green,
serrated leaves. Produces
white or yellow flowers.

Extraction Steam distillation
of the macerated flower
tops and leaves.

Appearance Pale yellow,
mobile liquid.

Odour M.♪ sweet, light,
fresh, lemon aroma.

Precautions May cause skin
sensitivity; use in low
concentrations.

Geographical source Europe
(France, Spain, Germany),
Russia, Middle Asia, North
America, North Africa.

Blends well with
Top: Citrus oils, ginger, basil
Middle: Geranium, lavender,
cypress, chamomile (r)
Base: Neroli, rose, vetiver

Home use
Inhalation – asthma, nausea
Burner – insomnia, insect
repellent, nausea

Main constituents – aliphatic aldehydes (approx. 50%)

Aliphatic aldehydes	Citronellal, citral
Alcohols	Citronellol, linalool, geraniol
Esters	Geranyl acetate, neryl acetate
Oxides	Humulene
Monoterpenes	Limonene
Sesquiterpenes	β-caryophyllene, cadinene

Properties – tonic	Use – soothing
Anti-depressant	Soothing for the body and soul, nervous tension
Anti-inflammatory	Calms skin and respiratory allergies
Anti-histaminic	Calms skin and respiratory allergies
Anti-spasmodic	Asthma, colic, period pains, calms breathing
Carminative	Nausea, morning sickness
Cordial	Heart tonic
Digestive	Colic, dysentery, vomiting, indigestion (particularly nervous)
Emmenagogue	Gentle action, dysmenorrhoea
Febrifugal	Fever-reducing
Hypotensive	Hypertension, palpitations
Nervine	Hypnotic effect, panic and anxiety
Sedative	Powerful sedative, insomnia
Sudorific	Increases sweating
Tonic	Heart, digestive and nervous systems
Uterine	Has a general affinity for reproductive system, fertility
Skin	Dry and mature

Myrrh *Commiphora myrrha* (family: burseraceae)

Origin Small tree or shrub growing to about 3 m. Branches have characteristic knots. Wood secrets a pale resin which flows from natural fissures in the bark.

Extraction Steam distillation of the crude myrrh resin. Solvent extraction is also available.

Appearance Pale yellow → reddish-amber oil. Very viscous; may need warming before use to mobilize.

Odour B.♪• warm, bitter and musky with a hint of camphor.

Precautions Do not use during pregnancy.

Geographical source Middle East (around the Red Sea), North East Africa, Southwest Asia.

Blends well with
Top: Coriander, mandarin, thyme, lemongrass, palmarosa
Middle: Cypress, geranium, lavender, juniper, pine
Base: Benzoin, cedarwood, jasmine, rose, ylang ylang

Home use
In creams for deep cracks and chapped skin
Inhalations – chest and upper respiratory infections
Bath – difficult, as it does not dissolve easily

Main constituents – sesquiterpenes (approx. 40%)

Aliphatic aldehydes	2-butanol
Alcohols	Myrrh alcohols
Aromatic aldehydes	Cinnamaldehyde, cuminaldehyde
Esters	Myrrrholic ester
Ketones	Methyl isobutyl ketone, curzerenone
Monoterpene	Limonene, dipentene, pinene
Phenols	Eugenol
Sesquiterpene	Elemene, heerabolene, cadinene, copaene, curzerene, lindestrene

Properties – see sesquiterpenes	Use – various
Anti-inflammatory	Arthritis, skin conditions (eczema, dermatitis)
Antiseptic	Prevents growth of micro-organisms (mouth infections, urinary)
Astringent	Contraction of tissues (digestive, weeping skin conditions)
Carminative	Diarrhoea, indigestion, flatulence, loss of appetite
Cicatrisant	Scar tissue, assists wound healing
Emmenagogue	Amenorrhoea
Expectorant	Asthma, bronchitis, catarrh, coughs
Fungicidal	Ringworm, athlete's foot
Genito-urinary	Thrush, leucorrhoea
Sedative	Calming (overactive thyroid)
Stimulant	Digestive, circulatory (white corpuscles)
Stomachic	Diarrhoea, flatulence, loss of appetite
Tonic	Immune system, uterine, digestive
Uterine	Uterine tonic
Vulnerary	Assists wound healing, chapped and broken skin
Skin	Ringworm (athlete's foot), chapped and cracked skin, mature skin, wrinkles, wet eczema and other weeping skin conditions

Neroli – orange blossom *Citrus aurantium var amara* (family: rutaceae)

Origin An evergreen tree with dark green, glossy leaves; grows to height of 10 m. Produces white flowers with an intensely rich aroma. The fruit is a little rounder and darker than the sweet orange.

Extraction Steam distillation of the freshly picked flowers.

Appearance Pale yellow liquid (darkens with age).

Odour B.♪ sweet and floral with a bitter undertone.

Precautions Phototoxicity and dermal reactions rare.

Geographical source Italy, Tunisia, Morocco, Egypt, France, USA.

Blends well with
Top: Coriander, clary sage, citrus
Middle: Chamomile (r), geranium, lavender
Base: Benzoin, jasmine, rose, ylang ylang

Home use
Burner – calming, emotional balancing

Main constituents – alcohols (approx. 40%)

Acids	Phenylacetic acid
Alcohols	Linalool, α-terpineol, geraniol, nerol, nerolidol, farnesol, benyl alcohol, phenylether alcohol
Esters	Methyl anthranilate, linalyl acetate, geranyl acetate, neryl acetate
Ketones	Jasmone
Monoterpenes	Limonene, β-pinene
Others	Indole

Properties – see alcohols	Use – emotional
Anti-depressant	Depression, PMT
Antiseptic	Destroy or inhibits the growth of micro-organisms
Aphrodisiac	Increases sexual desire
Bactericidal	Destroys bacteria
Carminative	Diarrhoea, colic, flatulence, nervous indigestion
Cicatrisant	Cell regenerator, scars, stretch marks
Cordial	Heart tonic
Digestive	Flatulence, diarrhoea
Hypertensive	Hypotension, stimulates the circulation, varicose veins
Nervine	Anxiety, depression, stress, PMT, shock, mild hypnotic
Sedative	Anxiety, peace-inducing
Tonic	Heart, nervous, circulatory, uterine
Skin	Scars, thread veins, stretch marks, mature (wrinkles) and sensitive skin

Niaouli *Melaleuca viridiflora* (family: myrtaceae)

Origin Bushy evergreen tree with pointed linear leaves and yellow flowers.

Extraction Steam distillation of the leaves and shoots.

Appearance Colourless or pale yellow, mobile liquid.

Odour T.♪ fresh, penetrating, sweet and camphorous.

Main constituents – oxides (approx. 60%)

Aliphatic aldehydes	Isovaleraldehyde
Alcohols	α-terpineol, viridifloreol nerolidol, globulol
Esters	Terpinyl valerate, terpinyl acetate, terpinyl butyrate
Oxides	1,8-cineole
Monoterpenes	Limonene, α-pinene, β-pinene
Sesquiterpenes	β-caryophyllene, viridiflorene

Precautions Mix with
sedating oils if using late in
the evening.

Geographical source
Australia, New Caledonia,
French Pacific Islands.

Blends well with
Top: Coriander, lemon,
orange, petitgrain
Middle: Fennel, juniper,
lavender, peppermint,
pine, rosemary

Home use
Diluted in boiled water to
clean wounds
Neat for burns or on sterile
gauze
Bath – antiseptic, douche
Inhalations – chest infections

Properties – cicatrisant	Use – cellular renewal
Analgesic	Muscular aches and pains, rheumatism
Anti-rheumatic	Rheumatism, gout
Antiseptic	Very powerful (skin, respiratory and urinary)
Anti-spasmodic	Muscular aches, coughs
Bactericidal	Skin infections and wounds, cystitis
Cicatrisant	Excellent skin rejuvenator for all skin wounds particularly burns, powerful tissue stimulant
Expectorant	Respiratory infections, nose, throat and chest, colds, flu, decongestant
Stimulant	Stimulates tissue renewal, stimulates immunity (antibodies), AIDS
Other	Non-hormonal cancers
Skin	Skin infections, cuts, wounds, burns, oily skin, acne

Orange – sweet *Citrus simensis* (family: rutaceae)

Origin Small evergreen
tree with shiny leaves
and bearing white flowers
and round orange fruits.

Extraction Expression of the
peel of the fruit.

Appearance Golden-yellow,
mobile liquid.

Odour T.♪ sweet, fruity,
warm, penetrating aroma.

Precautions Phototoxic.

Geographical source
Mediterranean (France,
Italy), California, Florida,
Israel, Cyprus.

Blends well with
Top: Lemon, clary sage,
coriander
Middle: Lavender, black
pepper, geranium
Base: Clove, myrrh, neroli

Main constituents – terpenes (approx. 95%)	
Aliphatic aldehydes	Decanol, citronellal, octanal
Alcohols	Linalool, α-terpineol, geraniol
Ketones	Carvone, α-ionone
Lactones and coumarins	Bergaptene, auraptene
Monoterpenes	Limonene (→ 98%), myrcene, sabinene, α-pinene

Properties – stomachic	Use – digestion
Anti-depressant	Dispels depression, sadness, lightens and cheers
Antiseptic	Destroys and prevents micro-organisms
Bactericidal	Inhibits the growth of bacteria
Carminative	Irritable bowel syndrome, constipation, indigestion
Digestive	Stimulates digestive system, promotes peristalsis
Hypotensive	Hypertension, palpitations
Sedative	Mild nerve sedative, insomnia, stress-related disorders
Stimulant	Stimulates lymphatic and digestive systems
Stomachic	Stimulates digestion, constipation
Tonic	Skin, emotional, disperses gloomy thoughts, obsession, fear, creates positivity
Skin	Dull complexions

Palmarosa *Cymbopogon martinii* (family: gramineae)

Origin Herbaceous fragrant grass.

Extraction Steam distillation of the partly dried grass.

Appearance Pale yellow or olive-coloured liquid.

Odour T♪ sweet, floral, rosy and geranium-like with earthy undertones.

Precautions Use sparingly as is an odoriferous oil.

Geographical source Africa, Brazil, Comoro Islands, India, Pakistan, Indonesia.

Blends well with
Top: Citrus, coriander, petitgrain
Middle: Chamomile (r), lavender, rosemary, geranium, rosewood
Base: Patchouli, sandalwood, frankincense, cedarwood

Main constituents – alcohols (approx. 85%)

Aliphatic aldehydes	Citral, citronellal
Alcohols	Geraniol, citronellol, farnesol, linalool, nerol, elemol
Esters	Geranyl acetate, geranyl formate, geranyl isobutyrate, geranyl hexanoate, neryl formate
Ketones	Methyl heptenone
Monoterpenes	Dipentene, limonene
Sesquiterpenes	β-caryophyllene

Several chemotypes

Properties – regulating	Use – skin regulator
Anti-rheumatic	Eases stiff joints
Antiseptic	Skin antiseptic, digestive
Bactericidal	Chest infections, cystitis
Cicatrisant	Stimulates cellular regeneration
Digestive	Anorexia, loss of appetite, digestive infections and upsets
Stimulant	Nervous exhaustion, circulatory, digestive
Tonic	Depression, stress, good for skin, uterine, cardiac systems
Skin	Regulates sebum productions (dry and oily), mature skin, wrinkles, encourages hydration, dry skin conditions, eczema

Patchouli *Pogostemon cablin* (family: labiatae/lamiaceae)

Origin A furry, perennial, bushy herb which grows up to 1 m in height. Sturdy stems with large fragrant leaves. Flowers are white with a purple tinge.

Extraction Steam distillation of the dried fermented leaves.

Appearance Dark amber, viscous liquid.

Main constituents – sesquialcohols (approx. 50%)

Alcohols	Guaiol, bulnesol, pogostol, patchouli alcohol ($\rightarrow$ 45%)
Ketones	Patchoulenone, isopaatchoilenone
Oxides	Guaiene oxide, bulnesene oxide, caryphyllene oxide
Monoterpenes	α-pinene, β-pinene, limonene
Sesquiterpenes ($\rightarrow$ 50%)	α-guaiene, patchoulenes, α-bulensene, scychellenes, cadinene, caryphyllene, aromadendrene

Odour **B.♪** persistent, earthy and musky, which becomes sweeter as the top notes wear off. Reminiscent of goats! Odour improves with age.

Precautions Highly odoriferous. Use sparingly as it has a persistent odour which can last for days.

Geographical source Malaysia, India, China, South America, Europe, USA.

Blends well with
Top: Bergamot, clary sage, petitgrain, palmarosa
Middle: Lavender, geranium
Base: Cedarwood, myrrh, neroli, rose, sandalwood, vetiver

Properties – see sesquiterpenes and alcohols	Use – various
Anti-depressant	Depression, stress-related disorders, obesity
Anti-inflammatory	Mild, cracked and weeping skin conditions
Anti-microbial	Resists and destroys micro-organisms
Antiseptic	Destroys and prevents micro-organisms, respiratory infections
Anti-viral	Respiratory viruses
Aphrodisiac	Dependent on whether the users find the aroma pleasing
Bactericidal	Inhibits the growth of bacteria (cystitis)
Cicatrisant	Promotes healing, sore and cracked skin, cell regenerator
Deodorant	Masks unpleasant odours
Diuretic	Cystitis, balances fluid retention
Febrifugal	Reduces fever
Fungicidal	Fungal infections, athlete's foot
Nervine	Nervous exhaustion, stress-related disorders, indecision, debility
Sedative	Anxiety, balancer
Stomachic	Constipation, diarrhoea, curbs appetite
Tonic	Uterine tonic, immune system
Skin	Stimulates production of sebum, dry skin, eczema, cracked skin, dandruff

Peppermint *Mentha piperita* (family: labiatae/lamiaceae)

Origin Small herb with dark green leaves with serrated edges and small purplish flowers.

Extraction Steam distillation of the leaves.

Appearance Colourless, mobile oil.

Odour **T.♪** sharp, piercing, strong, menthol fragrance.

Main constituents – alcohols (approx. 42%)	
Alcohols	Menthol (→ 48%) neomenthol, isomenthol, linalool
Esters	Menthyl acetate
Ketones	Menthone, isomenthone
Lactones and coumarins	Menthofuran
Oxides	1,8-cineole, caryphyllene oxide
Monoterpenes	Phellandrene, α-pinene, β-pinene, menthene, limonene
Sesquiterpenes	Germacrene, β-caryophyllene

Geographical source USA, Europe.

Blends well with
Top: Lemon, eucalyptus
Middle: Lavender, chamomile, geranium, rosemary, marjoram
Base: Benzoin

Home use
Inhalations – sinus congestion, colds, flu, bronchitis, asthma (apply to a tissue), nausea (travel sickness)
Burner – mental fatigue, nausea, colds, flu, chest infections/congestion
Compress – headache

Properties – stimulant	Use – fatigue
Analgesic	Sprains and strains, muscular aches and pains, colic, neuralgia
Anti-inflammatory	Swellings, dermatitis
Anti-microbial	Resists and destroys micro-organisms
Antiseptic	Powerful antiseptic, destroys and prevents growth of micro-organisms
Anti-spasmodic	Colic, irritable bowel syndrome, dysmenorrhoea
Anti-viral	Inhibits the growth of viruses, flu, fevers, herpes
Bactericidal	Inhibits the growth of bacteria (cystitis)
Carminative	Flatulence, nausea, indigestion, travel sickness, diarrhoea
Cephalic	Head clearing, head colds, migraine, mental fatigue
Cholagogue	Stimulates bile secretions
Cordial	Heart tonic
Emmenagogue	Dysmenorrhoea
Expectorant	Colds, flu, sinus congestion, dry cough, sore throats
Febrifugal	Reduces fever, colds, flu
Hepatic	Liver, tonic, jaundice, gall stones, cirrhosis
Hypertensive	Hypotension
Nervine	Mental fatigue, migraine, shock, stress, fainting, vertigo
Parasiticidal/insecticidal	Scabies, insect repellent
Stimulant	Mental, heart, ovaries, fatigue
Stomachic	Colic, flatulence, nausea, indigestion
Sudorific	Increases perspiration
Tonic	Heart, uterine, nervous
Vasoconstrictor	Constricts capillaries, varicose veins, bruises
Skin	Eczema, dermatitis, ringworm (tinea), scabies, lice, bruises, astringent, thread veins, decongests skin, acne

Petitgrain *Citrus aurantium* (family: rutaceae)

Origin The bitter orange tree.

Extraction Steam distillation of the leaves and *twigs*.

Appearance Hint of yellow → amber-coloured liquid.

Odour T♪ sweet and fresh with herbaceous undertones.

Geographical source North Africa, Paraguay, Haiti, France.

Blends well with
Top: Bergamot, clary sage, palmarosa
Middle: Lavender, geranium, juniper, chamomile, rosemary
Base: Jasmine, neroli

Main constituents – esters (40–80%)

Alcohols	Linalool, α-terpineol, geraniol, farnesol, nerolidol
Esters	Linalyl acetate, geranyl acetate, neryl acetate
Monoterpenes	Myrcene, limonene

Properties – neutral / Use – various

Properties – neutral	Use – various
Anti-depressant	Depression, insomnia
Antiseptic	Destroys and inhibits the growth of micro-organisms
Deodorant	Excessive perspiration
Digestive	Indigestion
Nervine	PMS, stress, nervous exhaustion, irritability
Stomachic	Flatulence
Miscellaneous	Good for children
Skin	Neutral oil, balancer for dry, oily, congested (spotty), acne

Pine (Scotch) *Pinus sylvestris* (family: pinaceae)

Origin Tall evergreen conifer.

Extraction Dry distillation of the pine needles.

Appearance Colourless → pale yellow, mobile liquid.

Odour M♪ strong, fresh and dry with camphorous undertones.

Main constituents – terpenes

Aliphatic aldehydes	Citronella, citral
Alcohols	Borneal
Esters	Bornyl acetate, terpinyl acetate
Monoterpenes (50–90%)	α-pinene, β- pinene, limonene, γ-carene, camphene
Sesquiterpenes	Cardinene

Precautions Use in low concentrations. Avoid using on sensitive skin.

Geographical source
Eastern USA, Europe, Russia, Scandinavia (Finland).

Blends well with
Top: Bergamot, citrus, eucalyptus, clary sage, tea tree
Middle: Juniper, lavender, marjoram, rosemary
Base: Cedarwood (other woods)

Home use
Burner – strong air antiseptic

Properties – see terpenes	Use – various
Adrenal cortex stimulant	Stress
Analgesic	Muscular aches and pains
Anti-microbial	Resists and destroys micro-organisms
Anti-rheumatic	Arthritis, rheumatism, gout
Antiseptic	Extremely good antiseptic (pulmonary, respiratory, urinary, hepatic)
Anti-viral	Colds, flu
Bactericidal	Cystitis, chest infections, pneumonia
Cholagogue	Gall stones
Deodorant	Excessive sweating
Expectorant	Respiratory problems (bronchitis)
Genito-urinary	Cystitis, antiseptic
Hypertensive	Hypotension, poor circulation
Insecticidal	Insect repellent
Pulmonary	Infections
Rubefacient	Dilates the superficial blood vessels, muscular aches and pains
Stimulant	Nervous (mental fatigue, to enhance concentration) and circulatory, digestive
Skin	Excessive sweating

Rose *Rosa damascena* (Damask rose) (otto)
Rosa centifolia (cabbage, Moroccan or Indian rose) (absolute)
(family: rosaceae)

Origin
Otto – small prickly shrub with pink, fragrant, many petalled flowers.
Absolute – hybrid between the pink *R. centifolia* and dark-red *R. gallica*.

Extraction
Otto – steam distilled in small quantities from the petals.
Absolute – solvent extracted from the petals.
Occasionally enfleurage may be used.

Main constituents – alcohols
Absolute/*otto

Other	Damascenone
Alcohols	Citronellol (18 → 40%), *(34–55%), phenylethyl alcohol (60%), *(3%), geraniol, farnesol, nerol
Esters	Citronellyl acetate, geranyl acetate, neryl acetate
Oxides	Rose oxide
Monoterpenes	Stearoptene

Complex composition with around 300 constituents

Appearance
Otto – pale yellow and semi-solid at room temperature.
Absolute – dark amber, reddish orange.

Odour B.♩
Otto – sweet, rich, deep floral and hint of vanilla and clove spice.
Absolute – heady aroma; sweeter than otto, floral, honey-like.

Precaution Use sparingly as it is a highly concentrated oil.

Geographical source
Otto – Bulgaria, Turkey, France.
Absolute – Morocco, Tunisia, Italy, France, China.

Blends well with
Top: Coriander, citrus oils
Middle: Lavender, clary sage, geranium, chamomile, peppermint
Base: Sandalwood, jasmine, cedarwood, patchouli

Home use
Bath – to purify the body, improve skin conditions
Burner – nausea, stress, tension

Properties – feminine	Use – female
Anti-depressant (potent)	Depression, insomnia, grief
Anti-inflammatory	Eczema, skin allergies, hay fever
Antiseptic	Very powerful, destroys and prevents growth of micro-organisms
Anti-spasmodic	Muscular aches
Aphrodisiac	Stimulates sexual desire
Choleretic	Stimulates production of bile, congestion of liver and gall bladder
Cicatrisant	General skin healing and scar tissue
Depurative	To purify the blood, remove toxins and purify the body
Digestive	Nausea, regulates appetite
Emmenagogue	Regulate menstruation, menorrhagia, oligomenorrhoea
Genito-urinary	Oligomenorrhoea, PMS, to aid conception, uterine disorders, leucorrhoea
Hepatic	Encourages bile flow, liver congestion
Homeostatic	Slows bleeding
Laxative	Constipation
Sedative	Palpitations, insomnia, nervous tension, stress
Tonic	Heart, stomach, liver, uterus, skin, circulation
Vasoconstrictor	Poor circulation
Miscellaneous	Headaches, excellent to use with children
Skin	Sensitive skin, thread veins, rosacea, dry and ageing skin, can ease dermatitis and eczema

Rosemary *Rosmarinus officinalis* (family: labiatae/lamiaceae)

Origin Evergreen aromatic shrub with silver-green, needle-shaped leaves and pale blue flowers.

Extraction Steam distillation of the fresh flower tops.

Appearance Colourless or pale yellow, mobile liquid.

Odour M.♩ strong, sharp, fresh, woody, herbaceous aroma with minty balsamic undertones.

Main constituents – oxides (up to 60%), terpenes (30%)

Alcohols	Terpineol, linalool, borneal
Esters	Bornyl actetate
Ketones	Camphor
Oxides	1,8-cineole caryophyllene
Monoterpenes	α-pinene, β-pinene camphene, ρ-cymene, limonene
Sesquiterpenes	Caryophyllene

Precautions Avoid during pregnancy, with high blood pressure, epilepsy (although small amounts have been used to treat this condition) and don't use with children.

Geographical source France, Spain, Tunisia.

Blends well with Spices
Top: Basil, petitgrain, coriander, citrus, cajeput
Middle: Lavender, peppermint, cypress, black pepper, marjoram, pine
Base: Frankincense, benzoin, jasmine

Home use
Burner – colds, antiseptic, coughs; to keep the mind alert and improve memory; insect repellent
Compresses – for muscular arches and pains
Hair – as a rinse for brunettes, for head lice on adults
Steam inhalation – respiratory problems
Massage – post-event, training or competing

Properties – stimulant	Use – warming
Adrenal cortex stimulant	Stress
Analgesic	Muscular aches and pains, muscle fatigue, headaches
Anti-microbial	Resists and destroys micro-organisms
Anti-oxidant	Prevents oxidization or deterioration
Anti-rheumatic	Rheumatism
Anti-spasmodic	Respiratory, asthma, coughs
Carminative	Colitis
Cephalic	Headache, migraine, giddiness, fainting
Cholagogue	Hepatic disorders, lowers cholesterol
Cicatrisant	Wound healing
Cordial	Heart tonic, poor circulation
Cytophylactics	Increases production of white blood cells to boost immunity
Digestive/stomachic	Flatulence, constipation
Diuretic	Fluid retention
Emmenagogue	Dysmenorrhoea (painful periods), muscular cramps
Expectorant	Sinusitis, colds, flu
Fungicidal	Athlete's foot
Hepatic	Tonic (gall bladder), hepatic disorders, jaundice
Hypertensor	Palpitations
Nervine	Stimulant and tonic, stress, depression, nervous exhaustion, debility, wasting diseases, e.g. multiple sclerosis
Parasiticidal	Head lice and other infestations
Rubefacient	Varicose veins
Sudorific	Induces perspiration
Vulnerary	To assist skin healing
Skin	To regulate oily or seborrhoea skin and hair

Rosewood *Aniba rosaeodora* (family: lauraceae)

Origin Tropical evergreen tree with red-coloured bark and heartwood.

Extraction Steam distillation of the heartwood chippings.

Main constituents – alcohols (approx. 90%)

Aliphatic aldehydes	Citronellal
Alcohols	Linalool, geraniol, nerol, α-terpineol
Oxides	1,8-cineole, *cis*-linalool oxide, *trans*-linalol oxide
Monoterpenes	α-terpinene, limonene, β-pinene

Appearance Colourless → very pale yellow liquid.

Odour M.♪ woody with floral, spicy and citrus undertones.

Geographical source Brazil and Peru (Amazonian rainforests), Guyana.

Blends well with Citrus, woods and floral
Top: Citrus, basil, coriander
Middle: Lavender, geranium
Base: Frankincense, sandalwood

Home use
Bath – deodorant
Burner – to steady nerves and clear head (pre-exams)

Properties – cephalic	Use – steadying
Analgesic	Mild in action, headaches
Anti-depressant	Depression, clears the mind, has a steadying effect, nervous stress and tension
Anti-microbial	Resists and destroys micro-organisms
Antiseptic	Destroys and prevents the growth of micro-organisms
Aphrodisiac	Stimulates sexual desire
Bactericidal	Destroys the growth of bacteria
Cephalic	Head-clearing, headaches, particularly if nausea is present
Deodorant	Body odour
Stimulant	Immune system and cellular
Tonic	Immune system, skin tonic and healer
Skin	Promotes cellular regeneration (wrinkles, ageing skin), deodorant

Sandalwood – (East Indian) *Santalum album* (family: santalaceae)

Origin Small evergreen, parasitic tree with leathery leaves and small pinky-purple flowers. Tree must be over 30 years old before it is harvested.

Extraction Steam or water distillation of the dried heartwood.

Appearance Resin. Colourless → pale yellow, viscous liquid with a green or brown tinge.

Odour B.♪ sweet, woody, balsamic with spicy oriental undertones.

Geographical source East India.

Blends well with
Top: Bergamot, coriander
Middle: Geranium, lavender, black pepper, pine, cypress
Base: Benzoin, jasmine, myrrh, frankincense, ylang ylang, rose, vetiver

Main constituents – alcohols (approx. 90%)	
Acids	Nortricycleokasantalol
Alcohols lanceol	α-santalol, β-borneol, *trans*-β-santalol, epi-β-santalene *cis*-
Ketones	Santalone
Monoterpenes	Limonene
Sesquiterpenes	α-santalene, β-sanalene, epi-β-santalene, curcumenes, farnescene

Properties – sedative	Use – calming
Anti-depressant	Depression, tonic, tension, PMT, helps to focus
Anti-inflammatory	Eczema
Antiseptic	Pulmonary and urinary infections (cystitis)
Anti-spasmodic	Hiccups, dry coughs, asthma, muscular aches, sciatica
Aphrodisiac	Impotence
Astringent	Constricts tissue (slight), good for acne and oily skins (healing)
Bactericidal	Pulmonary and urinary, cystitis, folliculitis (barber's rash)
Carminative	Nausea, diarrhoea, colic, irritable bowel syndrome

Home use
Compresses – warming, calming, chest infections
Burner – tonic, calming
Inhalation – chest upper respiratory infections

Properties – sedative	Use – calming
Cicatrisant	Promotes healing (sunburn), stimulates white blood cell production
Diuretic	Cystitis, fluid retention, decongestant
Expectorant	Catarrh, bronchitis, coughs (dry), laryngitis
Sedative	Insomnia, stress, nervous tension
Tonic	Strengthens the immune system, kidneys
Skin	Excellent emollient, dehydration, chapped, dry, mature skins, itching, sunburn, also acne and oily skins

Tea tree/ti-tree *Melaleuca alternifolia* (family: myrtaceae)

Origin Small tree with needle-like leaves. Grows in marshy areas.

Extraction Steam distillation of the leaves.

Appearance Colourless → yellow-green, mobile liquid.

Odour T.♩ sharp, fresh, spicy, camphorous aroma.

Precautions Possible skin sensitization in some individuals.

Geographical source Australia.

Blends well with Spices
Top: Eucalyptus, bergamot, clary sage
Middle: Lavender, thyme, rosemary, geranium, chamomile, marjoram, pine
Base: Myrrh, sandalwood, frankincense

Home use
Bath – no more than 3 drops; skin infections, thrush and candida
Neat application – spots, herpes, focus of sepsis; athlete's foot, verrucae (will take several weeks to clear), insect bites
Inhalations – respiratory infections
Burner – air antiseptic, insect repellent

Main constituents: alcohols (approx. 45%)

Alcohols	α-terpineol, terpinene-4-ol, *viridiflorance
Oxides	1,8-cineole (can be → 80%)
Monoterpenes (41%)	α-pinene, α-terpinene, γ-terpinene, ρ-cymene, limonene, terpineol
Sesquiterpenes	Cadinene, caryophllene, armoadendrene

*Rarely found in nature
Many chemotypes

Properties – see alcohols	Use – various
Anti-inflammatory	Skin infections
Antiseptic	General
Anti-viral	Herpes simplex and zoster, verrucae, glandular fever
Bactericide	General
Cicatrisant	Wound healing
Expectorant	Bronchitis, coughs, catarrh, sinusitis, asthma
Fungicidal	Athlete's foot, ringworm
Genito-urinary	Cystitis, thrush and other vaginal infections
Immuno-stimulant	Powerful stimulant of the immune system
Insecticidal	Insect repellent
Parasiticidal	Skin infestations, head lice
Vulnerary	Wound healing
Skin	All skin infections, infestations

Thyme – white/common

Thymus vulgaris
Thymoliferum (white)
Linanlolifermu or *geranioliferum* (common sweet)
(family: labiatae/lamiaceae)

Origin Small, perennial, evergreen shrub with aromatic grey-green leaves and pale purple or white flowers.

Extraction Steam distillation of partly dried leaves and flowering tops.

Appearance Pale yellow liquid.

Odour T♪ powerful aroma, warm, spicy, herbaceous. Sweet/common is fresher with hint of lemon.

Precautions Do not use during pregnancy, with hypertension or with young children. Restrict to professional use and then use with caution due to high amounts of phenols, which may be toxic. The use of common thyme is preferable due to its high alcohol content which makes it safer therapeutically.

Geographical source Algeria, France, Morocco, Israel, Spain, Tunisia, Turkey, USA, China.

Blends well with
Top: Bergamot, lemon
Middle: Lavender, marjoram, melissa, pine, rosemary

Home use
Compresses – rheumatism
Inhalation – respiratory infections
Bath – (well distributed) for insomnia or to revive; muscular aches

Main constituents –

Alcohols	*Borneol, linalool, *terpinene-4-ol **geraniol (30%)
Esters	*Linyalyl acetate, *terpinyl acetate
Ketones	*Camphor, *thujene
Oxides	*1,8-cineole, *linalool oxide
Phenols	*Thymol *carvacol
Monoterpenes	*ρ-cymene, *γ-terpinene, *α-pinene, *camphene, *myrcene, *limonene, *terpinolene
Sesquiterpenes	β-caryophyllene

Several chemotypes
*White thyme – phenols (approx. 40%)
**Common sweet thyme – esters (approx. 40%)

Properties – see phenols (w) and esters (s)	Use – to lift the spirits
Anti-microbial	Resists and destroys micro-organisms, colds, flu, infectious illnesses
Anti-oxidant	Prevents and delays oxidization
Anti-rheumatic	Rheumatic aches and pains, arthritis, gout
Antiseptic	Destroys and prevents the growth of bacteria (skin, intestinal, pulmonary and genito-urinary)
Anti-spasmodic	Muscular aches and pains, sports injuries, coughs
Anti-toxic	Counteracts the effects of toxins
Aperitive	Stimulates the appetite and digestion
Astringent	Contraction of tissues
Bactericidal	Destroys bacteria (colds and flu)
Carminative	Flatulence, diarrhoea, indigestion
Cicatrisant	Promotes healing
Diuretic	Fluid retention, cellulite, kidney tonic
Expectorant	Respiratory infections, catarrh
Genito-urinary	Cystitis, urinary antiseptic
Hypertensive	Hypotension
Immuno-stimulant	Stimulates the production of white blood cells

Properties – see phenols (w) and esters (s)	Use – to lift the spirits
Nervine	Insomnia (very effective although a stimulant; also acts to balance), stress, nervous debility, depression, stimulates the brain
Parasiticidal	Insect repellent, skin infestations
Rubefacient	Poor circulation, bruises
Stimulant	Circulation, immune system (white blood cells), digestion, fatigue
Sudorific	Induces sweating
Tonic	Used during convalescence to strengthen the body's resistance
Skin	Cellulite, sores and wounds, acne, bruises, eczema, dermatitis, insect bites, lice, deodorant

Vetivert (vetiver) *Vetiveria zizanoides* (family: poaceae)

Origin Tall growing grass with unscented leaves and fragrant roots.

Extraction Steam distillation of sun-dried and chopped rhizomes (roots).

Appearance Dark brown, viscous liquid.

Odour B.♩ rich, earthy with molasses undertones. When diluted there is a hint of lemon. Improves with age.

Geographical source India, Sri Lanka, Indonesia, Reunion, East Africa, Central America, Philippines, Java.

Blends well with
Top: Clary sage, petitgrain, grapefruit
Middle: Lavender
Base: Jasmine, rose, patchouli, sandalwood, ylang ylang, cedarwood, neroli

Home use
Bath – stress, relaxation, refreshing

Main constituents – alcohols (40%)

Acids	Vetivenic acid, benzoic acid, palmatic acid
Alcohols	Vetiverol
Esters	Vetiverol acetate
Ketones	Vetiverone
Sesquiterpenes	Vetivene, vetivazlene
Other	Furfural

There is a wide variation in the composition of chemotypes

Properties – sedative	Use – tranquillity
Anti-spasmodic	Rheumatism, arthritis, muscular aches and pains
Depurative	Detoxifying
Emmenagogue	Amenorrhoea
Rubefacient	Dilates superficial capillaries, muscular aches
Sedative	Deeply relaxing, insomnia, stress, nervous exhaustion
Stimulant	Poor, stimulates productions of red blood cells, liver
Tonic	Immune system
Skin	Acne, oily skin

Ylang ylang *cananga odorata* (family: anonaceae)

Origin Small tropical tree which produces large pink, mauve or 'yellow' (best) fragrant flowers.

Extraction Steam distillation of flowers, freshly picked early in the morning in summer. There are four grades of ylang ylang produced from successive distillates. Can also be produced by solvent extraction.

Appearance Colourless → pale yellow, oily liquid.

Odour B.♪ sweet intense scent with floral and spicy undertones.

Precautions Use in moderation due to heady scent (may cause headaches or nausea). Potential sensitizer.

Geographical source Madagascar, Reunion, Comoro Islands.

Blends well with Essences, which offset sweetness
Top: Bergamot, citrus
Middle: Lavender, melissa
Base: Rose, jasmine (with care), vetiver

Main constituents – sesquiterpenes (approx. 40%)

Acids	Pinenes
Alcohols	Linalool, geraniol (2–20%)
Esters	Geranyl acetate, methyl benzoate, benzyl acetate
Phenols	Methyl eugenol, ρ-cresyl, methyl ether
Sesquiterpenes	β-caryophyllene (5–10%), germacrene, cadinene

Properties – calming	Use – euphoric
Anti-depressant	Depression, panic, anxiety, PMS, promotes confidence
Antiseptic	Destroys and prevents the growth of micro-organisms
Aphrodisiac	Stimulates sexual desire, counteracts impotence
Euphoric	To lift spirits
Genito-urinary	Impotence
Hypotensive	Hypertension, palpations (tachycardia)
Nervine	Nervous shock, stress, panic, anxiety
Respiratory	Slows down breathing
Sedative	Stress, overwork, insomnia, PMS, anger
Tonic	Nerve
Skin	Oily and dry, has a balancing action on sebum

Knowledge review

1 What are the differences between top, middle and base categories?

2 Describe what is meant by the term synergy.

3 How would you ensure that your blend is synergistic and in harmony?

4 What oils would you avoid if you had a client with a history of skin sensitivity?

5 List four oils you could use to promote sleep. What advice would you give a client on how to use them at home safely?

6 Which oils could you recommend for use in a burner as a general room antiseptic?

7 Which oils would be beneficial to use on a client with a history of asthma?

8 Which oils could be used to treat a client with athlete's foot? How would you recommend their use at home?

9 It's a really hot summer's day, what precautions might you take both when blending oils and before the client leaves?

10 Why would you advise the client to leave the oils on the skin?

Website @

Visit the companion website at www.thomsonlearning.co.uk/ beckmann where you will find further case studies.

Case study

How would you treat the following client? Prepare a treatment plan. What carrier and essential oils would you use/not use. State your reasons why. What further advice could you give this client?

Client A
Male aged 45.
Client has the following notes taken during consultation.

● Complains of fatigue and feeling depressed. Some difficulty getting to sleep at night (but not during the day when he naps).

Has a history of raised blood pressure, but is not on medication (stress related).
Suffers with athlete's foot, which is quite severe, covering most of the soles of the feet.
Skin is dehydrated and dry.
Activity: cycles daily and has well-defined muscles in his legs as a result.
Occupation: works for blue chip company in a responsible position.
Consumes alcohol daily (beer).

12

Holistic facial

Learning objectives

This chapter covers the following:

- **what an holistic facial is**
- **skin types**
- **skin care products**
- **preparing for an holistic facial**
- **carrying out a skin analysis**
- **basic face reading**
- **cleansing**
- **facial massage**
- **adaptation to massage**
- **masks**
- **contra actions and after care**

This chapter will look at a useful addition to the treatment repertoire – a service that can be given when many others may be contra indicated for health reasons.

The holistic facial will improve the texture of the skin, increase circulation and encourage cellular activity and rejuvenation. It will both stimulate and soothe the nerve endings of the skin. It is also a wonderful way to relax and promote a sense of well-being. This facial uses technique rather than complex and expensive products; nevertheless it still achieves fantastic results.

What is an holistic facial?

This facial will improve the texture of the skin, increase the skin's circulation and encourage cellular activity and rejuvenation. It will both stimulate and soothe the nerve endings of the skin. It is also a wonderful way to relax and promote a sense of well-being. This facial uses technique rather than complex and expensive products but nevertheless it achieves fantastic results. It is a useful addition to the treatment repertoire, being a service that can be given when many others may be contra indicated for health reason.

What does the treatment include?

A simple consultation is completed prior to the start of treatment to ascertain the most suitable products for the client's skin type. The top of the chest, shoulders, neck, face and scalp are treated. The skin is then deep cleansed before a suitable massage medium is applied; this may be an oil, cream or a specially blended essential oil. The massage includes:

- pressure point massage to clear energy channels and to stimulate the muscles and nerve endings
- massage to generally improve the circulation and texture of the skin
- lymphatic drainage to assist the lymphatic systems in removing waste and encouraging healing
- on completion, the skin is toned and a suitable moisturizer applied.

Commercial timing: the treatment takes approximately 30 minutes (with no mask, or 45 minutes (with a mask).

To treat the skin effectively you will need to be able to diagnose the client's skin type and use suitable products.

Tip

Normal skin
Perhaps it is more appropriate to describe normal skin as being balanced. Normal may imply more of the population should have it! Only approximately 1 per cent of adults have a balanced skin.

If you want to know what a truly normal skin looks like look at a child's skin.

Skin types

Skin type	Texture	Colour	Characteristics	Cause
Balanced skin (normal)	• neither too fine nor too coarse	• healthy glow • even colour	• even distribution of secretions, neither dry nor oily • no blemishes • good skin elasticity and firm to the touch	• balanced secretions • healthy skin metabolism
Dry	• fine, slightly coarse • visible dry patches	• dull, prone to dilated capillaries which give the skin a ruddy tone • uneven pigmentation	• matt, flaky patches, creped, often highly vascular, parchment look to skin, may appear transparent • pores small and tight, no prominent pores • warm to touch	• insufficient oily secretions • after 25 years the skin starts to age and secretion of sebum decreases causing dryness • premature dryness may result from: excess exposure to ultra violet rays, hormonal imbalance, skin neglect, smoking, air conditioning, crash diets and illness

Skin type	Texture	Colour	Characteristics	Cause
Oily	• medium texture • may be tacky to the touch • may have coarse patches where dead skin adheres to sebum	• pale or sallow appearance • even pigmentation	• shiny relaxed, enlarged pores • comedones • flaky patches due to poor desquamation	• shows the signs of ageing more slowly than other skin types • hormonal (androgen), ethnic origin
Combination	• variable in different parts of the face	• dependent on skin type	• exhibits characteristics of a dry, balanced and oily skin, i.e. commonly oily T zone and dry cheeks and neck, but may be different	• combination of other skin types

Characteristics

Characteristics are found in conjunction with the four classic skin types. A skin can potentially have all three of the characteristics listed below; for example, a client could have dry, mature, dehydrated, sensitive skin

Sensitive	• may have coarse texture • or be delicate and fine	• prone to blemishes • has a ruddy or rosy appearance	• flushes easily • burns easily in the sun • rapid change in colour when exposed to temperature change • ages prematurely • often dry and dehydrated	• use of the incorrect skin care • inherited • may be sensitive to product ingredients and susceptible to allergic reactions

Reactive skins: skin suddenly becomes red and will settle after a few hours, possibly as a result of skin stimulation

Allergic skins: linked to an immune system response to antigens; effects may be adverse.

Dehydrated	• depends on skin type. Tip: squeeze skin between fingers to see fine lines	• skin will appear normal	• very fine lines around the eye area and jaw. • skin absorbs creams rapidly	• lack of moisture (water) • incorrect or harsh products, alkaline soaps
Mature	• thickened skin	• dull, lifeless • lack of colour or excess of colour	• changes start at around 25 years of age • lines, crepey, papery appearance, finer skin around jaw • loss of elasticity in the skin and tone in the muscles	• collagen depilation and reduction in cellular metabolism • menopause: reduction in oestrogen • post-menopause: loss of elasticity and changes in ability to retain moisture • collagen less resilient

Skin care products

Skin care product information

The table below is simply a guideline. Product companies will offer you the chance to train with them and learn about their specific products.

Cleansers

All skins will benefit from an effective cleanse.
Treatments are not effective if the skin has anything on the surface acting as a barrier. The purpose of a cleanser is to remove:

- dead skin cells, (these are continually being shed)
- surface pollution, dirt and grime
- excess natural secretions (sebum, perspiration)
- stale make-up.

A cleanser should be easy to use, economical and have a pleasant feel on the skin

Product	Description	Recommendation – skin type
Cleansing water	Liquid cleanser, applied to the skin using a cleansing pad.	All Not ideal for removing make-up
Cleansing milk	Light, very runny, place directly onto cotton wool or cleansing tissue. Has a higher water content than creams.	Young, oily, no make-up
Cleansing lotion	Texture of cream. Applied to skin and gently massaged in to dislodge surface grime and debris.	All, combination, normal, sensitive, dehydrated
Cleansing cream	Thicker than a lotion and usually comes in a pot. May be thick and liquefy on warming (e.g. cold cream).	Mature, dry
Soapless cleansers	Often gel-based. Water-soluble and easy to wash and go. Not ideal for removal of make-up.	Combination, oily
Complexion/cleansing bars	Look and feel like soap. Ideally, check that the product is alkaline-free and has a pH suitable for the skin.	As per product

Typical ingredients for cleansers are water, olive oil, stearic acid, glycerol, chloroxylenol (antibacterial agent). Higher level of oil in creams.

Eye make-up remover	Eye make-up remover can be a milk, lotion or cream but is designed specifically for removing eye make-up.	Ingredients are dependent on the type of make-up to be removed. Many contain oil to break down and dissolve eye make-up, particularly waterproof mascara

Exfoliants/scrubs

An exfoliant gives an enhanced, deeper cleanse, improving the appearance and texture of the skin. To exfoliate means to peel off the scales. There are different grades of peeling depending on the skin type being treated. All skins will benefit from regular exfoliating but care should be taken when exfoliating sensitive skins.

Product	Description	Recommendation – skin type
Exfoliants	May be applied as a mask and left to work, usually by an enzyme action. Product is smooth in texture. The main ingredient is usually white clay.	Sensitive, mature skin, (avoids unnecessary dragging)
	Alternatively, may be gritty in texture.	Suitable for deep cleansing on coarser skins
Facial scrubs/pore grains	Worked gently into the skin, gritty in texture. Not suitable for sensitive skins. Ingredients may include oatmeal, salt, nut kernels, silicon or synthetic grains.	Congested or skins in need of deep cleansing
Peeling creams	Work like masks. Clay ingredients draw out impurities. Product is applied in a thin layer and gently sloughed off using the fingertips. Small grains are formed during the process which act as an exfoliant.	Combination, normal, mature
	Alternatively, may be applied and left to work, then rinsed off. Ingredients may include white clay and kaolin in a water-soluble emulsion.	

Toners

Purpose of toners:

- remove traces of cleanser (if the cleanser is not water-soluble)
- restore the pH balance of the skin
- freshen the skin.

Product	Description	Recommendation – skin type
Toner or tonic	General term for a toner. Often between an astringent and a freshener. Ingredients may include sorbital, citric acid, lactic acid, hammalis water (witch hazel), orange blossom. May contain soothing agents such as azulene, chamomile and allontoin.	Combination Normal
Freshener/bracer	Usually has no alcohol content and is very light and gentle. For ingredients, see tonic.	Dry, mature, sensitive

Moisturizers, and barrier and protector creams

Moisturizers have several uses:

- to protect the skin and act as a barrier against the elements
- to replace, hold and attract moisture (humectants) to the skin
- to even out skin texture
- to provide a smooth base for make-up, acting as a barrier between the make-up and the skin underneath
- some contain natural moisturizing factors (NMFs), which mimic the complex substances of the skin cells
- many also now contain sunscreens (SPF).

Product	Description	Recommendation – skin type
Milks	Light, very runny, consistency of single cream. High water/low oil (if any) content.	Very young, oily
Lotions	Texture of pouring cream. Light and easy to apply. Can be either oil- or water-based, usually 85–90% (water): 10–15% (oil).	Young, problem or blemished skin, general combination

Product	Description	Recommendation – skin type
Creams	Thicker than a lotion and usually in a pot. May need to be liquefied by warming in the fingers before application. Higher oil (15–30%) content.	Dry, mature
Night creams	Very rich, nourishing creams. Texture of clotted cream. Often contain treatment ingredients.	Dry, mature

Typical ingredients for moisturizers are liquid paraffin oil, castor oil, almond oil, steraic acid, carnuba wax , tri-ethyl amine, collagen, elastin, water and glycerol

Neck creams

Rich products designed to compensate for neck neglect. Skin care for many means just the face but the neck is just as exposed and needs to be included in the skin care routine. Some neck creams contain firming agents.

Specialized products

These contain concentrated or active ingredients (e.g. essential oils), and once opened the ingredients deteriorate very quickly. Specialized products include serums and ampoules and are used in addition to the normal skin care routine. They are only used for short periods of time to boost or supplement the skin care routine.

Preparing for an holistic facial

Tip

The client should be encouraged to follow a simple skin care routine at home to gain the maximum benefits from the treatment.

The trolley

The trolley should be clean and tidy. Protect trolley surfaces with tissue. The tissue will make it easy to clean up any spillages – oil has a tendency to go sticky if left on a surface.

You will need the following items on your trolley:

- cotton wool/cleansing pads
- bowls
- spatula
- tissues
- cotton buds
- headband
- measuring jar
- blending stick.

Also useful is a selection of the following:

- cleansers
- exfoliant (if using)
- toners/floral waters
- moisturizers
- massage medium
- essential oils
- mask and brush (if using).

Tip

Labelling
Put labels on the back of the products to remind yourself of key ingredients, action and benefits. This will make you look knowledgeable to the client and creates interest in the products you are using. This is relaxed selling rather than the hard sell at the end of a treatment, which may be off-putting.

Tip

Hypersensitive skin
If a client revels that he or she has a sensitive skin you may find it useful to recommend that they try some of the products before they arrive for their facial. The client can either pop in or some samples can be sent to them of the products you are intending to use.

Tip

To make the client more comfortable, place a small support under the client's knees to relax the back and support the curves of the body.

Health & Safety

If working with the couch flat, check that the client does not have low blood pressure as this can make them feel light-headed.

Additional items include:

- mirror
- covered bin
- record card and pen.

Consultation

To ensure you are familiar with consultation techniques, go to Chapter 5, p.134.

During the consultation, in addition to taking the client's personal details, only those questions relevant to a facial treatment need to be asked.

- Do you have any problem areas?
- What products do you use?
- What is your current skin care routine (or lack of it!)?

Preparing the client

Give clear instructions to the client.

- As the scalp is included as part of an holistic facial it is advisable to ask the client to brush or comb through their hair before getting on the couch.
- Ask the client to remove any jewellery from the neck, face and ears.
- The client will need to remove their top (ladies can keep their bra on and the straps can be dropped down over the shoulder). This allows easy access to the décolleté area and avoids the risk of products marking clothes. Hold a towel in front of the client to preserve their modesty whilst they do this.
- Ask the client to remove their shoes.
- Settle the client on the couch. The couch should be raised very slightly at the head or their head should be placed on a small pillow or folded hand towel. There should be nothing obstructing the back of the neck; you should be able to comfortably put your hands behind the client's neck without them having to move.

Wrap or cover the client, checking whether they would like to keep their arms out or wrapped in. Leave the top of the décolleté open (bust covered in ladies) as you will be working across the top of the pectoral muscles.

Check the client is comfortable – you want them to be as relaxed as possible before you start.

Put on a headband, excuse yourself and wash your hands.

Explain what you are doing as you work so that the client is reassured. Warn the client if you are going to place anything cold or warm on the skin so that they do not jump.

Tip

Remember: as the body relaxes the body temperature will drop. Check that the client is warm throughout the treatment.

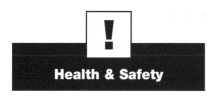

Health & Safety

Check whether the client is wearing contact lenses or not. These need to be removed before treatment to avoid the possibility of damage or products smearing the lenses.

Facial do's

- Use a clean spatula to remove products from jars.
- Where appropriate, apply products from the spatula rather than the back of your hand.
- Alternatively, place a small amount of product needed in a small clean bowl and apply from there.
- Warm products in the hands before applying to the skin.
- Headbands which fasten at the front are better than Alice bands. During treatment the headband will keep the hair out of the way and can be easily unfastened from the front to access the head without disturbing the client when necessary.

Carrying out a skin analysis

Why analyse?

- To check for contra indications.
- To ensure the client is treated with suitable products and/or essential oils.
- To identify specific areas for treatment.
- To ensure that a suitable treatment plan is provided.
- To build a rapport and gain a client's confidence.
- To check the progress of regular clients.

Look at the skin both before and after cleansing. Once you are happy that there are no contra indications, continue by cleansing the skin with either a generic cleanser or one suitable for the client skin type (see p.292, Cleansing). The cleanser should ideally be water-soluble so that the product does not form a barrier to any essential oils you might choose to use.

Look at the skin in a good light and preferably with a magnifier. Look at the skin on both the face and neck and consider each of the following points to help you decide the skin type and treatment plan.

- **Colour**
  (a) evenness of overall colour, pale, dark, olive
  (b) all skin has varying tones of skin tone so is it ruddy, sallow or clear
  (c) pigmentation – is there a tan, or just in patches, i.e. freckles, lentigens, etc.
- **pH balance**:
  (a) are there sufficient natural oils?
  (b) what is the moisture content?
  (c) is there excessive perspiration?
- Without looking, what does the skin feel like, what is its texture?
- How warm is the skin, or does it feel cool and clammy?
- Does the skin have good elasticity, muscle tone?
- The ageing process.
- Is there excess adipose tissue?
- Look at the bone structure.
- Are there any skin imperfections?
- Are there any skin abnormalities?

Tip

Skin elasticity
To see how good skin elasticity is, gently pinch a piece of skin between the fingers and release. Depending on how quickly the skin falls back into place indicates the level of elasticity. Quick retraction shows firm elasticity, slow retraction poor. A good activity is to try this on the back of the hand. Compare the skin of a young person to a very mature client.

Other factors to check for include the following.

- What is the client's occupation, and has this affected the skin in any way?
- Does their lifestyle affect their skin?
- History of the skin, origin, climate.
- Home care (or lack of it)/abuse! What is the client using and how suitable is it for their skin?
- Medication: some medication such as steroids can have an effect on the skin.

 Interesting fact

Free radicals
A young cell is a healthy cell; an ageing cell has free radical activity. Free radicals are atoms with unstable (i.e. not in pairs) electrons. The free radicals acquire electrons from other molecules around them causing a chain reaction. Anti-oxidants inactivate free radicals.

 Interesting fact

The 'smoker's face'
Half of all of smokers have this.

- A smoker's skin is between 25 and 40 per cent thinner than that of a non-smoker.
- Smoking causes vasoconstriction of arterioles thus hindering circulation.
- Free radicals build up, speeding up the signs of ageing.
- Small lines occur around the lips, especially upper lip (caused by frequent contraction of the lips) and eyes (squinting to avoid the smoke). Deeper lines may appear on the cheeks.
- Grey complexion caused by the smoke surrounding the face and entering the pores.
- Sunken cheeks (in body reading the cheeks relate to the lungs).

Basic face reading

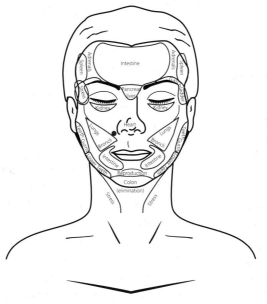

Zones of the face

Basic face reading

The face can reveal many weaknesses in the systems of the body. These can be used as guidelines for both choosing essential oils for the face as well as for guidance within other holistic treatments.

Skin congestion/blemishes	• forehead • bridge of nose • chin • groove of chin • sides of temples • by ears • along mandible • under jaw line and below ears	• digestion, stress • liver • intestine – toxic build up • cramped small intestine • related to nerves • back teeth, sinus, upper gums • lower teeth • lower teeth, glands, throat, stress
Eyes	• clear • yellowy whites • dull, lifeless, enlarged pupils	• good health • liver • tired, run down, poor general health
Sunken cheeks	• relates to lungs	• smoking, trauma and/or grief
Eye area	• look of smudged mascara under eyes • puffiness under eyes	• tired blood • poor excretion / kidney stress
Bridge of nose	• dry patches on bridge of nose	• problems with catarrh, sinuses, asthma
Base of nose and mouth	• pink skin around base of nose and/or sides of mouth	• deficiency in vitamin A, D, C, B groups

Cleansing

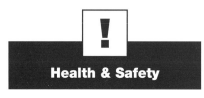

Health & Safety

If you prefer to use sponges, it is preferable to use new ones for each client as it is difficult to maintain hygiene between different clients. Chemicals and detergents may leave a residue in the sponges, which is not ideal when working on the delicate facial tissues.

Procedure for cleansing

Prior to massage, Indian head massage or aromatherapy, the skin will benefit from a simple cleanse, even if the client is not wearing make-up. A cleanse will remove any surface debris which may inhibit the penetration of the products being used. If the client is wearing make-up a deeper cleanse is advisable to ensure the skin is clean before applying products.

Cotton wool

- Damp cotton wool prevents dragging on the skin. It also makes the use of products more economical by preventing the cotton from wool absorbing excess product.
- Use large cotton wool pads. Small pads can make the treatment disjointed if there is a need to keep changing them.
- Small pads are good for cleansing the lips and eyes and for covering the eyes for relaxation.

Sponges

- Sponges should be soft and not coarse.
- Keep sponges in a gentle sterilizing fluid. Allow them to dry out once sterile and re-sterilize before use. Leaving them in chemical solutions will cause the sponge to deteriorate.

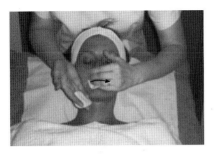

Cleansing the lips

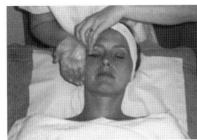

Cleansing the eyes

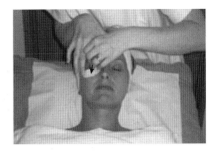

Cleansing the lashes

Health & Safety

Use the ring finger when working over the eye as this finger has the gentlest pressure. Never apply pressure over the eyeball.

Tip

If the client has stubborn eye make-up, place cleanser onto the two pads and place over the eye area. Leave this in place while you cleanse the lips. This will help to loosen the mascara

If the client is wearing lots of mascara, place a small piece of half moon-shaped cotton wool under the bottom lashes. Without the client opening their eyes, work the cleanser down the lashes onto the cotton wool; this avoids mascara marking the skin.

Cleansing the lips

Take two pads of damp cotton wool. Apply a little cleanser to one pad. Tell the client to keep their mouth closed. Support the face with one hand and wipe the lips with the cleanser. Wipe a second time with the clean pad. Alternate hands to cleanse and wipe until the lips are clean.

Cleansing the eyes

Tell the client to keep their eyes closed. Using the ring finger work over the eyelid of one eye towards the nose using gentle circular movements. Roll the finger down the lashes to loosen any mascara. Using a pad of damp cotton wool to remove the cleanser, wiping in to the nose and then down the lashes.

Ask the client to look up over your head. This will lift the tissue up below the client eye so that you can gently wipe under the eye. All make-up must be thoroughly removed

Repeat for the other eye.

Cleansing the face

For a simple, superficial cleanse

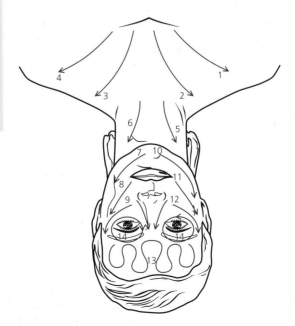

Superficial cleanse

Apply cleanser warmed in the hands to the décolleté, neck and face.

- Work across the chest using sweeping effleurage movements, take hands around the back of the neck and up around to the front of the neck.
- Use sweeping movements up the face to cleanse each side.
- Work cleanser across forehead using small circular movements.
- Circle fingers around both eyes.

Remove the cleanser with damp cotton wool, cleaning tissues or sponges. Use sweeping effleurage on the décolleté and neck. For the face, support with one hand and cleanse with the other, working up the face.

For a deep cleanse
Apply more cleanser with sweeping effleurage.

- Work across the décolleté with circular movements, effleurage up the neck and on to the face.
- Work over the mentalis on the chin using the thumbs. Work up to the corners of the mouth.
- With fingers on the chin, work out from the centre of the face with tiny circular movements to work the cleanser in. Work up the face to the eyes, working from the centre out (3 rows).
- Slide the thumbs alternately up the nose and work small circles around the nostrils and top of the lip.
- Slide middle and ring fingers up the nose and make a big circles around each eye ×6.
- Slide onto forehead and work in cleanser using small circles.
- Finish with finger on temples. Apply a little pressure and pause before lifting hands off.

Remove as for a superficial cleanse.

Procedure for toning

Place some toner onto damp cotton wool and follow the same sequence as for removal of cleanser. Not all cleansers require the use of toner. It does give the skin a fresh feeling after cleansing however.

Blot the skin dry using a tissue. Make a small hole in the centre of the tissue and place over the face, then neck, making sure that the skin is dry (especially under the nose).

Tip

The deep cleanse can be enhanced by using either a complexion brush or an exfoliating cleanser.

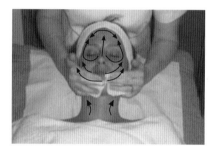

Toning the skin

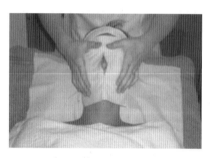

Blotting the skin

Facial massage

Before beginning this section review Chapter 8, Classification of massage techniques.

Facial massage is beneficial for the following reasons:

- it increases lymphatic and blood circulation to the skin and muscles
- it stimulates the removal of waste products and toxins from the tissues
- it increases cellular activity
- it relieves tension
- it improves the texture of the skin (desquamation)
- it promotes relaxation.

Preparing for a facial massage

Undo the headband (if used) to expose the hair.

Apply chosen medium to top of chest, neck and face with light effleurage. This may be

- a suitable carrier oil
- massage cream (non-mineral)
- blended aromatherapy oils (commercial blend or blended specifically for the individual).

Points to remember:

- Maintain contact with the skin at all times during the massage.
- Keep one hand in contact whilst you reposition the other.
- Keep the rhythm smooth and slow.
- Avoid sudden movements.
- Avoid being unduly repetitive with movements.
- Adapt pressure according the type of massage you are giving.

Commercial timing: 20 minutes is the maximum time the skin will continually absorb a medium through massage, therefore this is an ideal duration for the facial massage treatment.

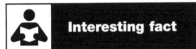

Interesting fact

During aromatherapy, parts 1 and 3 of the facial massage sequence are used to treat the client.

The massage sequence

Facial massage comprises three parts:

1 lymphatic drainage and pressure point treatment to the face, neck and décolleté
2 massage to décolleté, neck and face
3 pressure points, drainage and massage to the scalp.

Lymphatic massage and acupressure massage

(10 minutes)

Activity

Using the figure in Chapter 4, p.73, locate the position of the lymph nodes on a colleague's face and head.

- Drainage movements should be light, slow and precise, draining towards the nearest lymph nodes.
- Pressure point treatment should be slow and precise. The thumb, finger or fingers are used to apply pressure to a specified point. To apply this technique correctly, pressure should be applied as you breathe out. Working in time with your breathing will help regulate your movements. This routine uses generalized pressure points but more specific ones can be incorporated if appropriate.

1 Place hands over eyes and pause.
2 Place thumbs next to each other and apply pressure points from bridge of nose into hairline. Repeat ×3.
3 Slides thumbs along skin and up forehead along the same line. Repeat ×3.
4 Move thumbs out approx. 1 inch and repeat ×3. Repeat, moving out as far as the temples.
5 Using thumb pressure work outwards just above eyebrows. Repeat ×3. Repeat working across to cover the forehead.

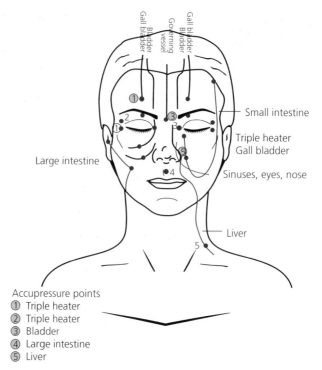

Accupressure points
① Triple heater
② Triple heater
③ Bladder
④ Large intestine
⑤ Liver

Accupressure point of the face

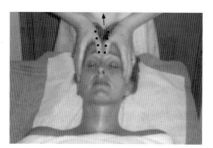

Thumb pressures

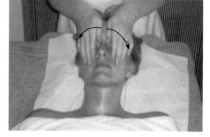

Palmar slide

6   Slide across forehead with flat palms. Repeat ×3.

7   Apply gentle pressure working along each eyebrow using a finger and thumb. Repeat ×3.

8   Using the thumb and finger slide along eyebrow to drain. Repeat ×3.

   With fingers (middle and index), apply pressure point along orbital bone. Repeat ×3.

9   Drain with the ring finger outwards along orbital bone. Repeat ×3.

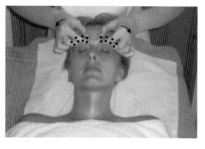

Pressure point around the eyebrow

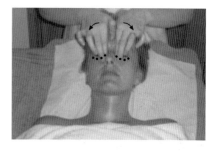

Pressure points around orbicularis oculi

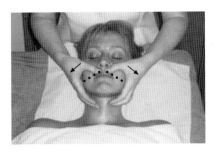

Drain along zygomatic bone

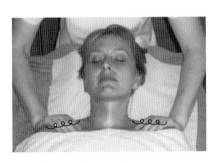

Pressure along mandible

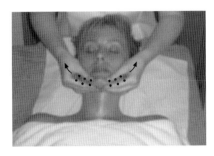

Thumb knead trapezius

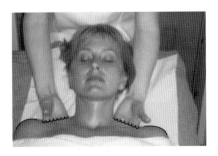

Knuckling around trapezius

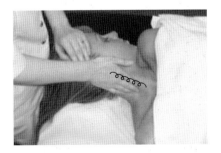

Sterno mastoid stretch

10 As above but alternate pressure then drain following first along zygomatic bone, then below (drain to ear in straight line).

11 Apply pressure point with the thumbs from under the nose out to ear.

12 Hook an index finger under the zygomatic bone (one each side), press and hold.

13 With the thumb and index finger, gentle squeeze and release along mandible. Repeat ×3.

14 Drain along mandible bone from the centre to the ears with tips of fingers and thumb. Repeat ×3.

15 Link the above movement with a palm slide across forehead creating one complete movement. Repeat ×3. Slide fingers down sternocleidomastoid on third movement to finish with fingers on the sternum.

16 Using the fingertips pump the skin above the top of sternum, across chest and under clavicle, gradually moving outwards towards axillary nodes (this is good for stimulating lymphatic flow into the lymphatic ducts).

17 Slide hands around to the back of the neck and apply pressure to base of occipital bone.

Neck and shoulders

(5–10 minutes)

1 Place hands on the top of the sternum with tips of fingers pointing down the chest. Effleurage across chest, hands divided. Take hands around top of the arms around the back of the neck to base of skull. Slide hands back around to front of the neck to sternum. Repeat ×4.

2 Divide hands; each hand effleurages out across chest. Thumb knead deltoids, turn hands and thumb knead along the trapezius up to occipital bone.

3 Repeat effleurage.

4 Knuckle across chest, from the centre out and back. Slide around deltoids and knuckle trapezius (this is good for stimulating lymphatic flow into the lymphatic ducts). *Avoid knuckling over bony areas as it is uncomfortable.*

5 Effleurage to link movement. Stroke up the back of trapezius using both hands alternately. Get the hands as far down the back as comfortable and draw the muscle up with the fingers. Stroke up the back of the neck.

6 Stroke with the fingertips along the base of the occipital bone. Support the base of skull at the occipital bone and 'ease' the spine with a gentle stretch. Do not lift the head up – it should stay flat – but the chin should tilt slightly. This should be a comfortable movement and if being performed correctly the toes should move slightly. *Avoid this movement with clients with a history of neck problems.*

7 Place fingers at the base of the occipital bone and vibrate with the fingers.

Face

(5–10 minutes)

1 Effleurage across the neck (platysma) with hands left to right. Repeat ×4. *Avoid pressure over the throat.*

2 Gently turn head to right and finger knead along sternocleidomastoid. Push shoulder down and *gently* stretch head to opposite side. Repeat for left side.

3 Effleurage along the mandible left to right. Repeat ×4.

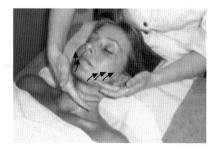

Rolling tapotemont

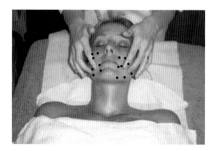

Raindrop tapotemont

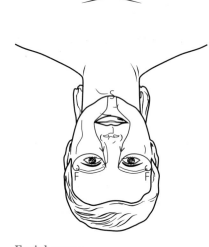

Facial sweep

4 Using alternate hands moulded to the mandible, vibrate along the mandible from left to right. Repeat ×4.

5 Knuckling under the mandible in the fleshy part behind the bone. Be careful not to touch the throat area. Repeat ×4.

6 Apply pincemont tapotement along the mandible. *Avoid on clients with vascular or sensitive skins.*

7 Thumb knead mentalis (chin).

8 Effleurage using the ring fingers around orbicularis oris, (mouth). Repeat ×4.

9 Using the ring and middle finger of both hand alternately apply a rolling movement to the lower cheek, left, then right. *Avoid on clients with vascular or sensitive skins. Good for improving skin tone along the jaw line.*

10 Apply raindrops tapotement over lower face and neck. *Avoid on clients with vascular or sensitive skins.*

11 Starting with fingers on chin, draw fingers up the sides of the nose to the bridge of the nose. Sweep hands across cheeks to temple and circle. Repeat ×4.

12 Fingers start on the chin. Draw fingers up the sides of the nose to the bridge of the nose. Fingers lift the skin or the eyebrows, slide down to the temples and circle fingers on the temples. Repeat ×4.

13 Link effleurage to slide hands to chin.

14 Corkscrew movement. Work up the face from the chin with small circles following mouth to nose line, sides of nose. Divide hands and effleurage across forehead, then slide the hands back to chin. Repeat ×4.

15 Steeple. Place hands together as if to pray. Slot hands over the chin, with fingertips pointing upwards. Move up the face and divide hands over nose, down cheeks to temples. Circle temples. Repeat ×4. On the fourth movement hands remain on temples.

16 Effleurage across the frontalis temple to temple. Repeat ×4.

17 Effleurage from the tip of the nose up the frontalis in a continuous movement, alternating hands. Repeat ×4 with each hand.

18 Scissors frictions across frontalis. One hand is placed on the temple to support the skin. The middle finger of the other hand is used to rub along the lines into the open fingers of the supporting hand. *Good for plumping up fine lines to reduce appearance.*

19 Petals. Using the ring fingers draw the shape of a petal over the forehead.

20 Divide the hands. One hand is placed on the temple to support the head whilst the other hand circles around the orbicularis oculi. Repeat ×4. Repeat for the eye.

21 Small drainage effleurage under the eye using alternate ring fingers. Repeat for other eye.

22 Place one ring finger on the left side of each eye. Circle the eyelids with the ring finger in a clockwise direction.

23 Divide hands across frontalis.

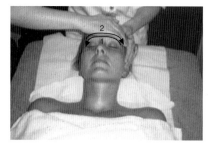

Effleurage across frontalis

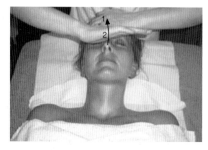

Effleurage up frontalis

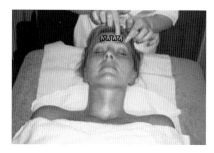

Petal shapes over frontalis

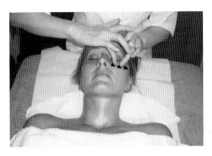

Finger drain under eye

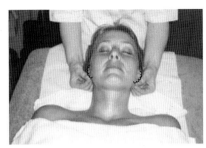

Knead ears

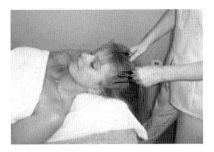

Stroking through hair

Scalp

Before beginning this section review Chapter 13, Indian head massage.

1   Slide fingers to the ears. Gently massage earlobes with fingertips, working up and around the ear cartilage.

2   From the top of each ear work the fingers onto the scalp. Using pressure point movements work over the scalp, pumping to stimulate the lymph nodes.

3   Shampooing. Massage the scalp as if washing the hair. Make sure you cover as much of the scalp as possible.

Completing an holistic facial

To finish your facial, run the fingers through the hair using a slow stroking action. Should the client not have any hair, place the hands on the head and pause.

Adaptation to massage

The routine above is for guidance. While lymphatic drainage and pressure point techniques are very similar in their routine, massage can vary enormously and there are many styles and techniques. All massage movements should be adapted to suit the client's skin type and needs.

Skin type and characteristics

● A client with a *greasy skin* will require an emphasis on calming and relaxing the skin to reduce skin activity. Avoid too much pressure, keep the pace slow and use light effleurage and minimal tapotement.

● A client with *dry skin* will require a more stimulating massage to stimulate skin activity.

● For those with *sensitive skin*, avoid overstimulation. The emphasis should be on effleurage and slow petrissage. Avoid tapotement and friction.

Age of client

Up to 20 – keep massage to a minimum, aim to relax the client; use pressure and lymphatic drainage.

20–40 – slow deep effleurage, sustained petrissage, vibrations and tapotement where indicated.

40+ – slow gentle petrissage and apply more tapotement to tone.

Gender

Male clients will need to be advised about shaving. Ideally they should shave a couple of hours before a facial so that the hair growth is minimal but the pores are not open.

Massage movements should include pressure and drainage movements. With massage, if there is facial hair you will need to work around this or alter the direction of your movement in the direction of hair growth to avoid irritating the skin.

Temperament

If the client is of a nervous temperament, keep the massage slow and rhythmic; avoid tapotement and any sudden movements.

Masks

This part of the facial is optional. A mask is not really necessary with this facial but it does provide the opportunity of further relaxation for the client. A mask can be applied to achieve virtually any effect you choose. Effects include:

- cleansing
- desquamation
- stimulation
- soothing
- nourishment
- peeling.

A mask can be classified as:

- *setting:* includes clays and plastic type masks – these are applied in an even layer and dry or set to form a firm layer on the skin.
- *non-setting:* includes biological fruit, etc. – as the name suggests these do not set and are soft in texture.
- *specialized:* includes thermal and warm oil – these may be setting or non-setting and usually offer more remedial properties.

Application of a mask

The most appropriate time to apply a mask will depend on the products being used. Traditionally the mask is applied after the massage, allowing the client time to relax. Some products may recommend application before the massage to deepen the effects of cleansing. The client should wear a headband to avoid getting mask products in the hair.

The type of mask being applied will affect the method used to apply it. Most masks can be applied with a brush in preference to fingers! This facilitates easy application and gives even coverage.

- If you are using a setting clay mask leave a good residue of massage medium on the skin as this will help make it easier remove the mask once it has set.
- Don't mix clay masks with your mask brush; use a spatula to avoid the bristles getting clogged up.
- Always apply the mask evenly, especially around the edges.
- Loosen masks with damp sponges by blotting over the face first. Once the mask is damp it will be easier to remove.

Tip

Place a piece of tissue across the hairline and fasten the headband. Fold the tissue back over the headband. This will help to protect the headband and facilitate removal of the mask.

The mask can be applied direct to the skin without removing the massage medium. Warn the client that you are about to apply their mask.

Apply the mask, working from the bottom of the neck, upwards onto the face. Apply to the face, leaving a gap around the hairline, nostril, mouth and eyes (unless the mask is suitable for application in the eye area). Cover the eyes with damp cotton wool discs and pull the towel or blanket up over the client's shoulders to keep them warm. Leave the client to relax.

Removing the mask

By the time it comes to removal of the mask the client may be in a deeply relaxed state or even asleep. You don't want to surprise them. Place one hand on the client so that they are aware you are there and then tell the client you are going to remove their mask. Start at the lowest point and work up the face. If you are using sponges, change the water frequently. Cleanse one final time with damp cotton wool and check that the entire mask has been removed (check nostrils, ears, under the chin and in the creases of the neck).

Finishing the facial

Freshen the skin with a suitable tonic; this will also make sure that the skin is clean and free from any traces of the massage medium or mask if used. Blot the skin dry with tissue. Apply a moisturizer suitable for the client's skin type as this will give the skin protection when the client leaves. To apply, warm the moisturizer a little in the fingertips and smooth onto the skin with light effleurage movements. Blot the skin with a tissue if there is any excess cream and in order to remove any shine.

Remove the headband if used and slowly sit the client up. Leave them to sit for a few minutes to adjust. You can use this time to give them some further treatment or home/after care advice.

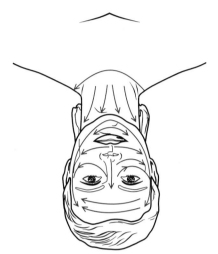

Application of a mask

Contra actions and after care

There are only a few adverse reactions to a facial.

If you have used the correct products for your client's skin you should have no adverse contra actions. If the client is sensitive to a product used they are more likely to react within 20 minutes than hours later. If the client complains of their skin feeling unusually hot or tingling (unless the product used indicates that this is normal), irritation or the skin becomes very red, remove the product. Use lukewarm water until all traces of the product have been removed. Do not continue with the facial as further stimulation may make the reaction worse.

If the skin is prone to spots and blemishes, a few additional spots may be noticed but these will come and go much quicker than normal.

To ensure you are familiar with general contra actions, go to Chapter 5, p.137.

After care, further treatments and advice

To ensure you are familiar with general after care, go to Chapter 5, p.141.

If the treatment is being carried out towards the end of the day the client need not do anything further to their skin. If the facial is carried out in the morning the client still needs to follow their skin care routine that evening.

Advise the client to leave the skin clear of any make-up for at least eight hours, and longer if possible. The skin has been cleansed and the circulation is active so you want to give the skin time to benefit from this. If you have a female client who insists on applying make-up tell them to restrict it to lipstick and eyes.

Advise the client about further treatments. This is a good opportunity to introduce them to other treatments as well as further facials.

The client should ideally have regular facials to maximize the benefits. Taking the client's financial constraints into consideration, recommend the following:

- treatment of a specific skin problem once a week for six weeks
- up to age 25, once a season
- 25+, minimum once a month.

Give them a simple skin care routine to follow at home and encourage them to follow it. To receive maximum benefits the client needs understand that they must look after their skin and that a facial is a supplement and boost to their routine, not an all damage and repair fix!

Treatment records

When you have completed your treatment, record in detail all the products you have used. This is important just in case the client has a reaction so that you can avoid the products in the future. It is also useful for follow-up treatments so that you know what to use again or, should the client fancy a change, what alternatives you can try.

Tip

If you have samples of products then give the client one to take home to use. Only offer samples that are suitable for the client's needs and ones that the client may be interested in purchasing. Make a note of the samples you have given them on the client's record card and follow this up on their next treatment by asking what they thought about the product.

Knowledge review

1 Compare and contrast the difference between an oily and a dry skin.

2 What is the difference between dry skin and dehydrated skin?

3 State the contra indications you would look for before starting a facial.

4 What hygiene precautions would you take before, during and after a facial.

5 How would you sell the benefits to your client of the following treatments:
   (a) cleansing?
   (b) moisturizing?

6 When and how would you adapt your massage techniques?

7 What precautions will you take while performing your facial massage?

8 Make a list of all the masks you have access to and:
   (a) state whether the mask is setting, non-setting or specialized
   (b) state what effect and benefit the mask has.

9 What after care and advice would you give a client after a facial?

Indian head massage

Learning objectives

This chapter covers the following:

- **a history of Indian head massage**
- **contra indications to Indian head massage**
- **preparation of therapist, client and treatment room**
- **physical and psychological benefits of Indian head massage**
- **oils used in Indian head massage**
- **the massage routine**
- **adapting the massage for different individuals**
- **specific after care advice**

In India, where Indian head massage is known as champissage, you can receive a head massage almost anywhere – on street corners, in barbers and hairdressers, on the beach, and particularly in the home where it is used for bonding and relaxation among family members.

In the West it is used more as a stress management treatment. Indian head massage is a relaxing and calming treatment which, as its name suggests, concentrates on massage to the head but also includes massage to the arms, shoulders and neck where we tend to accumulate the most stress and tension, and also incorporates a facial massage. Indian head massage is an extremely versatile, non-invasive treatment and as such is the perfect introduction to massage. It is performed seated in an appropriate chair with the client fully clothed.

A history of Indian head massage

Massage can be traced back through all cultures. The ancient Greeks and Romans used massage as their principal means of pain relief and healing. It is said that Julius Caesar was treated daily by being pinched all over to relieve neuralgia and headaches. In India, massage has been practised for over 4000 years and early Ayurvedic texts feature massage as one of the principles of Ayurvedic medicine (see Chapter 3, p.34). It promoted the belief that health results from the harmony within oneself, and produced a sacred book called the *Ayur Veda* – the Art of Life. The tradition of massage in India dates back to the beginnings of Hinduism, which has been the main religion of India for almost 2000 years. Massage in India is a way of life. Babies receive a daily massage until they are three years old to promote bonding between child and mother. This daily massage is reduced to two or three times a week until the age of seven at which age they start to massage their younger siblings, parents and grandparents. Massage in India is a family activity with everyone joining in, and is used for relaxation, bonding, and for ceremonial and social events.

Contra indications to Indian head massage

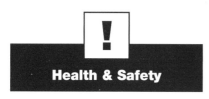

Health & Safety

Cross-infection
Cross-infection occurs when micro-organisms are transferred from one person to another, usually through personal touch. Cross-infection can happen if sterilization procedures are not carried out properly.

Contra indications to Indian head massage are similar to those for other massage treatments. It is important that you check thoroughly for these at the consultation stage, as inappropriate treatment may incur risk to the client, the therapist and other clients. The most common risk during Indian head massage is that of cross-infection so it is vital to identify any infections and/or contagious scalp conditions before beginning the massage.

It is important for a therapist to be able to recognize non-infectious and non-contagious skin conditions. See Chapter 4, pp.47–56, for further information on these conditions.

Preparation of therapist, client and treatment room

Tip

You do not want the client thinking the massage has finished when you are still working on the chakras, as this may spoil the total effect of the massage. Remember to advise the client at the consultation stage that you will be working with the chakras and that the massage is not complete until you come around to the front of the client and speak to them.

Therapist

Do as much as you can before your client arrives. Have a consultation card ready for completion, and have the selection of oils ready to show and discuss with the client. Make sure there is enough room to work comfortably. The client will be sitting in a chair but the therapist needs to be able to move around the chair as treatment positions are not only carried out standing behind the client, but also on both sides, and you need to come to the front of the client at the end of the massage.

Client

Carry out a full consultation to ensure there are no contra indications and that the client is suitable for treatment. Make sure the client is not only comfortable in the chair but that their feet can reach the ground. If they cannot, place a small cushion under the feet so they are not dangling. The client should not sit with crossed legs as this will disturb the flow of energy. Remove all jewellery before you start, particularly earrings, nose rings and necklaces, and place these in a safe and secure place, preferably in view of the client. If the client appears to have any hairdressing product on the hair, you may ask them to brush their hair to remove any residue. Glasses should be removed.

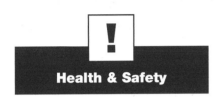

Health & Safety

Adjustable chairs
Many adjustable chairs have wheels fitted. If using a chair with wheels to perform Indian head massage, supervise the client when sitting down and standing up in case of movement.

Treatment room

As with any holistic treatment, the room should be warm, with dimmed lights and appropriate music (see Chapter 5, p.124). It is not recommended that you burn aromatherapy oils when carrying out an Indian head massage treatment. As stated below, leave the essential oils to an aromatherapy treatment. You may, with the consent of your client (and the salon manager), burn an incense stick to really set the scene. Have a small rolled-up towel to hand to place behind client's neck, ready for the facial massage. Have to hand also some water to offer the client immediately after the massage. An important factor in preparing the room for Indian head massage is the type of chair to be used. The best type of chair would be an adjustable one to suit the height of the client and therapist. A suitable chair would be one with a relatively low back and without arm rests, or with low arm rests. A *director's chair* is a good choice.

Physical and psychological benefits of Indian head massage

Physical benefits

- General feeling of well-being, calmness and relaxation.
- Improved blood circulation – massage increases the flow of oxygen and other nutrients into the tissues of the body and the brain, encouraging healing and better concentration.
- Helps improve muscle tone.
- Relieves muscular tension.
- Improves respiration by encouraging deeper breathing.
- Stimulates nerve endings which relieves muscular pain and fatigue.
- Softer and regenerated skin – sebaceous secretions are stimulated and the removal of dead skin cells (desquamation) is accelerated. The layers of the skin are stimulated, which improves their cellular function.
- Relieves physical and emotional stress.
- Helps to relieve eyestrain and tension headaches.
- Encourages hair growth.
- Helps relieve sinus problems.
- Stimulates lymphatic system.
- General relaxation – giving rise to better sleep and more concentration.

Psychological benefits

- ☙ The nature of the massage helps to relieve stress, anxiety and depression by its uplifting effect.

- ☙ Creates a balanced feeling in the whole body.

- ☙ Refreshes and revitalizes the mind and body.

- ☙ Emotional release may be experienced by the client.

Oils used in Indian head massage

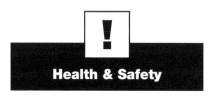

Health & Safety

Essential oils

Use only oils suitable for Indian head massage. Essential oils are not suitable for Indian head massage and should never be used undiluted on the scalp. Essential oils should only be blended by qualified aromatherapists for aromatherapy massage.

In traditional Indian head massage, oil is used by both men and women to keep the hair lustrous and in good condition. The oil is used on the scalp only and is applied directly to the scalp using the pads of the fingers in a 'shampooing' movement. The four main oils used in Indian head massage are almond, coconut, mustard and sesame. Olive oil can also be used, as it also has many beneficial properties, but its aroma is not as pleasant as the other oils and it can be described as a heavy oil. It is recommended that only these specially formulated organic vegetable oils be used for Indian head massage, as they are partially absorbed through the pores of the skin. Essential oils are not suitable for Indian head massage and should be used only during an aromatherapy body massage treatment.

The choice of oil is selected at the consultation stage – *remember to check for any nut allergies*. While using an oil is not compulsory they should be recommended not only for their therapeutic properties but to keep the massage as traditional as possible. Clients should be recommended to leave the oil on the scalp for at least 12 hours to gain the maximum benefit. If this is not possible, then even a couple of hours will be of some benefit. While all the oils have their own specific benefits, generally using an oil strengthens the hair. This is done partly by removing dryness, which is responsible for brittle hair and for some scalp disorders, and by softening the skin of the scalp, which promotes hair growth, slows down hair loss and encourages vibrant, shiny and healthy hair.

Almond oil

Almond oil is an excellent choice for Indian head massage. It is a light oil, high in nutrients and ideal for clients with either normal hair and scalp conditions or for clients who have dry hair as a result of chemical treatments.

Coconut oil

Coconut oil is very moisturizing and is a popular choice for Indian head massage. It is a medium to light oil with a wonderful aroma. As with almond oil above, it is excellent for use after chemical treatments on the hair, and also helps to relieve inflammation.

Mustard oil

Unlike almond and coconut, mustard oil is a hot, sharp and pungent oil, and an excellent choice for relieving pains and swellings, helping to relax stiff muscles and for clearing the sinuses. The effects of mustard oil are warming on the body and it is an excellent choice for use in winter. Take care when using mustard oil as its effects are very intense and stimulating.

Sesame oil

Sesame oil is a good general oil to choose for Indian head massage. It is said to be effective in preventing the hair from turning grey and there are claims that it can restore hair to its natural colour. This oil is very popular with Indian families practising champissage and helps to relieve swelling and muscular pain. Sesame oil is high in the minerals iron and phosphorus.

Olive oil

Olive oil is a heavy, strong-smelling oil, but is particularly beneficial for an excessively dry scalp. It has many stimulating properties which increase heat in the body, thereby helping to reduce swellings and alleviate muscular tightness and pain.

The massage routine

 Activity

Students: identify individual movements from the Indian head massage and put them into their appropriate categories.

The categories of massage used in Indian head massage are similar to those used for traditional body massage, full descriptions of which can be found in Chapter 8, p.186. These include effleurage, petrissage, tapotement, frictions and vibrations.

The massage is divided into six parts:

- shoulder massage
- arm massage
- neck massage
- scalp massage
- face massage
- balancing the chakras.

Length and frequency of treatment

Indian head massage is very versatile and can be offered as taster sessions of 15 minutes in a workplace environment or at health fairs. A 30-minute version of the massage seems popular if time is short, but by far the most benefits would be received from a whole treatment, including the chakra balancing, which could take up to an hour in total. The treatment described below consists of 40 minutes of hands-on treatment. If you require a shorter treatment time you can decrease the number of repetitions for each movement. You will need to add on consultation time at the beginning and after care, payment and re-booking time at the end.

If being used as part of a stress management programme, the massage should be performed between two and three times a week for maximum benefit. Offer clients a course of treatment at a specially reduced price. The frequency of the treatment may vary according to a client's time and financial circumstances but they should be encouraged to attend for treatments as often as possible. The massage should be tailored to suit individual requirements. You may wish to omit the facial massage and chakra balancing if clients are returning immediately to work and would probably choose to use no massage scalp oil on these occasions.

Indian head massage routine

 Tip

The therapist should take the opportunity of taking three deep breaths too, at the same time as the client, in order to prepare for and focus on the massage ahead.

Before commencing the massage ensure your client is sitting comfortably in an upright position on a straight-backed chair. Feet should be flat on the floor. The client may be more comfortable if shoes are removed and tight waistbands and collars loosened. The arms should be relaxed and the hands resting comfortably in the lap.

When you are ready to start, place your hands lightly on the client's shoulders as your initial contact, then, resting your hands very lightly upon your client's head, ask them to take three deep breaths in order to centre and prepare for treatment.

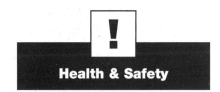

Health & Safety

The massage should always be appropriate to the client's needs and be carried out in a rhythmic and continuous sequence.

There follows a range of popular movements suitable for Indian massage, and the breakdown of timings given as an indication. However, there is no right or wrong way and the sequence of movements may vary from one therapist to another.

- Shoulder massage: 7 minutes
- Arm massage: 4 minutes
- Neck massage: 10 minutes
- Scalp massage: 10 minutes
- Face massage: 5 minutes
- Balancing the chakras: 4 minutes

Shoulder massage

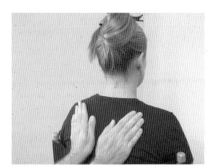

Effleurage

1 *Effleurage.* The massage commences with light effleurage to the shoulders. Using both hands and starting in the centre of the back, work from between the shoulder blades, up the centre of the back, out over the shoulders, returning to the centre and your starting position. Repeat approximately ×6.

2 *Heel rub.* With one hand resting on the client's shoulder, use the heel of the other hand in a side-to-side action to rub over the client's shoulder. Following the shape of the scapula, work down between the scapula and the spine, and around the bottom of the scapula before working back on yourself and to your starting position. You will be working in a large C shape around the scapula. Repeat ×3 before repeating for the other side.

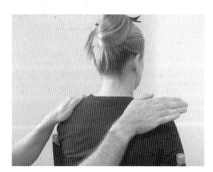

Heel rub

3 *Fingers rub.* Repeat the above movements with the pads of the fingers, using side-to-side movements. Repeat to other side.

4 *Effleurage.* Repeat as for step 1.

5 *Thumb pushes.* Use the thumbs only, with both hands together over the top of the shoulder (across the garment seam area) from the back to the front. Place your thumbs above the scapula, and gently push forward over the ridge of the trapezius muscle resting at the collor bone to the front. Repeat ×6, moving towards the base of the neck as you do so.

6 *Finger pulls.* Use the index fingers only, with both hands together over the top of the shoulder (across the garment seam area) from the front to the back. a reversal of the movement described above. Your thumbs can be placed behind the shoulder as an anchor, drawing your fingers towards them.

7 *Squeezing.* Having pushed forward and pulled back the ridge of the trapezius muscle, you are now going to pick up and hold the muscle. Using fingerpads and the heel of the hand (thumbs and fingertips

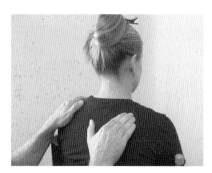

Fingers rub

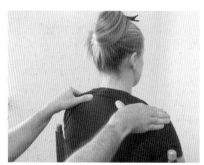

Thumb pushes

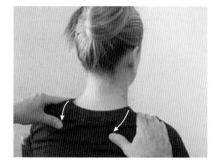

Finger pulls

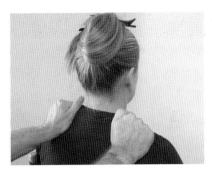

Squeezing

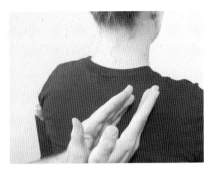

Hacking

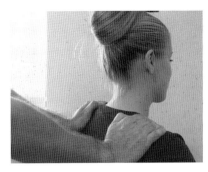

Hands resting before continuing
with next sequence

would pinch), pick up the muscle for a slow count of four before gently releasing. Repeat this ×4.

8 *Hacking.* Using traditional hacking movements hack over the entire area of the upper back and shoulder area, avoiding any bony areas and concentrating on the muscular areas.

9 *Effleurage.* As steps 1 and 4.

10 *Rest hands* gently upon the client's shoulders for a deliberate pause before moving on to the next part of the massage. Do not rush between sections.

Arm massage

1 *Squeezing to upper arm.* Standing to the side of the client, place your fingers to the front (around biceps) and your thumbs to the back (around triceps) and squeeze these two muscles together. Work from the top of the arm to the elbow, before sliding up to the top of the arm. Repeat ×4. Maintaining contact with the client, walk around the back of the client and repeat for the other arm.

2 *Heel rolls to upper arm.* Standing behind client, and working with both hands, place hands around the top upper arm of client and with the heel of your hand behind and your fingers in front. Roll the heel of your hand around the arm towards the fingers (as if you were pushing the triceps towards the front of the arm).

3 *Kneading the backs of upper arms.* Standing behind the client, knead the triceps. Fingers pointing downwards, and working from back to front and from the upper arm to the elbow.

4 *Ironing.* After the firm movements of the first three moves, gently iron up and down the arms. Using the palmar surface of the whole of your hand gently rub up and down, working both the anterior and posterior line of the upper arms. Use gentle pressure from the elbows up to the shoulders, releasing pressure as you go downwards.

Tip

Posture
Maintain a good working position at all times to prevent backache. Bend your knees! Do not bend from the waist!

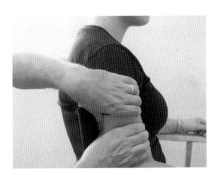

Squeeezing to upper arm

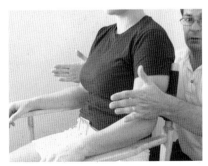

Heel rolls to upper arm

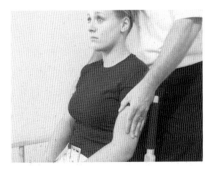

Kneading the backs of upper arms

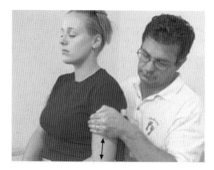

Ironing

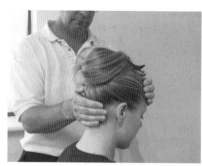

Head rocks

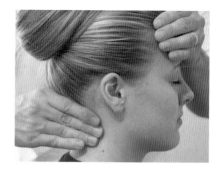

Kneading

5 *Rest hands* gently upon client's shoulders for a deliberate pause, before moving on to the next part of the massage. Do not rush between sections.

Neck massage

1 *Head rocks.* Standing to the side of the client, place one hand over the forehead/hairline of the client and the other hand across the nape of the neck. Gently rock the head forwards, backwards and return to the centre. Repeat ×3. The head should move quite easily but if it does not, you can take this opportunity to ask the client to take a further three deep breaths. Repeat the move and the head should move more easily. The more easily the head moves, the more the client is relaxed.

2 *Kneading.* Continue to stand at the side of the client with hands in same position as for step 1 above. Tip the head slightly backwards. This time knead the back of the client's neck with a 'grasp and pull back' motion. If the client is wearing a shirt/blouse with a collar, the collar may be put up and you can knead over it. Work down the length of the neck.

3 *Heel of hand rub.* Continue to stand at the side of the client with hands in same position – supporting the head at the front with head tilted slightly backwards. Use the heel of your hand to execute a vertical friction movement along the base of the occipital bone, working from ear to ear.

4 *Fingers extension rub.* As for step 3 but this time with three fingers extended, still working along the base of occipital bone, working from ear to ear.

5 *Soothing.* With working hand relaxed, gently soothe the back of the neck area.

Tip

Tipping the head slightly backwards keeps the upper part of the trapezius muscles relaxed, therefore making the movement more effective.

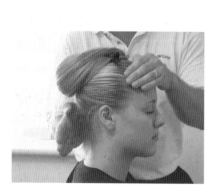

Heel of hand rub

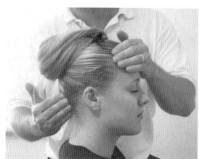

Fingers extension rub

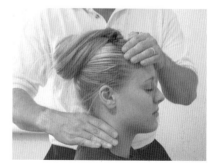

Soothing

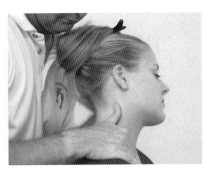

Thumb pushes to neck

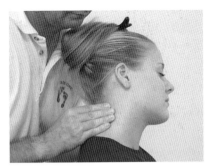

Finger pulls back

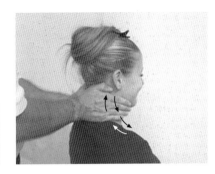

Smoothing down

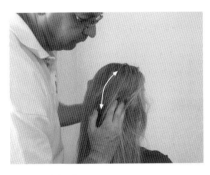

Heel rub frictions

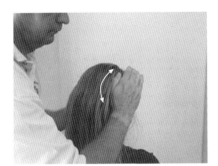

Finger frictions

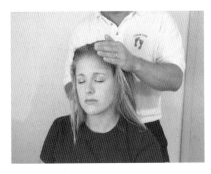

Heel rub frictions – half the head

6 *Thumb pushes to neck.* Standing behind the client, very gently tilt the head a little to the left, supporting with the left hand. The weight of the client's head should be in the therapist's left hand. Starting at the base of the neck, and using the thumb of the right hand, push thumb towards front of neck for a couple of inches, working up the neck to the top of the ear. Repeat from base to ear ×3.

7 *Finger pulls back.* With three fingers extended pull back the neck muscles towards the nape of the neck, starting at the base of the neck and working upwards to the top of the ear.

8 *Gently return head to centre.* Repeat steps 6 and 7 to the other side.

9 *Smoothing down.* Starting at the tips of the shoulders, use the whole of your palmar surface to make a long sweeping movement along the shoulder and up the neck until you reach the occipital bone, before returning to your starting point. Use gentle pressure on the upwards sweep, releasing it on the way down. The movement should be flowing and should be repeated ×4.

10 *Rest hands* gently upon client's shoulders for a deliberate pause, before moving on to the next part of the massage. Do not rush between sections.

Scalp massage

1 *Apply oil.* If you are using oil, now is the time to apply it. The oil will have been selected at the consultation stage and a very small amount placed in a small dish, close to your working area, ready for use. Dip pads of fingers into oil and transfer to other fingers before applying to scalp area in gentle shampooing movements. Try to do this without leaving contact with the client.

2 *Heel rub frictions.* Standing behind the client, supporting the head with your non-working hand, use the heel of your working hand to make short side-to-side movements from the front hairline, working back around the ear to the nape of the neck. Lift hand and replace gently in starting position and repeat ×4.

3 *Finger frictions.* Do not change your position. Repeat step 2 using the pads of the fingers, again making short side-to-side movements from the front hairline, working back around the ear to the nape of the neck. Lift hand and replace gently in starting position and repeat ×4.

4 Repeat steps 2 and 3 for the other side.

5 *Heel rub frictions –.* As for step 1. This time you are working on half of the client's head. From an imaginary centre parting, work side to side from parting to ear, and from the front of the head to the back. When you reach the back of the neck, lift your hand and replace at the front and repeat ×4. Repeat for the other side of head, working 'half the head' to the other side.

6 *Whole head sweep.* Stand at side of the client and with your non-working hand on the client's forehead as support, use the whole of the

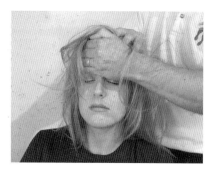

Whole head sweep

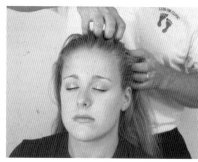

Raking the scalp

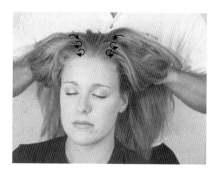

Shampooing

Tip

The purpose of the ruffling movements is to gently but deliberately keep the client's hair off the face.

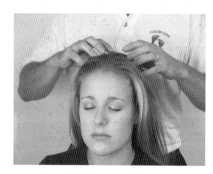

Tapping

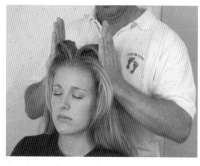

Squeeze and lift

palmar surface of the hand to sweep from the front of the head to the back, with your hand touching both ears as you move over the whole of the head. Lift hand and replace at front and repeat movement ×4.

7   *Raking the scalp.* Using both hands in alternating movements, 'rake' the fingers through the hair, bringing the hair back into some kind of order. This move can be made any time the hair needs tidying up.

8   *Shampooing.* Holding the hands in a claw-like shape and using the pads of your fingers, make circular movements with your fingers as you work over the whole scalp. Apply medium pressure during this movement and imagine that you are massaging the oil you applied earlier into the scalp.

9   *Tapping.* Using a light drumming action, and starting at the front hairline, gently cover the whole head, working with both hands at the same time.

10 *Squeeze and lift.* Standing behind your client, place your hands on either side of the head, just above the ear. Thread your fingers through the hair if necessary, to ensure that your hands are resting on the scalp – your fingers should be pointing towards the ceiling. Using both hands together, gently squeeze the head and move the scalp upwards. Hold the squeeze for a couple of seconds before gently releasing. Repeat the same movement at the temple areas and just behind the ear. You may have to adjust the angle of your hands to get a 'grip'. The scalp should actually move when you are carrying out this movement. Carry out the movement ×3 for each area.

11 *Circular temple frictions.* Using the pads of the fingers, circle around the temple area. For the best effect the circles should go upwards as you pass over the temple, and downwards and you come through the hair. There should be no movement of the client's skin – your fingers are just skimming the surface with this calming and soothing movement and it should be done with very little pressure.

12 *Rest both hands* on head to complete scalp massage.

Face massage

Before commencing the face massage, you will need to stand very close to the back of the client's chair. You may need a small rolled-up towel to place behind the client's neck, before gently tilting the client's head back onto your chest. Take care not to tilt the head back too far as this will be uncomfortable for the client. You will not be able to see the whole area of the face you will be working on, so you will have to rely on your sense of touch.

1   *Palmar placing.* Before commencing the facial massage, gently touch the areas of the face you will be working on.

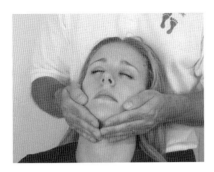

Palmar placing (a)

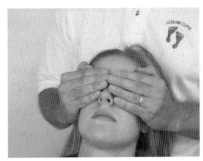

Palmar placing (b)

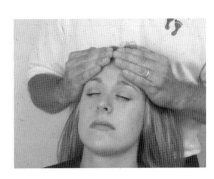

Palmar placing (c)

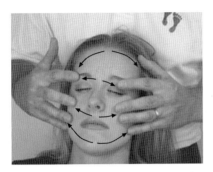

Feathering

(a) Start by placing the heel of your hand gently over the ears, and cup the lower jaw bone with the rest of your hand. Your fingertips should just touch the centre of the chin.

(b) Swivel your hands gently round until the fingers lie over the closed eyes. Your fingertips should now be just touching at the bridge of the nose.

(c) Move your hands upward to cover the temples and the forehead area.

2   *Feathering.* Using your fingerpads and feather-light strokes, work from the mid-line of the face towards the ears, then from the forehead down to the chin.

3   *Pressure points: the forehead.* With the client's head resting on your chest, and using the pads of the index or middle fingers, your starting point is at the centre of the forehead. You will be working three lines from the eyebrows to the hairline. The movement is 'press, release and slide'. When you press, you are applying medium pressure, holding for approximately four seconds before releasing and sliding up to the next position. Move up the forehead in a straight line, towards the hairline. Once at the hairline, lift fingers and replace in the centre of the eyebrows, to start the second row up towards the hairline. Finally, lifting fingers again once you reach the hairline, replace fingers at the outside edge of eyebrows to work a final line up towards the hairline.

4   *Pressure points: the eye sockets.* Return to your starting position of in between the eyebrows. This time you are going to work over the eyebrow from the middle to the outside continuing with your 'press, release and slide' movements, using both hands. Once at the outside edge, continue working under the eye, still around the eye socket, taking care not to stretch the skin. Once at the inside edge of the eye, slide fingers up towards the bridge of the nose and repeat the movement ×3.

5   *Pressure points: the cheekbones.* Linking the above movement to follow on smoothly from the last movement, glide your fingers down the sides of the nose to the indent at the sides of the nostrils. Feel for a point at the end of the cheekbone and slightly under it. Continue to use the

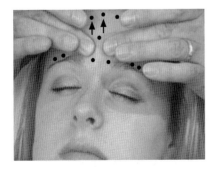

Pressure points – forehead

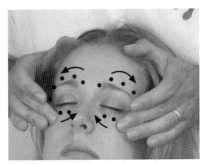

Pressure points – eye sockets

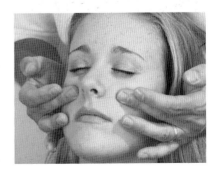

Pressure points – cheekbones

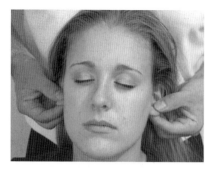

Massaging the ears

pads of either your index or middle fingers for these movements, still using the 'press, release and slide' as for the previous facial movements. Complete the movement by sweeping lightly along the cheekbones towards and behind the ear for draining purposes.

6 *Circular temple frictions*. Repeat step 11 from the scalp massage.

7 *Massaging the ears*. Beginning with the ear lobe, and using the thumb and fingers and small circular movements, work your way up and around the ear. Work up and down the ear a few times, gently squeezing and pulling and generally twiddling.

8 *Return head to upright position*. Gently return head to the upright position, removing the small towel, and complete the facial massage by resting both hands on the head. The massage may finish here or you may continue with chakra balancing.

If the massage ends with the facial massage, the hands would be returned to the shoulders, and the massage would be completed by some gentle kneading of the back of the neck and some effleurage movements to the back, before coming to the front of the client to quietly tell them that the treatment is complete.

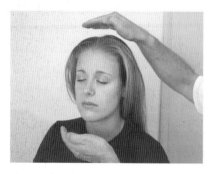

Chakra balancing – the base Chakra

Chakra balancing

While not compulsory, balancing the chakras at the end of an Indian head massage treatment gives depth and completeness to the treatment. Many books on Indian head massage will recommend you work with the three higher chakras only at the conclusion of a massage – these are the throat, brow and crown. However, for the extra few minutes it takes, it is highly recommended that you work with all seven of the major chakras, starting with the base and completing at the crown. This will not only help restore harmony and energy to the client but will also serve to ground the client before they leave the salon to continue their day.

For further information see Chapter 3, p.30.

Adapting the massage for different individuals

As with other forms of massage, all clients are treated as individuals and have different needs. As such you may need to adapt the massage to suit different people. Here are a few examples how to do this:

Men generally need a firmer massage than women do. Their muscles tend to be larger and firmer. The therapist may need to use more of their body weight to achieve the required result.

Clients who are thin and bony will need the pressure alleviated and tapotement movements avoided, otherwise the massage may become extremely painful and uncomfortable.

For *clients with tight and contracted muscles*, tapotement movements should be avoided. The movements should be slow, with a slight pressure applied to try and stretch the muscles, making the area more supple.

For *clients with slack muscles*, such areas require the stimulating tapotement movements to increase circulation and help tone up the area.

Those *clients who are returning to work* should not be made too relaxed to return to a working environment. You may decide not to use scalp oil, or not to massage the face (so as not to disturb any make-up being worn). You may decide not to do the chakra balancing. You would end the massage with more stimulating movements than usual to invigorate the client before returning to work.

As stated at the start of this chapter, Indian head massage is an extremely versatile, non-invasive treatment. Use your imagination to adapt the massage to suit all clients.

After care advice for Indian head massage

Immediately after the treatment offer the client a glass of water, and encourage sitting quietly for a few minutes before gently standing up. Recommend oil is left in hair for next 12 hours, or as long as practicable.

Evaluating the treatment is of great importance for you as a therapist. Feedback should be recorded on client's record card, and the treatment plan revised as necessary.

Knowledge review

1 What is the Indian word used to describe Indian head massage?

2 Describe the sitting position of your client that will allow him or her to gain maximum benefit from the treatment.

3 Why should the client not sit with crossed legs?

4 Name four physical benefits of Indian head massage.

5 Name four psychological benefits of Indian head massage.

6 What is the benefit of the deep breathing before commencement of massage?

7 When carrying out the 'grasp and pull back' movement on the neck, what is the head position of the client and why is it important?

8 What is the main purpose of the 'raking' movement?

9 What should you do before commencing the facial massage?

10 At which stage of the massage do you apply the oil?

11 Name three benefits of using oils for scalp massage.

12 For which oils must you carry out an allergy test?

13 Which oil would be suitable to use on a cold day for a client suffering with sinusitis?

14 Why are organic vegetable oils preferred for treatments?

15 What after care advice should you give your client at the end of the treatment? healing crisis?

16 How might you adapt the massage to suit the following:
(a) an elderly, thin and bony woman?
(b) a strong, muscular man?
(c) areas of slack muscles?
(d) on clients returning to work?

14 Reflexology

Learning objectives

This chapter will cover the following:

- **a brief history of reflexology**
- **what reflexology is and how it works**
- **mapping the feet**
- **reading the feet**
- **treatment techniques**
- **preparing for treatment**
- **contra indications to reflexology treatment**
- **a reflexology treatment**
- **treating the hands**

Before reading this chapter review the following chapters:

- Chapter 4, Anatomy and physiology
- Chapter 5, Client care
- Chapter 8, Classification of massage techniques.

Chapter 14 will introduce you to reflexology, a divine treatment that uses pressure techniques on a small area of the body achieving profound results. It will help to restore the body's equilibrium and balance the mind and spirit. This chapter will take you through the treatment process, from mapping the foot (and hand) to treatment techniques and practices, so that you can offer a safe and effective reflexology treatment.

A brief history of reflexology

Massaging feet like so many other therapies is an ancient art dating back 2500 years. Egyptian hieroglyphics and papyrus show hand and foot treatments. The Chinese have used pressure point techniques for even longer, even though these were incorporated in full body treatments such as acupuncture and shiatsu. Even the Cherokee Indians have passed down treatment techniques for healing using the feet.

Reflexology as a treatment in its own right is still new. Its development into the treatment we know today began at the turn of the twentieth century when Dr William Fitzgerald, an American ear, nose and throat specialist, developed zone therapy. He discovered that applying pressure to certain parts of the body, in particular the hands and feet, could give pain relief. He divided the body into ten zones, each zone linked organs and the energy flow between the zones. Fitzgerald further refined his findings before a colleague, Dr Riley, and Riley's wife added the three transverse zones.

Eunice Ingham, a physiotherapist, joined the Rileys and moved away from zone theory to develop a foot map pinpointing the bodies, organs and systems of the feet. This is the basis of reflexology as we know it today. Doreen Bailey, a student of Ingham, bought the theories to England in the 1960s.

There are now several variations of the foot map produced by different schools of training – this only goes to demonstrate that our feet, like each of us, are individual.

What is reflexology and how does it work?

Reflexology is an holistic treatment that works on the feet and/or hands to balance the whole body. It includes both massage and pressure point techniques to have an effect on the energy pathways or reflex zones of the body. Each part of the foot corresponds to a part or an area of the body. Our anatomy and physiology of the human body can fit neatly into the shape of the feet. The points on the left foot correspond to the left side of the body and those on the right to the right side.

Energy may be deficient, stagnated or in excess, and reflexology aims to create balance and harmony in the systems of the body. Where there is congestion or imbalance these can be detected through changes in the feet or hands.

Like so many other therapies there are some vague scientific explanations as to how the treatment actually works but little research has been carried out to date. Part of the scientific issue for those who are broadminded enough is that we do not currently have the technology to prove these theories!

The benefits and effects of reflexology

- Reflexology has an holistic approach it balances energy in order to return the body to a state of equilibrium on a mental and emotional as well as physical level.
- Circulation is increased, particularly micro-circulation, even though only the feet are physically massaged. Stimulation of the circulatory points encourages a more effective circulation.

- The lymph system is boosted, improving immunity and the removal of toxins and impurities from the tissues.
- The treatment encourages the body to eliminate toxins and impurities and this can be seen by an increase in the activity of the kidneys and digestive system.
- It is deeply relaxing, relieving mental and physical fatigue.
- In a deeply relaxed state the body initiates it own healing forces (reflexology doesn't heal, the body does).
- Reflexology has far-reaching effects, more so than working on the external area of the body.
- The treatment creates a feeling of well-being as endorphins are released.
- It eases pain as the pressure on the points acts to confuse the body pain receptors and interrupt the pain cycle.
- It both stimulates and soothes the nervous system.
- There is a balancing effect on the endocrine system.
- Reflexology has been shown to affect blood pressure, having a normalizing effect.

Although benefits are often felt after a single session, regular treatment will maintain the effects.

Interesting fact

Disease is often a direct consequence of our mental state and our physical actions. Poisonous thoughts create a poisoned body. Energy flow is often suppressed by negativity and medication.

The signs of imbalance

There are several different changes that can be detected in the feet. Some of these can be experienced by the client while you work; others may only be detected by your skill and touch.

Sensitivity varies enormously from one person to the next; it is subjective and is not always a sign of something medically wrong. For example, a client who has had a rich meal and several drinks the night before a treatment is quite likely to show changes in the digestive organs, especially the liver.

Sensations during treatment

Pressure: For much of the treatment the only sensation will be that of pressure. However, a client may experience increased sensitivity when working over a specific point or area.

Sensitivity: Sensitivity when working a specific point may be experienced in the following ways:

- as if the skin is sore or tender
- the area feels bruised
- the area feels sharp as if a nail, splinter or sharp object is pushing into the skin.

Pain: There will be occasions when the pain is so intense that the specific point cannot be worked. The pain is caused by a deviation in the normal pathway of energy along the reflex zones and the organs that they correspond to.

Crystals: The area may feel gritty and distinct crystals may be felt under the skin's surface. The client will also be aware of these crystals as you work over the point. There are debatable theories as to the nature of these crystals:

- they are caused by a build up of calcium deposits which it is believed collect at the nerve endings in the feet
- the crystals are formed from uric acid which collects at the peripheral capillaries in the feet.

It may even be a combination of these things. Both theories agree that crystals

- are the result of faulty cellular metabolism and are a form of toxic waste
- occur as a result of gravity working against the natural return of the peripheral circulation making it sluggish
- may also be affected by constraint from shoes.
- can be dispersed by massage and removed by the circulation.

Travelling sensations: These may be experienced as tingling or sharp shooting sensations that travel around the body. They are experienced as the energy pathways are cleared, allowing energy to travel along a meridian line.

Sensations in the body: Sensitivity may also be experienced in another area of the body. This may correspond to the point being worked or to a cross reflex. This is not uncommon where there is injury or internal scar tissue.

Other sensations: Other common sensations experienced during treatment are a feeling of light-headedness, a general tingling feeling, twitching legs and a rumbling tummy (very common).

The zone system

- The feet can be divided into a longitudinal and transverse map.
- There are five longitudinal zones running vertically on each side of the body either side of a central line. The zones begin in the head and end in the feet. These lines run all the way through so the body can be divided neatly into sections.
- There are three transverse zones that divide the body longitudinally.
- The transverse and longitudinal zones provide a 'grid-like' map.
- These grids help to map the position of various reflex areas. By locating the organ in the body grid you can map its expected location of the feet.

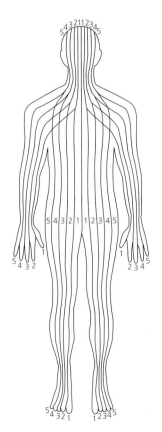

Zones of the body

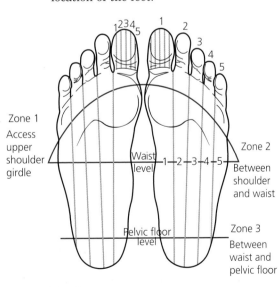

Zones of the feet

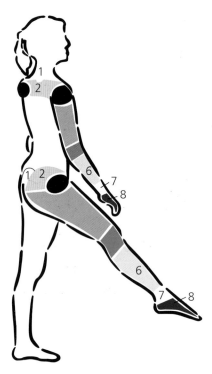

Cross reflexes

Cross reflexes and related areas

A cross reflex is the crossover between the opposite area within the zone framework. This connection is used to link the energy flow from the upper and lower body. If one area or organ is out of balance the whole zone may be affected.

Cross reflexes are useful as they can be worked when you are unable to work a specific point. Sometimes the point may be very painful, there may be a contra indication to the point (e.g. verrucae) or it may not be advisable to work a specific point as it may aggravate a condition, as when there is inflammation. Note that an imbalance may also be sensitive on the cross reflex rather than on the specific point.

Tip

- If there is a contra indication for the area of the point use the hand point instead.
- The cross reflexes can also be used to supplement treatment of a particular area.

Referral area

- Toes treat fingers
- Feet treat hands
- Ankle treats wrist
- Calf treats forearm
- Knee treats elbow
- Thigh treats upper arm
- Hip treats shoulder

Mapping the feet

Website @

Refer to the website www.thomsonlearning.co.uk/beckmann for activities to help you become more familiar with footmapping.

Having an understanding of the systems of the body is vital if your treatment is to succeed. An awareness of how the organs function and work with each other is an integral part of reflexology treatment.

Once you have a good knowledge of anatomy and physiology it becomes increasing clear that the feet are mini maps for the rest of the body. The spine for example clearly follows the shape and formation of the medial side of the foot.

The body can be clearly divided both in relation to its structure and position within the feet:

1 head and neck → the toes/fingers
2 thoracic region → ball of the foot (joint between phalanges and metatarsals/metacarpal)
3 abdominal area → arch of the foot
4 pelvic area → heel of the foot (calcaneum).

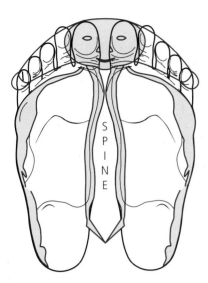

Body map, the body into the feet.
Divide the foot into sections to
help you. The head corresponds to
the big toe, but also extends out
over the toes, so that the ears
correspond with the little toes.
Limbs run down the sides, spin
down the medial line

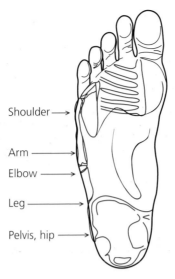

Foot map for the shoulder and
pelvic bones

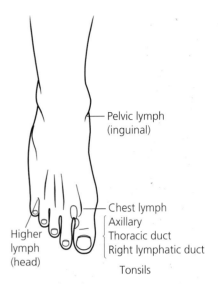

Foot map for the lymphatics dorsal
surface

Other easily defined areas are

5 spinal column → medial side of foot

6 shoulder and pelvic girdles → lateral side of foot

7 reproductive organs → around ankle

8 circulation, chest/breasts → top of the foot.

Meridians of the feet

To ensure you are familiar with meridians go to Chapter 3, p.21.

The meridians are mirrored on the feet. These are useful reference points
because sometimes you can note a reaction along a meridian (e.g. travelling
sensations). Unlike with the zone theory meridian lines may run in curves
or zigzag across the body.

Preparing for the treatment

Reflexology may be carried out on a couch or in a comfortable chair.
As with other treatments the area should be covered with clean couch roll.

You will need the following:

- talc
- massage oil
- tea tree oil/wipes
- antiseptic wipes
- additional towels to keep the feet warm during treatment
- a record card and pen
- a glass of water for the client.

Consultation

To ensure you are familiar with consultation techniques go to Chapter 5, p.134.

A full consultation should be carried out prior to the first treatment. This should be reviewed at the beginning of each consecutive treatment and updated accordingly.

Along with all the general information your consultation should include an in-depth medical history and details of the client's general health and energy levels.

Tell the client about the treatment and what to expect. Remember, it is a balancing treatment to create harmony and equilibrium in the body not a diagnostic procedure. The client must be clear about this.

Record keeping

It is useful to make notes about the feet during your initial observations. You may choose to use an assessment checklist or use diagrams and label them according to your findings. A visual record is often quicker, especially for referring to on subsequent treatments.

You should record in detail all your findings during treatment. During training you may be encouraged to do this as part of the learning process. However, this may be distracting to the client, breaking the continuity of treatment, and so should be phased out as you become more proficient. Complete your records at the end of treatment – there will be adequate time while the client is relaxing.

Preparing the client for treatment

Ask the client to remove their shoes and socks/tights and any restrictive leg wear and get them comfortable on the couch or in a chair. The body needs to be well supported. If using a couch, put the client in a semi-reclined position so that you can see their face. It is important that you watch for non-verbal communication (NVC).

Place a cushion or support under the knees, and if on a couch one under the ankles as well. This will allow you easy hand access under the feet. Cover the client with a towel.

Excuse yourself to wash your hands. Wipe the feet with an antiseptic wipe and check for contra indications. Observe the feet carefully while you are doing this.

Washing hands

How well do you wash your hands? I am sure you have seen surgeons scrub up before surgery. You don't need to go to quite the same lengths. However,

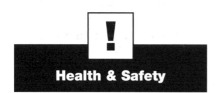

Health & Safety

Never prescribe or tell a client to alter their medication and/or to stop taking it. Refer them back to their GP.

Tip

It is important to communicate with your client:

- give them a brief overview of what the treatment involves
- let them know when you are going to start your treatment.

Tip

Place a large towel on the end of the bed so that it hangs down at the sides. This should be covered with tissue. Fold the towel over the feet so that one side covers one foot and tuck it around the feet. This will keep the feet warm and cosy during treatment.

be aware that bacteria collect between the webs at the base of the fingers and under the fingernails, and that these two areas are often neglected in everyday hand washing.

Do spare a thought for the process: I am always amazed at the amount of therapists who don't wash their hands on completion of a treatment and then go and eat their lunch!

Contra indications to reflexology treatment

To ensure you are familiar with contra indications go to Chapter 5, p.137.

As well as the general contra indications listed, there are a few other specific points that need to be considered.

- Steroids: use your judgement but be aware that long-term use of steroids thins the skin making it very transparent and prone to bleeding.
- Active shingles: do not treat as it may trigger the infection along the nerve pathways. Wait for at least 2 weeks after the spots have gone.
- Pregnancy: never treat if there is a history of miscarriage. Treatment may be carried out during the later stages providing the client is well.
- Serious eye problems.
- Varicose veins: do not work over varicose veins (working up the Achilles).
- Heavy medication: because the treatment has a balancing effect it may increase the side effects of medication.
- Diabetes: do not treat acute diabetes because the balancing effect may adversely affect the condition.
- Menstruation: do not work on the uterus as it will increase uterine flow. Treatment can be given on the point until menstruation begins.
- Presence of an IUD: be careful when working the uterus so that you do not stimulate the area.
- Be cautious also when treating children going through puberty. Treatment during puberty can be beneficial but take extreme care when working on the endocrine system.

Reading the feet

 Activity

In order to look at the bone structure of the feet make some footprints using paint. This is a good exercise for detecting flat feet and high arches.

Before you begin your reflexology treatment, observe the feet. There is much to learn from the condition of the feet even before treatment has begun. Often problems with the feet relate to disharmony in the body. Unfortunately which came first can be more difficult to determine.

Foot posture and bone structure

Weight distribution in the foot will depend on general posture. Poor posture can cause pressure on different points of the feet. In some cases this can be reflected in the organ or system to which it corresponds.

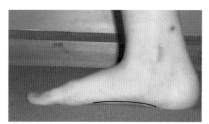
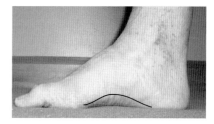

A flat foot   Foot with high arch

- Fallen arches indicate the client is walking on the chest points.
- Flat feet can affect the spine.
- Highly arched feet are often stiff and less mobile.

Shape and size

Look at the shape of the feet. Like the bodies they carry, feet come in all shapes and sizes. Carefully locate the positions and zones of the feet.

Condition of the skin

Feel the texture of the skin, look at the general skin condition and note the skin temperature.

- Dry skin: may be an indication of neglect or poor circulation.
- Corns and calluses: an imbalance in one of the systems may make certain areas of skin more sensitive, and as a consequence corns or calluses can occur.
- Flaking peeling skin: may be an indication of a fungal infection.
- Cracked skin: dietary deficiency (B group), poor circulation, wearing of open shoes, flip-flops, etc. which encourages the skin to toughen up.
- Inflammation: what is the cause? Ingrowing toenails? Or habitual picking of the feet?
- Scar tissue: any operations (bunions, toe straightening)?
- Fungal infections: look at digestive points (candida), urinary system and foot hygiene.
- Excessively moist and sweaty feet: may indicate kidney stress.

Condition of the nail

Check the nails for ingrowing toenails, usually caused by improper cutting of toenails, any signs of fungal infections, bruising or lifting of the nail plate.

Puffiness or swelling

Look for puffiness and swelling on the foot. These will be subtle and need to be observed carefully.

- Around the bladder: may indicate either a full bladder or bladder retention.
- Lymph and chest problems: may indicate puffiness on the front of the foot.
- Around the ankles and particularly under the fibula bone and above the cuboid bone: may indicate pelvic congestion (menstruation or menopausal uterine problems).
- Around the hip point: may indicate pelvic and postural problems.

Tip

Athelete's foot
If the client has athlete's foot make a note of where it is and whether it corresponds to any meridian lines. The common place to find this is the fourth and fifth toes which relate to the bladder meridian. The third and fourth toes relate to the gall bladder meridian.

Skin colour

Note any discoloration of the skin.

- Cold, bluish, mottled or white feet indicate poor circulation.
- Yellowish tone: possible elimination problems including kidneys and liver.
- Very pink feet: (not necessarily hot) may indicate that the kidneys are stressed, salty diet, excessive urine production, presence of medication.
- Pinky/orange tinge to metatarsal or metacarpal pads: may indicate the use of recreational drugs.

Odour

- Sweaty feet may indicate a hormonal problem or kidney stress.
- Cheesy feet: usually associated with poor foot hygiene.
- Acetone: due to incomplete breakdown of fatty acids, linked with diabetes and anorexia (starvation diets).
- Rotting flesh: athlete's foot has a distinctive odour which you will soon learn to detect.

Oedema

- Check for fluid behind the nails (finger and toes) and around the ankles

Temperature

- Cold feet (common in women) indicate poor peripheral circulation. Coldness only in isolated areas of the feet may indicate a lack of activity and imbalance in the corresponding area of the body.
- Hot feet, stimulated circulation (common in men): if the heat is specific to areas of the foot this may be mirrored within the body and indicate an imbalance.

Palpation skills

You will over time develop strong palpation techniques so that not just the obvious changes such as crystals can be felt. Like the body the feet suffer tension, but the changes are much more subtle than those felt in the large muscles. Stiffness and slight swelling over a point are common.

Tip

Press each toe below the nail. The quicker the white patch disappears, the better the circulation.

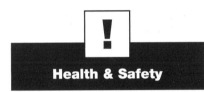

Health & Safety

Posture
Check your posture while you are working. It is just as important for you to be as comfortable as the client. If you are fidgeting it will detract from your treatment. Make sure your back is straight and your feet are flat on the floor.

Tip

Grounding
Keeping your feet flat on the floor while you are working will not only help your posture but will also keep you physically grounded.

A reflexology treatment

Commercial timing: the treatment should last approximately 45 minutes to 1 hour; the initial consultation will add a further 15 minutes.

A standard routine to follow is:

- warm-up massage
- reflexology treatment
- relaxation massage.

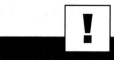

Warm-up foot massage

Apply sterilized talc to both feet. Talc is used to facilitate contact and soak up any excess moisture. Place a *small* amount on the tissue between the feet in case you need some additional talc later in your treatment. Introduce your hands to the feet by gently stroking both feet together.

It may be advisable to give a gentle first treatment to introduce the client to reflexology – the last thing you want to do is put the client off. My experience is that this is one of the most powerful treatments and as such should be treated with great respect. Gradually build the treatment up, increasing your techniques and specific point work.

Although reflexology is a good indicator of changes in the body it must never be used to diagnosis a client's aliments. Only those medically qualified to do so should undertake a medical diagnosis. You must never claim to treat a specific condition.

The feet always respond better than any other part of the body if they are warm and relaxed.

For the right foot:

Support foot in your left hand.

1 *Foot rotation*. Hold the foot firmly and rotate at the ankle, clockwise and anticlockwise.

2 *Leg stretch*. Very gently lift leg and pull very gently towards you. Place leg down.

3 *Gastrocnemius pinch*. Run fingers down the muscle applying a slight pinch between the fingers as you come down towards the foot. Repeat.

4 *Ankle stretch*. Hold the heel in one hand and stretch the leg from the ankle.

5 *Shaking*. Hold the foot between the ulna side of the hands and shake the foot. This will help to loosen the ankle.

6 *Foot roll*. Hold the foot between the hands and roll from side to side between your palms.

7 *Spinal twist*. Place your hands together on the medial side of the foot with the elbows straight. Using alternate hands very gently twist the side of the foot as if wringing out a cloth. This is to work down the spine to relax and loosen the back.

8 *Kneading*. Clench the hand into a fist and using the phalanx surface below the knuckles, place it below the toes and press. Move the hand down a little and repeat until all the foot has been treated.

9 *Toe rotation*. Rotate each toe clockwise and anticlockwise.

(Note that many of these techniques can be found illustrated in either Chapter 9, Body massage or Chapter 10, Aromatherapy).

10 *Opening the chest*. Place the thumbs on the solar plexus and draw the fingers out over the top of the foot (open lungs).

Cover the foot and repeat for the left foot.

When both feet have been massaged:

11 Supporting the feet, place a thumb on the solar plexus point on each foot and ask the client to take three deep breaths. Press into the point and push the feet gently forward as the client breathes in. Time the movement to their breathing pattern. Make sure the client breathes in through the nose (providing they do not have any nasal problems) and out through the mouth.

Treatment techniques

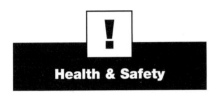

Health & Safety

Because you are using the tips of the thumbs and fingers, any length of free edge on the nail will inhibit your technique. Nails must be short and well manicured to avoid scratching or breaking the client's skin.

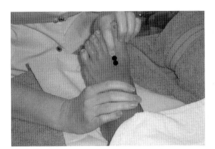

Finger walking

Reflex point treatment

When holding the foot the hands support each other as they work:

- the working hand is the one which applies the pressure
- the supporting hand supports or pushes the foot, or pushes towards the pressure.

Pressure techniques

Thumb walking or the caterpillar walk

Thumb walking is a continuous movement. Bend the thumb at the first joint so that it is at a right angle, then relax. This is the basis for the movement. It is applied to the skin so that only the tip of the thumb makes contact, presses and releases with the thumb remaining in contact, moving and repeating the pressure. The pressure is applied with a slight pull back action.

Finger walking

As for thumb walking but using one or more fingers.

Hook in and back up

This movement is used to work a specific point. The pressure is very deep and so the technique should be used with care. The thumb walks to locate a point. The thumb is flexed and hooks into the point; a slight pull back is applied.

Rotating

This movement is used to work a specific point. The thumb is usually used, rotating may also be applied with a finger. The digit is placed on a point and gently rotates or pivots with deep pressure in the point. The pressure can be enhanced by applying pressure in front from the supporting hand behind.

Rocking

As for rotating but the digit rocks from side to side.

Pinch grip

This movement uses the thumb plus one or two fingers to pinch into an area without nipping the skin. It is a pressure movement and should not be hurt. Often used for the soft web of skin at the base of the toes and fingers.

Finger press

Light pumping movements using the fingertips.

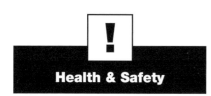

Many clients are interested in what you are doing. This is natural but be careful that you don't mislead them. Remember to emphasize that sensations in an area are not always negative and can simply be due to normal activity. Where possible encourage the client to relax and avoid giving them a detailed rundown on what area you are working on.

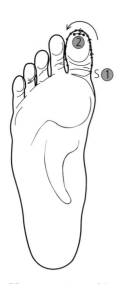

Movement 1 working over the head
Movement 2 working across the brain and top of the head

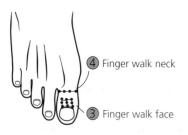

Movement 3 and 4 working the neck and face

Treatment procedures

There are different procedures for treating the feet.

- Both feet may be worked at the same time, i.e. working on alternate feet, a system is used for one foot then the other. This method tends to break up the continuity of treatment and may not be so relaxing. It is beneficial, however, for working some systems, e.g. the digestive system where to work the organs systematically you need to work across both feet.

- The feet are treated one foot at a time, starting with the right foot and working through the treatment and concentrating on specific points in response to what is found.

- As above but the treatment is more superficial. The sequence is then repeated for both feet paying particular attention to areas requiring balancing.

Zones have been given for guidance to help you locate the reflex point. However, use your intuition and palpation skills. There are a few specific individuals whose organs are in unusual places!

The following routine works each foot individually.

The treatment begins with the *right foot*. Follow the same procedure for each foot working those only those organs mirrored on the respective foot. Organs located only on a particular foot are marked with a *.

> Key
> L = longitudinal zone
> T = transverse zone

Right foot

1 Technique: thumb walk
   Area of the body: side of head, hypothalamus, pineal gland, brain, ear area and occipital region
   Part of foot: up the medial side, over and down the lateral side of the big toe
   Zones: L1 T1

2 Technique: thumb walk using side of the thumb
   Area of the body: brain
   Part of the foot: across tip of big toe
   Zones: L1 T1

3 Technique: finger walk
   Area of the body: mouth and teeth
   Part of the foot: 3 rows down front of big toe
   Zones: L1 T1

4 Make a beak with thumb and index finger
   Technique: thumb supports finger walks
   Area of the body: front of neck
   Part of the foot: front of big toe midway down 2nd phalanx
   Zones: L1 T2

5 With finger and thumb still in beak position, supporting the big toe with the finger
   Technique: thumb walk
   Area of the body: back of neck
   Part of the foot: back of base of toe and walk 2 lines one above the other
   Zones: L1 T1

6 Technique: thumb or finger walk 3 small points
Area of the body: occipital region
Part of the foot: inside of big toe
Zones: L1 T1

7 Technique: locate and rotate
Area of the body: pituitary gland
Part of the foot: off centre of big toe
Zones: L1 T1

Tip

Finding the pituitary point
Look at the print pattern of the big toe. Find the centre of the swirl (as you
would for fingerprints). This is just off centre from the middle of the toe.
Feel gently for a small pea shape in the skin – this is the pituitary point.

8 Technique: finger walk
Area of the body: sinuses
Part of the foot: up the side, over and down the other side of each toe
Zones: L1–4 T1

9 Use the thumb of the supporting hand to pull the pad under the toes
down to make access
Technique: thumb walk
Area of the body: ear and eye points

- left foot, left eye and ear
- right foot, right eye and ear

Part of the foot: across base of toes, walk 2 lines one in each direction
Zones: L1–4 T1

10 Technique: locate and rotate using the index finger
Area of the body: eyes

- left foot, left eye
- right foot, right eye

Part of the foot: between the 2nd and 3rd toes
Zones: L4–5 T1

11 Technique: locate and rotate back using the index finger
Area of the body: ears

- left foot, left ear
- right foot, right ear

Part of the foot: between the 3rd and 4th toes
Zones: L2–3 T1

12 Technique: pinch
Area of the body: Eustachian tube
Part of the foot: top of foot in web of skin at base of 4th and 5th toes
Zones: L4–5 T1

13 Technique: locate and press
Area of the body: balance
Part of the foot: base of 4th toe on top of the foot
Zones: L4 T1

14 Supporting hand pulls toes back
Technique: thumb walk once in each direction (medial to lateral, lateral
to medial)
Area of the body: diaphragm
Part of the foot: underpads of foot (base of proximal phalanges and top
of metatarsals)
Zones: L1–5 T1

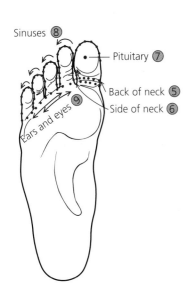

Movement 8 and 9 working across
the sinuses and general points for
the ears and eyes

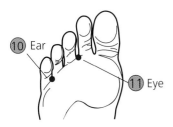

Movement 10 and 11 location of ear
and eye specific points, and rotate

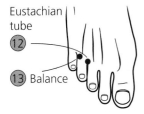

Movement 12 and 13 location and
rotation of the Eustachian tube and
point of balance

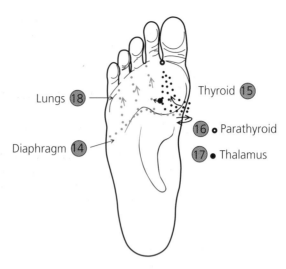

Lungs (18)
Thyroid (15)
(16) Parathyroid
Diaphragm (14)
(17) Thalamus

Movement 16 and 17 locate and rotate the parathyroid and thalamus points
Movement 18 work the lung area

 Interesting fact

Shivering may be experienced when working the thyroid.

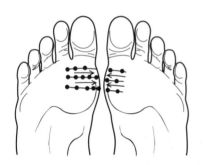

Movement 19 work the cardiac region

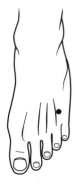

Movement 20 locate the heart reflex (left foot only)

15 Technique: thumb walk
Area of the body: thyroid
Part of the foot: around the base of the proximal phalanx of the big toe and up the lateral side to the base of the big toe. Repeat ×3 slowly moving up and into the bone
Zones: L1 T2

16 Technique: locate hook up into the big toe at 45°
Area of the body: parathyroid
Part of the foot: between the big toe and 2nd toe at the base
Zones: L1 T2

17 Technique: locate and rotate
Area of the body: thalamus
Part of the foot: halfway down between the proximal phalanx of the big and 2nd toes
Pressure towards the little toe
Zones: L1 T1

18 Open the toes by placing fingers on supporting hand between toes
Technique: thumb walk
Area of the body: lungs

- left foot, left lung
- right foot, right lung

Part of the foot: between proximal phalanges from diaphragm to base of each toe, 4 columns
Zones: L1–5 T2

19 Technique: thumb walk
Area of the body: cardiac region
Part of the foot: across proximal phalanges from diaphragm to below the toes, 3 rows
Zones: L1–3 T2

20 *Left foot only*
Technique: pinch
Area of the body: heart reflex
Part of the foot: dorsal foot, push up from the under the foot to make the point visible. On 4th metatarsal head
Zones: L4 T2

21 *Right foot only*
Technique: thumb walk
Area of the body: liver

Part of the foot: under diaphragm, in line with base of 2nd toe medial to lateral 3 rows in 2 rows back
Zones: L2–5 T2

Tip

The liver
The liver is responsible for detoxifying the body. It may be wise to work this very gently on a first treatment as the client may feel nauseous. Where there is a toxic build up in the liver this may take several treatments to release.

!

Health & Safety

Never work on a client with suspected gallstones or kidney stones until the stones have been passed. Only after this can you work on elimination points to prevent further recurrence.

22 *Right foot only*
Technique: hook in and back up
Area of the body: gall bladder
Part of the foot: under diaphragm, under 3rd toe. Hook in and apply pressure towards the little toe
Zones: L3 T2

23 Technique: thumb walk
Area of the body: stomach and pancreas
Part of the foot: under diaphragm, 3 rows to medial edge
Zones: right foot L1–2 T2; left foot L1–3 T2

24 *Left foot only*
Technique: thumb walk
Area of the body: spleen
Part of the foot: beneath diaphragm zone 4/5, walk 3 rows
Zones: L4–5 T2

25 Technique: thumb walk
Area of the body: small intestine
Part of the foot: 4 rows from zone 2 medially, then 3 rows from end of heel diagonally across sole
Zones: L2–5 T3

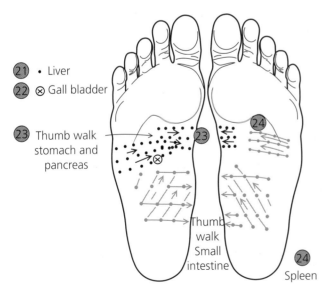

21 • Liver
22 ⊗ Gall bladder
23 Thumb walk stomach and pancreas

Movement 23 work the stomach and pancreas (larger area on left foot)
Movement 24 work over the spleen region (left foot only)

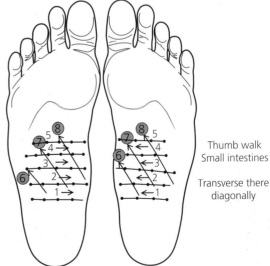

Thumb walk Small intestines

Transverse there diagonally

Movement 25 work the small intestine region, four lines medially and three lines diagonally

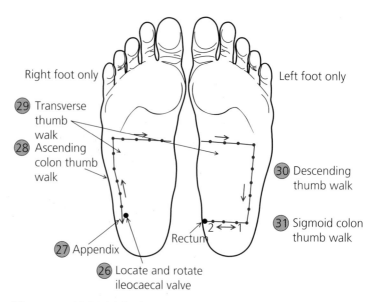

Right foot only

Left foot only

29 Transverse thumb walk

28 Ascending colon thumb walk

30 Descending thumb walk

31 Sigmoid colon thumb walk

Rectum 2 ↔ 1

27 Appendix

26 Locate and rotate ileocaecal valve

Movement 26–31 (right foot) locate ileocaecal valve, walk up ascending colon, across transverse colon (left foot) start medially and walk across transverse colon, down descending colon, across sigmoid colon to rectum at medial point.

Tip

Finding the ileocaecal point
Once in position the ileocaecal valve can be felt as a tiny circle under the skin.

Tip

Finding the transverse colon point
The transverse colon can be pinpointed roughly two fingers' width down the foot from the diagram point.

26 *Right foot only
Technique: hook in and back up
Area of the body: ileocaecal valve
Part of the foot: sole of foot in zones 3–4 (approximately in line with base of 4th toe)
Zones: L3–4 T3

27 *Right foot only*
Technique: thumb walk from point up and join next movement
Area of the body: appendix
Part of the foot: just below ileocaecal valve, above pelvic floor area, on 4th tarsal
Zones: L4 T3

28 *Right foot only*
Technique: thumb walk
Area of the body: ascending colon
Part of the foot: up side of foot, lift wrist to turn
Zones: L4 T3

29 Technique: thumb walk
Area of the body: transverse colon
Part of the foot: continue transversely across foot at approximately waist level
Zones: L1–5 T3

30 *Left foot only*
Technique: thumb walk
Area of the body: descending colon
Part of the foot: work down the plantar surface with right hand down lateral side of foot
Zones: L4/5 T3

31 *Left hand only*
Hold toes with right hand
Technique: thumb walk
Area of the body: sigmoid colon, rectum
Part of the foot: continues from descending colon across zones. Walk in from medial edge to meet descending colon
Zones: L1–4 T3

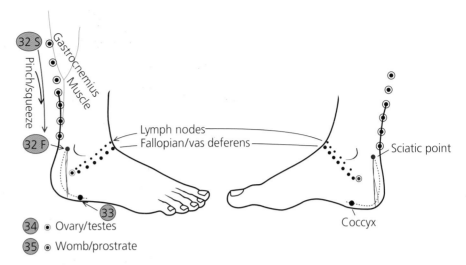

Movement 34–37 locate and rotate ovary/teste, locate and rotate uterus/ prostrate walk from ovary point over ankle along fallopian/vas deferens.

Tip

Measuring for the ovary/testes point
Place three fingers: one on the back of the heel, one on the fibula bone, letting the middle finger drop – this is the ovarian/testes point.

Tip

The uterus is usually very tender just prior to menstruation. You may also notice the point is slightly swollen at this time.

32 Technique: pinch grip
Area of the body: haemorrhoids, constipation, rectum, sciatic points
Part of the foot: work down from middle of the gastrocnemius down the Achilles tendon and the calcaneum bone

33 Technique: locate and rotate
Area of the body: coccyx
Part of the foot: medial border of distal calcaneum
Zones: L1 T3

34 Turn foot medially
Technique: locate and rotate
Area of the body: ovaries/testes

- left side corresponds with the left ovary/testes
- right side corresponds with the right ovary/testes

Part of the foot: lateral side of foot midway between the middle and back of the calcaneum
Zones: L5 T3

35 Turn foot laterally
Technique: locate and rotate
Area of the body: uterus/prostate
Part of the foot: medial border of foot between middle and back of calcaneum
Zones: L1 T3

36 Technique: finger or thumb walk
Area of the body: fallopian tubes/vas deferens

- left foot, left fallopian tube/vas deferens
- right foot, right fallopian tube/vas deferens

Part of the foot: push foot up holding the toes to see crease of ankle. Walking lateral to medial over crease of the ankle. (Ovary cleared into uterus. Testes cleared into prostate)
Zones: L1–5 T3

37 Technique: finger or thumb walk
Area of the body: lymphatic nodes in pelvis
Part of the foot: push foot up holding the toes to see crease of ankle. Change hands to walk medial to lateral just above the previous line over the crease of the ankle
Zones: L1–5 T3

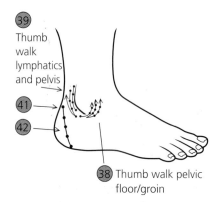

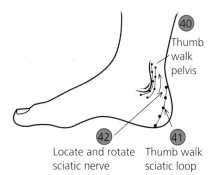

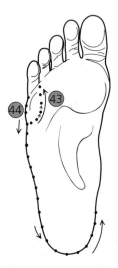

Movement 38 and 39 work pelvic area, medial and lateral ankle

Movement 40–42 walk sciatic loop working from one side of the foot along the plantar surface (42b) and up the other side to the opposite sciatic point

Movement 43 walk the shoulder area

38 Technique: thumb walk
Area of the body: groin, pelvic floor muscles

- right side of pelvis, right foot
- left side of pelvis, left foot

Part of the foot: below lateral malleolus (projection at end of the bone) of the fibula and above talus bones, work space below in 3 decreasing rows
Zones: L5 T3

39 Technique: thumb walk
Area of the body: inguinal lymphatics and pelvis
Part of the foot: behind lateral malleolus of fibula (outside of foot), 3 lines
Zones: L5 T3

40 Technique: thumb walk
Area of the body: pelvis
Part of the foot: behind medial malleolus of tibia (inside of foot), 2 lines upwards
Zones: L1 T3

41 Technique: locate and rotate
Area of the body: sciatic nerve
Part of the foot: top of tallus bone on either side of the foot on Achilles tendon
Zones: L1 and 5 T3

42 Technique: thumb walk
Area of the body: sciatic loop
Part of the foot: support the foot. Walk in from sciatic point at a diagonal to the fibula down and under heel at about a third from the back of the heel. Walk across heel changing hands midpoint then up the other side to the opposite point. Avoid the uterus/prostate and ovary/testes points
Zones: L1–5 T3

43 Technique: thumb walk
Area of the body: shoulder

- left shoulder, left foot
- right shoulder, right foot

Part of the foot: around base and up medial side of 5th proximal phalanx
Zones: L5 T1/2

44 Supporting hand, foot supported with fingers over the toes
Technique: thumb walk
Area of the body: shoulder, arm, elbow, lower leg, knee, hip, lower back
Part of the foot: lateral edge from base of little toe, down lateral edge, following edge of 5th metatarsal up to feel along the cuboid bone and across on to the calcaneum. Follow round, changing hands to finish on the medial edge at the end of the calcaneum (coccyx point)
Zones: L5 T1/2 shoulder; T2, upper arm, elbow; T2/3, knee, hip; T3, lower back

45 Rest heel into working hand
Technique: locate and press, thumb walk
Area of the body: bladder
Part of the foot: small pink puffy or shiny area under navicular bone
Walk across the bladder in 3 rows, or in lines radiating from the centre of the bladder point
Zones: L1 T3

46 Technique: thumb walk
Area of the body: ureter

- left foot, left ureter
- right foot, right ureter

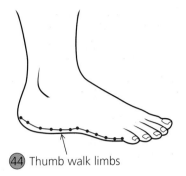

(44) Thumb walk limbs

Movement 44 and 45 walk from the base of the little toe, to work over shoulder point, down arm, and up the leg

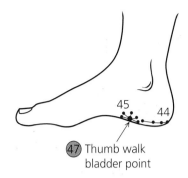

(47) Thumb walk bladder point

Go around the back of the ankle to end on the coccyx point on the medial side of the foot. Work over the bladder area in radiating lines working from the centre

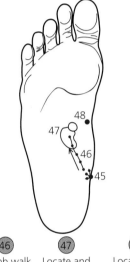

(46) Thumb walk ureter (47) Locate and rotate kidney (48) Locate and rotate adrenal

Movement 46–48 from the centre of the bladder work up the ureter to the kidney, locate and rotate. Locate and rotate adrenal gland

Part of the foot: move 3 points in to the foot then walk up diagonally from L1 across to L2/3 to approximately waist level. Remember to pull back with the walk to clear the ureter
Zones: L1–3 T2/3

47 Technique: locate and rotate
Area of the body: kidney

- left foot, left kidney
- right foot, right kidney

Part of the foot: as you come to the top of the ureter you should feel a slight change
Zones: L2/3 T2/3

> **Tip**
>
> **Finding the kidney point**
> When locating the kidneys, if you are in the correct position walking up the ureter, at the top you should feel a tendon, and under that tendon is the kidney point.
>
> Note: as the feet mirror the body the left kidney is slightly higher than the right.

48 Technique: locate and rotate
Area of the body: adrenal

- left foot, left adrenal
- right foot, right adrenal

Part of the foot: like the body the adrenal are located on top of the kidney. From the kidney point lift your thumb and place to the right of previous position
Zones: L2 T2

49 Supporting hand holds foot by the ankle. Working hand is palm to the sole of the foot; fingers cover toes so that the thumb is in line with the big toe
Technique: thumb walk
Area of the body: spinal column – 7 cervical, 12 thoracic, 5 lumbar, 4 sacral, coccyx

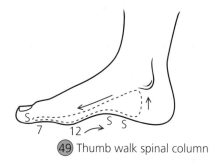

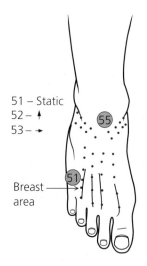

(49) Thumb walk spinal column

Movement 49 walk from base of big toe along spinal points, follow lines of bones and return

51 – Static
52 – ↑
53 – →

Breast area

Movement 52 apply finger pressures to chest, circulatory and lymphatic areas
Movement 53 apply transverse finger pressures across the dorsal region for the chest
Movement 55 finger pump around the pelvic lymphatics

Part of the foot: start at the joint between the 1st and 2nd phalanx. Thumb walk in tiny movements counting each of the vertebrae of the spine as you walk down the medial edge. Follow the line of the bones. Walk down to the edge of the navicular bone; walk up under the bottom of the tibia. Change hands; walk down back towards the medial edge at an angle back up to the big toe
Zones: L1 T1–3

50 Technique: index finger pressure
Area of the body: lymphatics
Part of the foot: place index finger between metatarsal 1/2, press and release, working up between metatarsal bone. Repeat between each metatarsal – 2/3, 3/4, 4/5
Zones: L1–5 T2/3

51 Technique: finger locate and feel gently for changes
Area of body: breast
Part of foot: dorsal surface in area about two finger widths down from 4th and 5th toes
Zones: L3–5 T2

52 Technique: finger pressure
Area of the body: chest, pulmonary, circulatory and lymphatic congestion
Part of the foot: dorsal surface. Fingertips positioned between 1/2 and 4/5 metatarsal joints. Press twice and stretch outwards and upwards using the thumbs underneath the foot to add pressure. Repeat, moving up the metatarsals towards the toes. Move fingers to 2/3 and 3/4 metatarsals and repeat
Zones: L1–5 T2–3

53 Technique: finger pressure
Area of the body: chest, pulmonary, circulatory and lymphatic congestion.
Part of the foot: dorsal surface. Fingers tips positioned between 4/5 metatarsal joints. Fingers spread. Press several times then move across to next zone. Move fingers to 4/3, 3/2 and 2/1 metatarsals and repeat
Zones: L1–5 T2–3

54 Technique: rotation and pinch
Area of the body:
Part of the foot: gently rotate each of the toes in both directions holding them at the tip. Pinch the toe with the finger placed at the base of the fleshy bulb and flick your fingers off
Zones: L1–5 T1

55 Technique: finger pumping
Area of the body: lymphatics
Part of the foot: make a V shape with the hands, pump with the fingertips around the ankle joint
Zones: L1–5 T3

Cover foot with a warm towel and begin left foot

Relaxation massage

The treatment should be concluded with a foot massage. This draws the treatment to a close and adds further opportunity for relaxation.

Oil or cream may be applied at this point should you choose. This has the added benefit of conditioning the skin after treatment but should be used sparingly.

Any massage can be used on the feet for completion of treatment. Each foot should take no longer than five minutes. The movements below are for guidance.

Slippery feet
If you have used oil or cream on the feet make sure you blot any excess off before the client gets off the couch otherwise they may slip. Get them to stand on a piece of couch roll while they put on their shoes.

Completion of treatment

- To bring the client back from a deeply relaxed state, maintain hand contact and talk to them quietly. Once they are back with you ask them to repeat the breathing that you got them to do during the warm-up treatment.

- Stroke towards the clients to finish, or take your hands away from the feet and move to the floor. Flick your fingers so that you do not take on any negative energy.

- (In your head thank the client and wish them well.)

- Give the client a glass of water.

Treatment adaptations

Unlike many other treatments there are not many occasions when adaptations are required as the treatment itself is modified to meet the client's individual needs. There are occasions when the hand may be treated instead of the feet (see below, p.338, Working the hands).

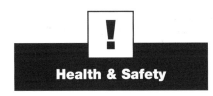
Interesting fact

Parental consent
Remember that to treat a minor, i.e. anyone under the age of 16, for any treatment you must have parental consent. It is suggested that you obtain this verbally and that the parent or guardian signs something to acknowledge their agreement to the treatment taking place. Ideally, the guardian should remain for the duration of the treatment.

Treating the very young

Treatment involves stroking and massage, ensuring that the feet have been covered. The problem is usually keeping a young child still for long enough. Because the feet and hands are so small it is difficult to locate many points exactly.

Young children

As children get older they are often very receptive to having their feet massaged. Use only very light pressure and remember that the reflexes will be sensitive. Keep the treatment short – around 20 minutes – as children are often more responsive. Reflexology is useful for alleviating the symptoms of hay fever and asthma.

Puberty

Reflexology is a wonderful treatment for balancing. However, during puberty the body is changing. Extreme care must be taken to avoid stimulating endocrine activity. Again keep treatment shorter and only use very light pressure over the endocrine and reproductive organs.

Contra actions and after care

To ensure you are familiar with contra actions and after care go to Chapter 5, p.137.

More so than any for other treatment, with reflexology the client is likely to experience some form of contra action. Thus, it is important that you advise the client as to what these might be and what to expect. You must do so without causing alarm however. Be tactful – the client does not want to return home under the impression that they are about to feel ill. Remember the power of suggestion. If you tell the client they might experience something, chances are that they will convince themselves they are going to experience what you have suggested.

Give the client an after care leaflet with contra actions listed. Advise the client, should they have any queries, to call you.

Foot hygiene

Recommended points for maintaining foot hygiene:

- wash daily and dry well between the toes
- wear cotton socks and change them daily
- change shoes regularly, preferably alternate shoes so that the same shoe is not worn two days running as this gives time for the sweat that we all produce to evaporate
- in the summer try to wear open shoes as much as possible
- use tea tree or a medicated product or spray to treat fungal infections
- spray shoes regularly with an anti-fungal deodorizing spray
- give the feet a pedicure – keep toenails cut straight across (this prevents ingrowing toenails), use a foot scrub, pumice or rough skin remover and moisturize the feet.

Follow-up treatments

When the client returns for consecutive treatments always ask them about their previous treatment. Do not prompt them for an answer or make suggestions.

Remember that:

- three treatments are generally needed to balance basic problems before a client will start to feel the lasting benefits
- old injuries can be more problematic as can long-term stress.

Treatment can be carried out twice a week initially, then once a week, moving to once a month for maintenance.

Working the hands

Interesting fact

Personal zone
The personal zone is the space around our bodies; it usually comprises a margin of around 75 cm from the body. We allow only those people whom who we really like into this space. When people get too close we can feel threatened or intimidated. Many of our treatments, not just reflexology, place us in people's personal space and it is important you are aware of this. Once you are this close, it takes a lot of trust for someone to relax.

It is beneficial to work the hands in the following instances:

- if is structural damage to the bones of the feet
- injury
- infections which contra indicate treatment
- hypersensitive or ticklish feet
- severe arthritis
- amputation.

The *advantages* of such a treatment are as follows:

- hands are more accessible than feet
- back up treatment at home or/or a quick fix
- can be performed anywhere; no need for a couch.

The *disadvantages* are:

- some points on the hands are not so easy to locate
- the client is usually seated and so may not be fully relaxed

- treatment is performed at a much closer proximity than a foot treatment and as a result you will be sitting in the client's 'personal zone' so be clear about your treatment boundaries
- the hands are more mobile than the feet and so your technique must be firm and controlled.

Nevertheless, working the hands is of great value.

Procedure for hand treatment

The procedure for treating the hands is an adaptation of the same procedure as for working the feet.

- You may choose to sit opposite the client with their hands placed on a couch or cushion (or both) to support them.
- Or sit the client in a comfortable upright chair and support the arm of the hand you are working on with a large cushion.
- Alternatively, you may choose to lie the client down but this does not give the best treatment position, as it can be an awkward position for you to work comfortably in. It puts you at an angle to the client and the client's hands and arms are not fully relaxed.
- Cleanse the client's hands with an antiseptic cleanser.
- Follow the routine for the feet but work the hands. Use the zones for guidance.

Guidance for hand treatment

- Work the hands the opposite way to the feet as they will be upside down; this may take a while to become accustomed to.
- Use a firmer technique to locate the reflexes as these are often deeper than for the feet.
- Bear in mind that the hands are less reflex-sensitive than the feet.
- The skin is more mobile on the hands so you may find you need to adapt slightly your walking technique.
- You may feel more comfortable using the index finger to walk some of the smaller areas or for point location.

Remember to follow up your hand treatment with your usual after care and advice. You may also wish to include some points that the client can use to supplement their treatment.

Activity

Using the treatment routine for the feet, modify this and write down a routine for the hands.

Tip

Tips for locating some confusing points on the hand:

- *bladder:* palms of hand over medial carpal bones extending round to the back of the hand
- *ovaries/testes:* lateral border of the hand just above the wrist on back of the hands
- *uterus/prostrate:* medial border of the hand just above the wrist on the back of the hands
- *sciatic loop:* across end of the palm just below wrist.

Knowledge review

1   What are the different techniques that are used during a reflexology treatment and give one example of when you would use each?

2   What are cross reflexes?

3   Briefly describe what sensations a client might experience during treatment.

4   What contra actions might the client experience?

5   What after care will you advise your client to follow?

6   Why is it important to carry out a comprehensive consultation? What information will you require to perform a safe and effective treatment?

Website @

Visit the companion website at
www.thomsonlearning.co.uk/
beckmann where you will find
further case studies.

Case study

For the following client write a treatment plan indicating

- what further information you would ask
- what points you may choose to pay more attention to
- how many treatments you would recommend, giving your
  reasons.

Client A

Client A is 68 years old. She is very underweight but has a good diet.
She had her duodenum removed 10 years previously as a result of
cancer, but was given the all clear 5 years ago. Her feet are very
tender and the skin is tight around the middle of the feet. She has a
little arthritis in the big toe but this does not bother her.

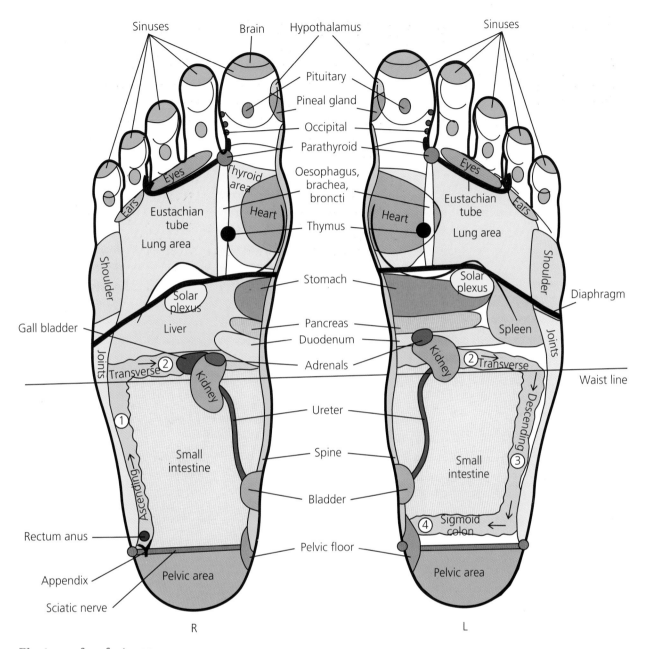

Sinuses   **Brain**   **Hypothalamus**   **Sinuses**

Pituitary

Pineal gland

Occipital

Parathyroid

Sinuses

Eyes

Thyroid area

Oesophagus, brachea, broncti

Eustachian tube

Ears

Heart

Heart

Eustachian tube

Lung area

Thymus

Eyes

Ears

Shoulder

Lung area

Shoulder

Solar plexus

Stomach

Solar plexus

Diaphragm

Gall bladder

Liver

Pancreas

Spleen

Joints

Duodenum

Joints

Transverse ②

Adrenals

② Transverse

Kidney

Kidney

① Ascending

Ureter

Waist line

Small intestine

Spine

Small intestine

③ Descending

Bladder

Rectum anus

Sigmoid colon ④

Pelvic floor

Appendix

Pelvic area

Pelvic area

Sciatic nerve

R

L

Planter surface foot map

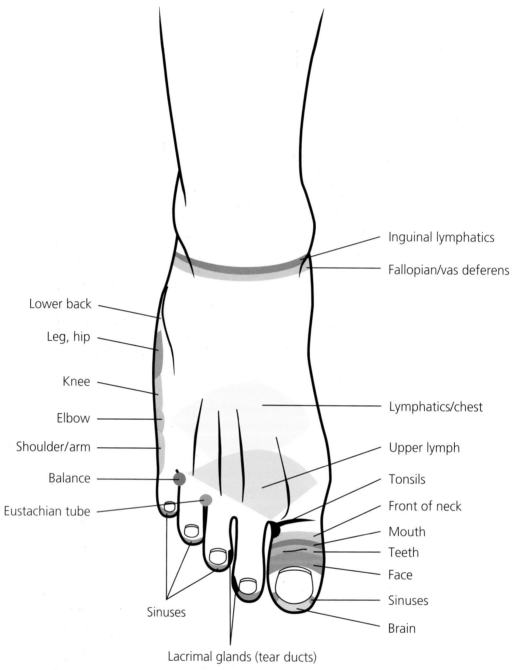

Inguinal lymphatics

Fallopian/vas deferens

Lower back

Leg, hip

Knee

Elbow

Shoulder/arm

Balance

Eustachian tube

Lymphatics/chest

Upper lymph

Tonsils

Front of neck

Mouth

Teeth

Face

Sinuses

Brain

Sinuses

Lacrimal glands (tear ducts)

Dorsal surface

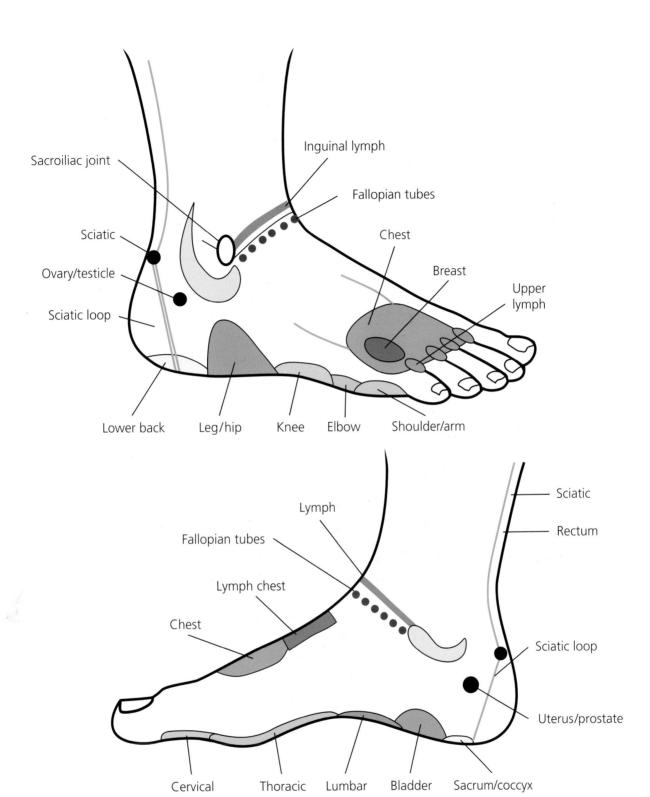

Sacroiliac joint

Sciatic

Ovary/testicle

Sciatic loop

Inguinal lymph

Fallopian tubes

Chest

Breast

Upper lymph

Lower back   Leg/hip   Knee   Elbow   Shoulder/arm

Lymph

Fallopian tubes

Lymph chest

Chest

Sciatic

Rectum

Sciatic loop

Uterus/prostate

Cervical   Thoracic   Lumbar   Bladder   Sacrum/coccyx

Medial foot

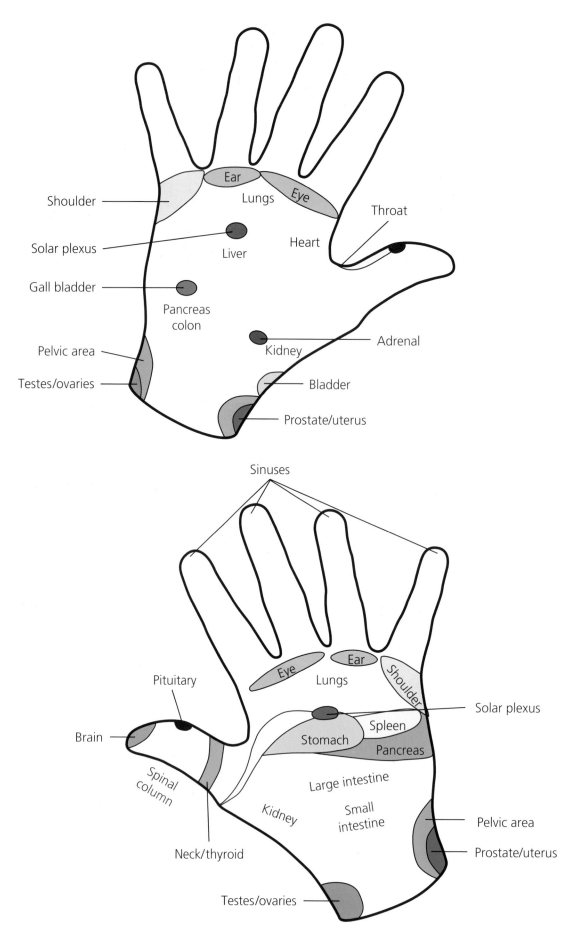

Map of the hands

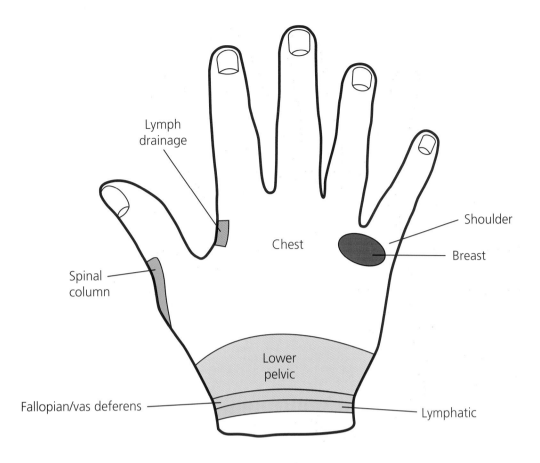

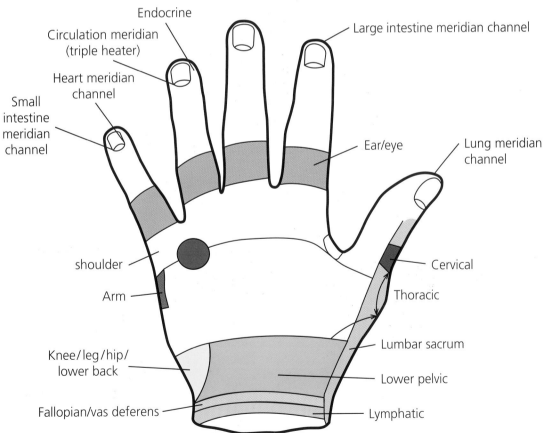

Map of the hands

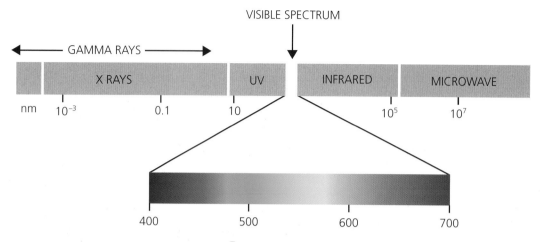

Wavelengths

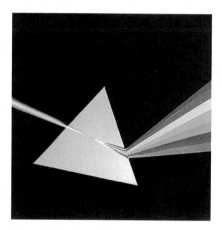

How light is refracted

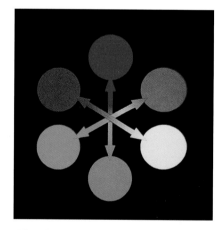

Wheel of colour

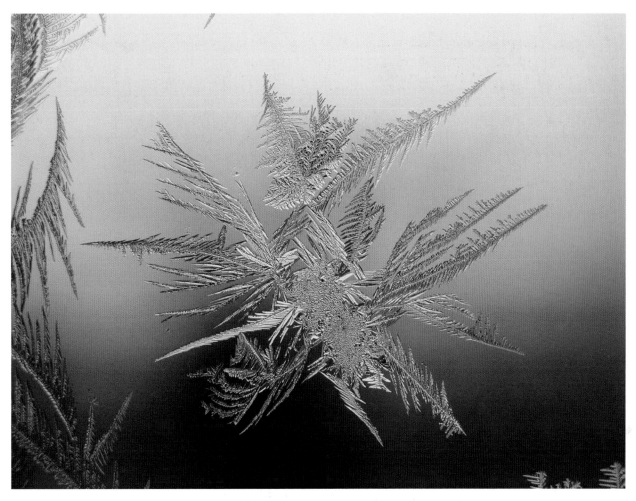

Ice crystals

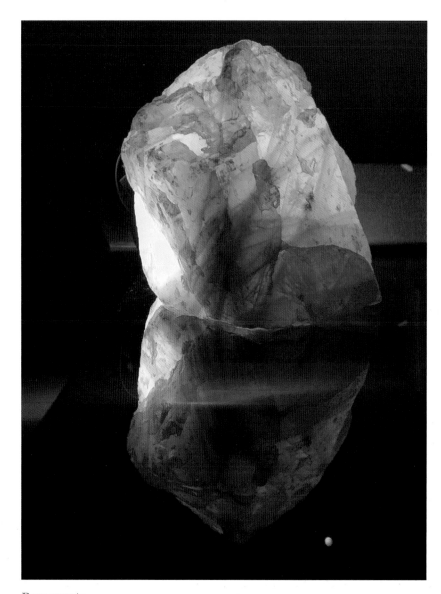

Rose quartz

Stress management

Learning objectives

This chapter covers the following:

- **what stress is**
- **environmental, emotional, chemical and nutritional stress**
- **the causes of stress**
- **the symptoms of stress**
- **the stress response**
- **how to reduce and/or manage stress**

Stress has been described as one of the most serious health problems of the twenty-first century. It is not necessarily a bad thing, despite its negative image, as stress can be positive as well as negative. Stress is an inescapable part of being human and is a normal response to challenge. The body is constantly trying to maintain internal stability and will do what it can to return to stability if that state is altered. This is called homeostasis. If it's a very hot day, your body will cool itself by perspiring. To repair a cut, the body creates a scab, which helps heal the wound and protects the skin from further damage. If you eat foods that are acid-forming the body will take calcium from bones in order to neutralize the acid. Every minute of every day the body responds to stress with a complex series of biochemical changes that attempt to bring the body back into its pre-stressed state. However, this can be an uphill struggle for our systems if we continue to bombard ourselves with 'stress'. Stress comes in many guises – environmental, emotional, chemical and nutritional stress being the most widely researched. We talk about stress constantly, often referring to someone as 'stressed out' or 'burned out' but few people really understand the gravity of a highly stressed body. A life without any challenge, with too little to do and too much time, can be as great a source of stress as too much work and too many deadlines. So what exactly is stress and how can we manage it? This chapter will answer these questions for you.

What is stress?

Stress has been described as the pressure we experience in situations
that threaten our well-being or tax our resources. Much of the time it is
a positive force: it prompts us to get out of the way of a runaway car,
for example, or to revise hard for examinations. However, stress can be
a problem for those who feel overwhelmed and unable to cope with the
challenges faced. An individual's perception of a situation and the amount
of stress already being handled is important: two people faced with a
stressful event, such as being late for an important appointment, may
react completely differently.

Environmental, emotional, chemical and nutritional stress

Environmental stress

Environmental stress concerns our everyday activities. How we react to
the 'environment' around us. This could be our travelling to and from
work, going on holiday, trains, buses, cars, traffic jams, accidents and
breakdowns. Environmental stress can also include moving house, having
a new job, an old job with too many tasks to fulfil in a working day or
moving from one school to another. All these activities in our lives are
'stressors', and the more we put upon ourselves, the more difficult we
may find it to cope.

Emotional stress

Emotional stress is caused by problems within relationships. For example,
relationships between parents and children; siblings; children and teachers;
bosses and their employees, working colleagues; or husbands and wives.
Any imbalance or unhappiness in these relationships is a cause of emotional
stress. Emotional stress also includes bereavement. As individuals everyone
responds differently to the loss of a loved one. Some people show their
emotions openly by crying and 'letting out' their emotion, while others
'bottle it up'. On the death of a loved one some people keep every last
possession of that person, while others dispose of everything immediately.
Some people can't understand the actions of others in such cases, but
depending on current levels of stress, our coping abilities differ. A death
may be expected, in the case of illness, or may be unexpected in cases of
accidents. All these factors play a huge role in the way we react to the
event. Happy events such as marriage brings with it stressors too. Getting
married is a big step in anyone's life, bringing with it many changes, and it
is only natural that the stress response is activated. Pregnancy and divorce
are other major events where stress is inevitable.

Chemical and nutritional stress

Chemical and nutritional stress is when the body receives a continued
intake of harmful substances (chemicals) and/or deficient quantities of
beneficial substances (nutrients from food). Chemicals such as caffeine,

nicotine and alcohol all have a detrimental effect on the endocrine system, resulting in a condition known as 'hormones in havoc'. With continued intake of any of these substances, the body doesn't have time to recover between each cup of coffee, cigarette or drink or combinations of these resulting in a continued and permanent state of alert. All nicotine, alcohol and caffeine should be avoided in people suffering with stress, anxiety or panic attacks. Synthetic chemicals (pesticides) found in processed foods, fish and plastics should also be avoided as these cause internal stress to the endocrine and nervous systems. One chemical group in particular is of concern – PCBs (polychlorinated biphenols).

Increased smoking

The repetitious ritual-like behaviour each smoker employs while smoking acts as a temporary tension reducer. Rituals bind anxiety and can be useful in dealing with tension. However, when the ritual is associated with behaviours having health-damaging side effects the potential health hazard overshadows any benefit gained. Large amounts of nicotine also serve to depress the central nervous system, creating a sense of relaxation. Ironically, the overall effect is to elevate blood pressure, cholesterol and noradrenaline. All of these are physical stressors endangering health. Thus, the more you smoke, the more stressed you become; so you smoke more, which creates more stress and so on in a never-ending circle!

Increased alcohol consumption

Alcohol is an effective central nervous system depressant. It results in increased muscle relaxation and clouded thinking which reduces mental tension. Precisely because it works so well it is a major danger during stressful periods. The potential for alcoholism and alcohol abuse during periods of excessive stress demands proper vigilance and control.

Increased caffeine intake

An increased intake of caffeine may be an indicator of coping with burn-out. Caffeine serves two purposes in countering stress. The stimulant effect counteracts the lethargy from depression and the ritualistic activity of consumption reduces tension. Unfortunately, caffeine is also a physiological stressor. The average cup of coffee contains between 100 and 150 milligrams of caffeine. As little as 250 milligrams of caffeine has been implicated in nervousness, insomnia, headaches, sweaty palms and ulcers. Another vicious cycle is predictable.

Interesting fact

Common sources of caffeine include:

- tea
- coffee
- cola
- energy drinks.

The causes of stress

Both positive and negative events in one's life can be stressful. However, major life changes are the greatest contributors of stress for most people because they place the greatest demands on us for coping.

Environmental

- Moving house
- Going to college
- Transfer to a new school
- New job
- New lifestyle
- Being fired from your job
- Time pressure
- Competition
- Financial problems
- Noise
- Disappointments

Emotional

- Death of a loved one
- Marriage
- Pregnancy
- Divorce
- Relationship problems

Chemical and nutritional stress

- Excess of caffeine
- Excess of alcohol
- Excess of processed and refined foods
- Vitamin and mineral deficiencies
- Excesses of nicotine
- Drugs and manufactured synthetic compounds such as PCBs

The symptoms of stress

There are many signs and symptoms associated with people suffering from stress. These fall into four categories: feelings, thoughts, behaviour and physiology.

Feelings

- Feeling anxious
- Feeling scared
- Feeling irritable
- Feeling moody

Thoughts

- Low self-esteem
- Fear of failure
- Inability to concentrate
- Easily embarrassed
- Worrying about the future
- Preoccupation with thoughts/tasks
- Forgetfulness

Behaviour

- Stuttering and other speech difficulties
- Crying for no apparent reason
- Acting impulsively
- Easily startled
- Laughing in a high pitched and nervous tone of voice
- Grinding your teeth
- Increased smoking
- Increased use of drugs and/or alcohol
- Being accident-prone
- Losing your appetite or over-eating

Physiology

- Perspiration/sweaty hands and/or feet
- Increased heartbeat
- Trembling
- Nervous tics
- Dryness of throat and mouth
- Tiring easily
- Urinating frequently
- Sleeping problems
- Diarrhoea/indigestion/vomiting
- Butterflies in stomach
- Headaches
- Pre-menstrual tension
- Pain in the neck and/or lower back
- Susceptibility to illness

The stress response (stressed out/burnt out)

We could probably all cope with a few of the above-mentioned symptoms. But what happens if we experience five of the symptoms, or ten or twenty or more? With ever-increasing stress, our coping skills begin to deteriorate. As coping skills deteriorate, vulnerability to stress multiplies and a vicious cycle ensues, which can result in failing mental and physical health. The above symptoms are early warning signs you can become aware of, and the more symptoms a client has, the more chance the client is approaching burn out from too much stress. The official terms for burn out are either adrenal stress or a nervous breakdown – when the body just cannot cope any more and the body literally collapses in desperate need of rest and restoration.

The body's reaction to any emergency (a 'stressor') is known as the 'fight or flight' response. Fighting or running away (fight or flight) are natural *physical* reactions to the stressor. During this response stress hormones flood the system, the heart pumps faster, muscles tense ready for action and the breathing rate increases. This reaction anticipates *physical activity*, which dispels the stress hormones. Unfortunately, in our modern life, this physical activity doesn't happen, resulting in the responses to stress – the stress hormones, heart pumping faster etc. – flooding our system and not subsiding but building up in the body. The strain of being in this constant state of alert, without the release physical action brings, leads to problems such as back pain, headaches, raised blood pressure, indigestion, sweating, palpitations, irritability, anxiety and insomnia. In addition, stress contributes to, or directly causes, a variety of complaints, from cold sores to heart disease. Stressors can be environmental, emotional, chemical, nutritional or any combination of these. Stressors can also be described as '*external*' – events over which we have little control, for example traffic jams, financial hardship or bereavement; or '*internal*' – our personality traits and emotions. Our reactions to these external and internal pressures are governed by the amount of control we feel we have.

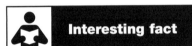

Interesting fact

It is estimated that 80 per cent of visits to the doctor are for stress-related complaints.

The stages of adaptation

Dr Hans Selye researched the effects of stress on health during the 1950s and identified three stages of adaptation to describe how the body copes with short-, medium- and long-term challenges.

1 The body's first reaction to a challenge, shock or stress is the alarm or 'fight or flight' response. Stress hormones such as adrenaline are produced; tension builds around the head, neck, lower back, chest and abdomen; thoughts focus on escape or attack. If the stress is removed, the body returns to normal functioning.

2 If the stress continues, the body copes by maintaining resistance or 'adapting'. Although the body begins to feel normal again, and may have adapted to deal with the stress, the process drains energy from the structural, biochemical and psychological realms of the body. Over time, this will affect the body's ability to function efficiently.

3 If stress is long-term, the body becomes exhausted. Reserves needed to keep adapting to ongoing stress are depleted, and one or more of the body's systems breaks down. The body becomes run down and fatigued, with recurring minor illnesses and psychological burn out. Symptoms may worsen and disease may develop, depending on the organs or systems affected. Eventually, and even if the stress is withdrawn, the body may be irreversibly damaged.

One example we can use is smoking. Most people try a cigarette at least once in their life, induced by either curiosity or peer pressure. With the first few intakes of nicotine, you may feel sick, dizzy and weak. The heart rate will increase, and generally the body will react to the 'challenge' you have given it – the challenge being a dangerous chemical taken into the body. When the cigarette is finished the body will recover quite quickly, probably in about an hour. However, if the stress continues, in other words, if you continue to smoke, the body will adapt to this continued stress and will appear to function efficiently. Eventually, with long-term use of the stressor (cigarettes), one or more of the body's systems will become very weak. In smoking it is usually the lungs that suffer either with chronic bronchitis or lung cancer. (With alcohol it may be the liver that will be affected and with chemical and nutritional stressors it may be the large colon that will suffer.) The body can only cope for so long.

Responses to stress

- Adrenaline is released into bloodstream; heart rate and blood pressure increase.
- Liver releases energy stored as glycogen; blood sugar and cholesterol levels increase.
- Increased breathing; increased metabolic rate.
- Muscular tension; increased production of lactic acid.
- Gastric acid increases or decreases; digestive enzymes and peristalsis inhibited.
- Perspiration increases.
- Increased levels of cortisol; immune system inhibited.
- Emotional tension as attention focused on emergency reaction.

Long-term effects of stress

- High blood pressure; anxiety; insomnia; irritability.
- High cholesterol levels.
- Breathlessness; hyperventilation; palpitations.
- Muscular aches and pains, including headaches and back pain.
- Nausea; indigestion; constipation; ulcers; food intolerances.
- Skin rashes; eczema.
- Raised cortisol levels increase the risk of problems with the immune system.
- Emotional outbursts; depression.

Responses to relaxation

- Decreased adrenaline levels; lower blood pressure; less stress on cardiovascular system.
- Decreased blood sugar and cholesterol levels.
- Slow breathing; improved lung function and metabolic rate.
- Relaxed muscles; less lactic acid in muscles.
- Improved digestive process.
- Improved physiological stability.
- Increased activity of immune system; less susceptibility to illness.
- Emotional calm; increased alertness and energy.

Depression, anxiety, insomnia, back pain and appetite disturbance

The above five conditions are the result of too much stress being placed upon the body. As many clients present with these symptoms, each one is described briefly below.

Depression

Depression can be both caused by stress and worsened by stress. If at least three or more of the symptoms listed below have occurred over a period of the last two years, or have recurred episodically, it would be recommended you refer your client to a stress management specialist.

1 Insomnia (trouble sleeping) or hypersomnia (excessive sleeping).
2 Low energy levels or chronic tiredness.
3 Feelings of inadequacy, loss of self-esteem, low self-appreciation.
4 Decreased effectiveness or productivity at school, work or home.
5 Decreased attention, concentration or ability to think clearly.
6 Social withdrawal.
7 Loss of interest in, or enjoyment of, activities which normally produce pleasure.
8 Irritability or excessive anger.
9 Inability to respond with expressed pleasure to praise or rewards.
10 Less active or talkative than usual, or feeling slowed down or restless.
11 Pessimistic attitude towards the future, brooding about past events, or feeling sorry for oneself.
12 Prolonged crying and/or unexplained tearfulness.
13 Recurrent thoughts of death or suicide.

Anxiety

Anxiety is the mind's natural response to an unknown but anticipated danger. When no effective response to the anticipated danger is possible, or known, anxiety itself becomes the danger since it leads to physical debilitation and psychological immobilization. A referral to a stress management specialist is recommended when there are symptoms from three of the following four categories:

1 *Motor tension:* shakiness, jitteriness, jumpiness, trembling, tension, muscle aches, fatigue, inability to relax, eyelid twitch, furrowed brow, strained face, fidgeting, restlessness, being easily startled.

2 *Autonomic hyperactivity:* sweating, heart pounding or racing, cold, clammy hands, dry mouth, dizziness, light-headedness, tingling in hands or feet, upset stomach, hot or cold spells, frequent urination, diarrhoea, discomfort in the pit of the stomach, lump in the throat, flushing, pallor, high resting pulse and respiration rate.

3 *Apprehensive expectation:* anxiety, worry, fear, obsessive thinking and anticipation of misfortune to self or others.

4 *Vigilance and scanning:* hyper-attentiveness resulting in distractibility, difficulty in concentrating, insomnia, feeling 'on edge', irritability, impatience.

Insomnia

Insomnia is characterized by:

- the inability to fall asleep
- walking and not being able to go back to sleep.

Insomnia can be a symptom of anxiety and depression, as well as excessive stress. Periodic insomnia is not abnormal and, while usually associated with excitement or concern (both are types of stress), it commonly goes away when the stressor is removed. However, chronic (of long duration or frequent recurrence) insomnia is a danger sign and indicates excessive stress. Clients should be recommended to visit their doctor for guidance.

Pain in the back or neck

The symptom of pain in either of these regions may be related to unconsciously tensing these muscles in a stressful situation. When chronically tensed they may become painful.

Appetite disturbance

Over-eating or under-eating can be responses to stress. Under-eating results from a loss of appetite owing to excessive rumination (repetitious thinking on the same subject) and concern. Over-eating is prevalent because over-eating causes large amounts of blood to be diverted to the stomach and intestines to facilitate digestion. This reduces blood flow to the brain causing a slight tranquillizing effect. Since eating tends to relax a person, people under stress tend to eat more. It is also a form of self-nurturing, with undesirable side effects. Gaining or losing weight unintentionally may be a sign of excessive stress.

How to reduce and/or manage stress

Reducing stress

Many stresses can be changed, eliminated or minimized. Here are some things you can do to reduce your level of stress.

- Become aware to your own reactions to stress.
- Reinforce positive self-statements.
- Focus on your good qualities and accomplishments.
- Avoid unnecessary competition.
- Develop assertive behaviour.
- Recognize and accept your limits – remember that everyone is different.
- Get a hobby or two; relax and have fun.
- Exercise regularly.
- Eat a balanced diet daily.
- Talk with friends or someone you can trust about your worries/problems.
- Learn to use your time wisely:
  - evaluate how you are budgeting your time;
  - plan ahead and avoid procrastination;
  - make a weekly schedule and try to follow it.

- Set realistic goals.
- Set priorities.
- If studying for examinations, study in short blocks and gradually lengthen the time you spend studying. Take frequent short breaks.
- Practise relaxation techniques.

Managing stress

Tip

Don't forget to check out the qualifications of the various teachers you meet – you only want to recommend to your clients well-qualified and insured therapists.

There are many treatments and self-help options that can be undertaken to relieve stress-related conditions. Not all treatments and options are suitable for everybody, however, and an efficient therapist should know about the many options available in order to make suitable recommendations to their clients. Rather than just casually suggesting yoga, meditation or swimming to your stressed-out clients, it is recommended that *you* attend a yoga or meditation class and that *you* go swimming. It is much easier to recommend these stress-relieving treatments if you practise what you preach! You can also put some marketing and managing skills into practice here by introducing yourself to the teachers of these classes, so you can refer clients to each other. Don't just go to one class; try a few until you find a class you really enjoy.

Exercise

Research has revealed that exercise can improve mood, lift depression, boost self-esteem, lessen anxiety and generally enable us to cope better with stress. It encourages sound sleep, improves the immune function and helps us live longer.

Exercise is nature's anti-depressant. Physiological changes in the body and brain can induce elation when we exercise, and depression and anxiety when we do not. During exercise the body temperature rises by two or three degrees, giving a sense of warm relaxation; endorphins, the body's natural opiates, are released; and the alpha brain waves associated with relaxation become more dominant. Sustained exercise burns the stress chemicals accumulated during an inactive day and after exercise the body's natural relaxation response returns body and mind to a regenerative state. It might take 6–8 weeks for exercise to change the body and improve body image, but it can change your mood at once. Vigorous activity is usually followed by between 60 and 90 minutes of calm and euphoria, and higher self-esteem may be reported after only one session. Aerobic exercise such as brisk walking, jogging or cycling or weight bearing exercise like swimming is best for mood enhancement. Co-ordinating your movements with your breathing helps to stop you overexercising and may even help to induce a state of 'relaxed awareness'.

Breathing

Breathing is involuntary and automatic, but since it can also be consciously controlled, it forms a bridge between mind and body. In Traditional Chinese Medicine (TCM), good health is said to depend on the harmonious interaction of Qi (life energy) in the air with the Qi in the body, through the medium of the lungs. Therapies such as Qigong involve breathing exercises to control Qi. Indian yogis practise Pranayama to steady the breathing and calm the body and mind. Conventional medicine does not recognize the concept of 'life energy' but does acknowledge the important role of efficient breathing in dealing with stress. When stress triggers the body's 'fight or flight' response, breathing becomes quick and shallow, reinforcing the messages of alarm being sent to the brain. If this 'overbreathing' continues, too much carbon dioxide is removed from the blood, which then loses its proper acidity. This directly affects the nerves and muscles, prompting symptoms such as faintness, palpitations and panic attacks. Slow, abdominal breathing, often practised in conjunction with muscle relaxation and visualization, may alleviate conditions such as these. These techniques calm both body and mind, and help to 'turn off' the flight-or-flight response, thus enhancing well-being throughout the whole body.

Relaxation

Many people find relaxing a very hard thing to do, with lifestyles more stressful than ever. However, relaxation is vital for good health; it helps to combat stress and gives the body time to replenish its energy. It is also essential to relax before, during and after meditation in order to get into and maintain the alpha state. Here are some suggestions to help you relax

- listen to gentle music
- lie in a warm, scented bath
- have a massage
- join a yoga class.

Exercise – progressive muscle relaxation

1   Adopt the lying down posture, close your eyes and breathe naturally. You may want to place a small towel under your head for comfort.

2   Starting with your feet, focus your attention on your feet, ankles, lower legs and knees, and 'relax' them. You should be able to feel the muscles relax and 'let go' as you direct your focus on each part of the body.

3   Move your focus to your thighs and buttocks and again 'relax' the muscles. You should immediately feel your body getting heavier. Do the same with the lower back, shoulders, arms, hands and neck.

4   Continue working up the body. There is no particular sequence, just move around the body in whatever way feels right, ending at the face and head. Notice any tension here and 'relax' and let it go. All the time be aware of your breathing. The face, head and neck carry a lot of tension, so concentrate on each part individually – the forehead, scalp and eyes. Focus, relax and let go.

5   Be aware of your whole body – now relaxed – and continue breathing slowly for a few more minutes. You may want to return to the feet and work up the body again, relaxing more each time. It will get easier the more you do it. The whole exercise should take no less than 10 minutes – the longer the more benefit it will have.

Meditation

Meditation is much more than simply relaxation: during relaxation the mind wanders uncontrollably, whereas during meditation the mind stays alert and focused. By using meditation to restrain the wanderings of the mind, we can bring ourselves back to full awareness and experience things as they really are. Clinical trials show that regular meditation induces a state of deep physical relaxation and mental awareness. It also reduces stress, as measured by a slower pulse rate, lower blood pressure, lower levels of stress hormones in the blood and an increase in alpha brain waves, associated with relaxation. The word meditate comes from a combination of the Latin word *meditor*: to think, reflect upon, and consider; and the Sanskrit word *madh-a*: wisdom.

There are many different ways to meditate and there are thousands of different meditation exercises. However, they all have one thing in common – they all start with a period of relaxation, then the mind is given one point of focus and concentrates on this and nothing else. Every time the mind tries to stray onto something else, it is gently but firmly brought back to the point of focus. There are two main choices for meditation:

Tip

This exercise can also start with the face and work down the body. Try to keep focused on each individual part of the body and on your breathing. You can also do this exercise while lying in the bath to enhance the effects of the warm water.

Tip

You can mix different methods and approaches. For example, you may start off by focusing on the breath (inner focus) while at the same time concentrating on a candle flame (outer focus).

- the *inner focus technique*, frequently used in yoga exercises, involves using something within the self – usually the breath or an inner sound or image – as the core of the exercise
- the *outer focus technique*, often found in Zen Buddhist exercises, involves using something outside the self – looking at a candle flame or a flower for example.

Meditation helps to restore balance between the left and right sides of the brain. The left side of the brain deals with thinking, speaking and writing. When we are awake and in a busy, thinking state of mind, the brain emits faster electrical patterns called 'beta' waves. In this state we are able to rationalize and think about the past and future. The right side of the brain deals with intuition, imagination and feeling. When we are sensing something, such as listening to music, and we are in a receptive rather than an active state, the brain emits slower electrical patterns called 'alpha' waves. In the alpha state we are more passive and open to our feelings. The alpha state is most likely to happen when we let ourselves live in the present rather than in the future or the past. It often happens just before or after sleep (but not during sleep as when we are sleeping the brain emits other waves called theta and delta). When we are awake we are usually in beta most of the time, and spend only about an hour in the alpha state. Meditation helps to restore the balance by increasing our time spent in alpha: it helps us to recover feeling and to experience the world directly in the present, before the sensations are 'interpreted' by the left side of the brain. The table in the margin lists the difference between the two types of wave.

Many people use the excuse that they have no time for meditation, but even if you lead a very busy life with a heavy workload and family commitments, often all that is needed is a little planning and reorganization (time management) to help you incorporate meditation into daily life.

Correct posture and breathing are essential for good meditation practice. Meditation should be enjoyable, so make sure you are comfortable – that way you can meditate uninterrupted for any length of time. There are many different meditation postures to choose from: try them all until you find one that really suits you:

- seated posture
- cross-legged posture
- kneeling posture
- lying down posture.

For the *seated posture* you can use a straight-backed chair, although you will not be leaning against it. Sit up, with your back straight, holding your head and spine in alignment. Rest your hands comfortably on your knees, or rest on the arms of the chair. Your thighs should be parallel to the floor. If you are indoors, shoes may be removed to help grounding, but you can meditate outdoors too – just remember to keep your spine straight.

For the *cross-legged posture*, simply sit on the floor and cross your legs, feet tucked under your legs. Sit upright, back straight, with your head and spine in alignment. Rest your hands on your knees. You can sit on a cushion if it means you are more comfortable.

For the *kneeling posture*, kneel on the floor, knees together, buttocks on your heels and toes almost touching. Keep your back straight, head and spine in alignment, and rest your palms on your thighs. Put a cushion on the backs of your heels and rest on this if you find this more comfortable.

The *lying down posture* is knows as the Savasana posture or 'the corpse' posture in yoga. Simply lie down on your back on a carpeted floor, rug or towel. Your legs should be straight but relaxed. Let your arms rest comfortably by your sides. The lying down posture is not ideal for meditation because it is much easier to fall asleep in it. However, it can be useful if you are feeling particularly stressed and need to relax or if you are very tired.

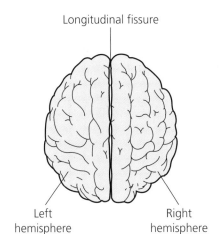

Longitudinal fissure

Left hemisphere

Right hemisphere

Left and right brain

Characteristics of alpha and beta waves

Alpha	Beta
Receptive	Active
Intuition	Thought
Present	Past/future
Relaxed	Tense
Being	Doing
Listening	Talking
Imagination	Calculation

Simple meditation exercise – inner focus

Counting the breaths is one of the easiest and best-known meditations. Do it for as long as feels comfortable. A few minutes may be all you can manage at first, but try to build up to about 20 minutes if you can.

1   Choose a position from those mentioned above. Close your eyes, relax your body and breathe normally for a few breaths.

2   Focus your attention on your breathing. After each exhalation, but before breathing in, count silently as follows: 'One' (inhale, exhale), 'Two' (inhale, exhale), and so on until you reach Five', then start again from 'One'.

3   Feel the air going in and out as you breathe. You will soon notice how your mind tries to distract you from counting, with all manner of thoughts. Just bring it gently back each time you realize you have been side-tracked. When you have finished, come back from the meditation slowly and open your eyes.

Simple meditation exercise – outer focus

1   Sit in a straight-backed chair at a table and light a candle which should be placed safely in front of you. Do not close your eyes, but relax your body and breathe normally for a few breaths.

2   Look intently at the candle flame, but without straining your eyes. Keep your eyes and eyelids relaxed. Be aware of the movement of your breath in your abdomen. During the entire exercise, stay aware of your breath, and keep observing the candle flame. Do not think about the candle flame, just look at it attentively, as if it were the most interesting thing you have ever seen. As outside thoughts come into your mind, bring your attention back to the candle flame and your breathing.

Tip

Try each exercise a couple of times, and you will then know if you prefer to use an inner or an outer focus for your meditation sessions.

Visualization

Visualization is an extremely powerful technique that uses the imagination to create particular states of mind and being. It can be used for a wide variety of purposes:

- to cope with stress
- to improve the concentration
- for training the mind
- to increase self-confidence
- for problem solving
- to activate the body's self-healing processes.

It is unclear precisely how visualization works, but it is said to encourage activity in the right hemisphere of the brain, which relates to creativity and emotions. Visualization can be used as a self-help technique or can be practised on a one-to-one basis or in a group, often as part of psychotherapy or hypnotherapy.

Visualization goes far beyond just the imagination. Although it uses the imagination to create mental images of things, it goes much further because it involves all the senses, and not just sight, smell, touch, hearing and taste, but the emotions as well. Think of or 'visualize' something you really do *not* like. This could be spiders, mice or rats, heights or water. Really 'imagine' using all your senses. For example, if you are afraid of spiders, imagine one jumping onto your hand or into your hair. If you visualize this clearly enough, or you can recall a past experience, or *feel* the spider moving in your hair, you will find that your body responds to this stress and you will notice some physical reactions taking place. For example, you will probably tense up and your pulse rate will increase. You might also find that you are breathing more rapidly. If the stress is strong enough you might even find yourself sweating or shivering. The reason your body is responding in this way is that our bodies do not distinguish between things we visualize and reality itself. So if the situation you are visualizing is stressful enough it will trigger the body's 'fight or flight' mechanism. So just by imagining the spider (or mouse or height or water or whatever) your body will shut down all the systems that are not essential to immediate survival. Adrenaline and anti-inflammatory agents will be pumped into the system and your body will be poised for a potentially life-saving 'fight or flight' response.

Why visualize about something we don't like? Change the situation around and visualize positive events and thoughts and they become real, as the mind cannot distinguish between real and non-real events. Thus positive thoughts and images can become real with determined and continual practice of the visualization technique.

The benefits of visualization

Visualization can be used for many beneficial reasons:

- to combat stress
- to achieve success
- to fight illness
- to increase self-confidence.

When we think about something that makes us happy, the brain produces endorphins and other pleasure-giving chemicals and our bodies experience the physical sensations of happiness. We can use visualization to achieve the same effects in what might otherwise be a stressful situation.

To combat stress:

- Visualize a beach – where you can relax and unwind. Feel the warmth of the sun and the texture of the sand, hear the waves and smell the sea air.
- Visualize a tropical waterfall – this may help calm your mind. Listen to the sound of rushing water and mentally explore the banks of lush plants and fragrant flowers.
- Visualize a mountain scene – this can promote a sense of harmony. Imagine the space and light around you and the sensation of filling your lungs with fresh clean air.

Initially try to find a quiet place, lie down or sit in a comfortable chair, and close your eyes. Breathe slowly and relax before focusing on your chosen mental image. Try to repeat the exercise three times a day. With continued practice, you will be able to do these exercises anywhere. While walking down a busy, fume-filled street, while travelling on overcrowded transport, waiting in queues or in any stressful situation.

To achieve success:

- Fear of public speaking can be overcome by imagining yourself speaking calmly to a room of people. Imagine the audience is smiling and hanging onto every word you say. Imagine enjoying the experience and feeling very calm and comfortable. Hear the applause as you finish.
- To prepare for interviews, visualize yourself calmly greeting the panel of interviewers and dealing confidently with their questions.
- Before a sports event, motivation can be boosted by mentally rehearsing the precise sequence of events required for a successful performance.

Imagine a situation in which you hope to succeed. Tell yourself that you are confident and in control. If you feel that you are becoming tense at the thought of a particular difficulty, breathe slowly, relax and detach yourself from the scene.

To fight illness:

- Create a mental picture of your illness: some people have described pain as an iron bar or a red-hot needle. Envisage any treatment you are receiving as eliminating pain and strengthening your self-healing powers. Imagine yourself healthy again.

- *Dial* – imagine a dial the indicator of which is registering your pain. Turning down the imaginary dial can be visualized as 'turning down' the pain. This may help you to feel in control of pain and able to cope more successfully with short or long-term illnesses.

- *Box* – locking worries, pain or illness in a mental box where they can be contained and shut away has proved effective in some cases.

If you keep on visualizing these positive situations eventually the right side of the brain will come to associate the thought of public speaking, interviews, the sports event, controlling pain, or whatever the situation you are visualizing, with pleasure or comfort and your fears disappear. So visualization is not just all in the mind. Although it starts in the mind, it can have profoundly physical effects.

To cure an addiction:

- If you want to cure an addiction, perhaps to give up smoking, drinking caffeine, or you would like to increase your self-confidence, you can use visualization to help with that too.

The main thing to bear in mind with visualization is that you should endeavour to do it as clearly and in as much detail as possible. You also need to *keep* doing it, in order to reinforce the message you are giving to the right side of your brain. This side of the brain, you will recall, is the side that deals with feelings and intuition rather than thinking and speaking. It will receive your visualizations without question and transform them into feelings, once you get them past the left side of the brain. Practice and repetition will help you achieve this.

Exercise – visualization skills using meditation

Although you can practise your visualization skills anywhere, practise initially in a quiet place where you know you won't be disturbed.

1 Get comfortable using one of the postures described above. Breathe naturally and close your eyes.

2 Choose an item you are going to visualize. This can be a flower, a piece of favourite clothing, a coin, a building or someone's face. Let's say you chose a rose. Try to visualize the rose. Try to see in it your mind's eye as though it really exists. See it in as much detail as you can. Notice everything about it – its colour, shape and texture, notice every petal, turn the rose over in your mind, and study the other side and look inside the rose. Is it the same colour all over or does it get paler in the centre? If you can bring in the other senses so much the better. Smell the rose, feel the delicate petals, the stem, the needles that may prick you. What do the petals feel like? Are there any leaves? What do they feel like? What colour are they?

3 Open your eyes. Write down every sensation and detail. Repeat this exercise with other objects. A leaf, a strawberry, a £5 note, anything you like. The more you can develop your skills of visualization on everyday items, the more successful you will be when visualizing events. Don't forget to use all your senses.

Yoga

Best known in the West as a form of gentle exercise consisting of body postures and breathing techniques, yoga is in fact a complete system of mental and physical training, originally developed as preparation for spiritual development. It has been practised for thousands of years in India as part of Ayurveda and has now become popular around the world. In the West it is valued more for its physical than spiritual benefits, such as its ability to increase suppleness and vitality and to relieve stress.

The benefits of yoga and its main uses

- To combat stress and fatigue.
- To reduce headaches and migraines.
- To alleviate depression.
- To improve circulatory disorders.
- To improve asthma and bronchitis.
- To improve rheumatoid arthritis.
- To improve digestive disorders.
- To relieve back pain.
- To reduce menstrual problems including PMS.
- To improve mobility.

A 1990 study in the medical journal *Lancet* showed that yoga breathing reduced the frequency of asthma attacks, while in 1993, psychologists at Oxford University found yoga breathing more effective for restoring energy than either relaxation or visualization. In the *British Journal of Rheumatology,* a 1994 study indicated that yoga therapy could benefit people with rheumatoid arthritis.

The relaxation response

The 'relaxation response' is a quick and easy exercise devised by Dr Herbert Benson, a cardiologist from Harvard Medical School. The changes the exercise bring are distinctly different from the physiological changes experienced when you just sit quietly or sleep. The relaxation response is the physiological opposite of the fight or flight response, as it decreases the activity of the sympathetic nervous system. It also decreases metabolism, heart rate, the rate of breathing, blood flow to the muscles and blood lactate levels (which are associated with muscular fatigue), but increases the alpha brain waves, associated with feelings of relaxation and well-being.

Exercise – the relaxation response

What you need:

- *A quiet environment*. This can be anywhere but must have no loud noises or distractions.
- *A mental device*. This is equivalent to using a mantra while meditating. It is a single-syllable sound or one word that you repeat silently or in a quiet tone. It helps you to remove yourself from logical thought and distractions. The word 'ONE' is often used in exercises of this kind.
- *A passive attitude*. This sounds simple and it should be, but people sometimes make too much of it, defeating the purpose. A passive attitude means not focusing on how well you're doing in the exercise or whether you're getting the correct response. When either of these thoughts occurs to you, let it go and focus instead on repeating your chosen word.
- *A comfortable position*. You want to reduce any awareness of your muscles as much as possible. A comfortable chair that supports your head is good. It's even better if you can lie down.

Now:

1   Sit in a comfortable position in a quiet environment.

2   Close your eyes.

3   Relax your muscles, beginning with your feet, then your calves, thighs, lower torso, chest, shoulders, arms, neck and head. Pay special attention to the muscles in your neck and face, which get very tense.

4   Breathe through your nose, paying attention to your breathing. As you exhale, say aloud or just think about your chosen word.

5   Do this for at least 10 minutes – 20 minutes if you have the time. You can gently open your eyes to check the time, but it is strongly recommended that you *do not* use an alarm.

The exercise is most effective when performed in the middle of the day. It is recommended that you practise the relaxation response at least once, or even better twice, every day. You, and your clients, will be amazed to find that such a simple exercise that takes so little time can have such an important effect on your body and mind. It helps in bringing stress levels down, leaving you feeling calm but invigorated, and enabling you to work more efficiently and effectively.

Knowledge review

1   What is stress?

2   What is environmental stress? Give three examples.

3   What is chemical and nutritional stress?

4   Give four examples of chemical stressors.

5   What are PCBs?

6   There are four main categories that cause stress – what are these?

7   There are four main categories of symptoms for stress – what are these?

8   What happens during the stress response?

9   What is anxiety?

10   Give eight examples of how to reduce stress.

11   List five benefits of exercise.

12   What happens to breathing when stress triggers the fight or flight response?

13   What is the difference between relaxation and meditation?

14   What are the two main techniques used in meditation?

15   What does meditation actually do?

16   What is the difference between beta and alpha waves?

17   What is visualization?

18   Give five examples of the benefits of yoga.

19   What is the 'relaxation response'?

20   A 'mental device' is required for the relaxation response. What is a 'mental device'?

Crystal therapy

16

Learning objectives

This chapter covers the following:

- **a history of crystal therapy**
- **what are crystals**
- **grounding**
- **recommendations for a basic set of crystals**
- **types of crystal**
- **self-treatment**
- **chakra balancing**
- **using crystals with other therapies**
- **specific after care advice**

The beauty, power and healing abilities of crystals and other stones have been used for thousands of years, from the encrusted golden mask of Tutankhamun to the modern masterpieces of Cartier and Fabergé. Due to awarding bodies introducing qualifications in crystal therapy, their use and acceptance has grown in popularity amongst therapists. They can be used alone but are usually used in conjunction with visualization or meditation, and often involve working with chakras, acupressure points, meridians or auras. Methods vary widely, but all tap into the 'healing energy' stored within the crystals. Crystals can also be used to increase the effectiveness of other holistic therapies. Crystal therapy offers deep relaxation, relief from stress, mind and body balance, and abundant energy. They are used to enhance the process of healing in the treatment of any physical or emotional condition. Different crystals have different abilities: some crystal energy can be used to heal, while the energy of others is used to unblock and revitalize the body and mind. Just one crystal can be used or a combination of crystals selected according to the client's needs, just as you would select essential oils for an aromatherapy treatment. They can be used everywhere: as jewellery, or in the home, the office or classroom, the garden or the treatment room, to create balance, vitality, energy or calmness. Their uses are limited only by the confines of your imagination. Learning to trust your intuition is also an important aspect of crystal therapy.

A history of crystal therapy

There does not seem to be a concise history of the use of crystals. Looking back there is evidence that ancient cultures including the Aborigines, the Native Americans, the Mayans, the Tibetans, the Celts, the Egyptians and the Aztecs, effectively used and had great respect for crystals for power, influence or healing. There are also many books on the legends of Atlantis, the people of which are reported to have used crystals for many purposes including communication.

Crystals have also been used throughout the centuries by royalty and the church as a sign of wealth and power. Today they are just a sign of wealth, but in years gone by there may have been a deeper reason for using crystals and precious gems. It has been suggested that certain crystals and certain combinations of crystals and gemstones helped with a leader's power, helping them increase their natural intuition and psychic powers to protect and control the people! We hear of the *crown* being fought over, not the ruler; it is the *ring* that signifies the bishop, not the person; and even today there are coronations where the monarch is presented with a crown and other symbols covered in gemstones and crystals.

Interesting fact

The Bible mentions crystals over 200 times, with many particularly notable references. One describes the breastplate of the high priest (Exodus 28:17.20) which was decorated with sardius, topaz, garnet, emerald, sapphire, ligure, agate, amethyst, beryl, onyx and jasper.

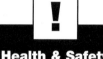

Health & Safety

Never hit crystals with hammers – or try to break them. The amount of energy that could be released by the act of hitting and breaking crystals was well known in ancient societies. It would not be enough to do any harm, but it may give you a bit of a jolt!

What are crystals?

There are three kingdoms on this Earth: the elemental kingdom, the plant kingdom and the animal kingdom. The elemental kingdom is believed to be the first kingdom on Earth, and from the four elements – air, fire, water and earth – come things composed of these elements, for example stones, crystals and magma. It is considered the most independent of the three kingdoms because it can exist alone.

Any substance in which the atoms are arranged in a geometric, symmetrical, 3D pattern is called a crystal. The Earth is covered by variety of rocks, many of which are made up of minerals, of which there are approximately 2000. Virtually all minerals contain atoms arranged in this geometric fashion; this pattern is called crystalline. The word 'crystal' derives from the Greek for 'ice', and refers to the early belief that crystals were simply water which had frozen so solid that they were beyond thawing. As late as the eighteenth century some scientists maintained that clear rock crystal was simply fossilized ice!

Of course scientific knowledge then was not as advanced as it is now. Today we know that one atom of any mineral is the replica of another atom of the same type. Gold atoms, for example, are all identical – and this is the basis of chemical classification. A chemical that is composed solely of one type of atom is called an element, but most minerals are composed of a variety of different sorts of atoms, glued together by electrical forces to produce

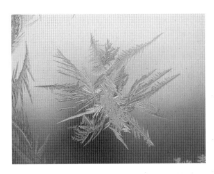

Ice crystals

molecules. A molecule of water, for example, is composed of the atoms of two elements: hydrogen and oxygen. The crystal form of water is ice, a solid substance in which the atoms of hydrogen and oxygen are arranged in ordered geometrical patterns.

We see the natural shape of water crystals in the snowflakes that drift from the sky in the freezing winter. They grow, floating on the breeze, by collecting more and more molecules of water, which arrange themselves according to the characteristic hexagonal pattern of their atomic structure.

Minerals can change their state. In nature water can exist as a solid and as a liquid depending on the environment, e.g. the North Pole. Ordinary rocks are no different except that the temperature at which they melt (change state) is very high; it is usually attained in active volcanoes. Because of the high temperatures involved, many crystals are formed deep in the Earth or in volcanoes, where mineral-rich liquids slowly solidify in fractures in the Earth's crust. It is because different minerals crystallize at different temperatures that we find such a wide variety of spectacular crystals. Not all crystals rely on volcanic heat to form. Some minerals are soluble (salt, for example, dissolves readily in water) and when the mineral concentration in the liquid is high enough, the atoms start to stick together, forming crystals. Selenite, which can form distinctive desert roses, is the first of various minerals, including salt, to crystallize when sea water evaporates.

To further complicate the story of how crystals grow, it is worth noting that many minerals can crystallize in a variety of different shapes and forms. Some minerals have a cube as their basic building blocks, some have a pyramid formation, others are patterned on a hexagon – it is the wide variety of forms and shapes that makes crystallography such a fascinating subject. At first glance the graphite 'lead' in a pencil bears no relation to the glittering diamond in a ring, but they are actually the same atomic element – carbon. What has happened is that the diamond has been subjected to enormous pressure underground and its atomic structure has been crushed into a more compact crystal lattice.

How do crystals obtain their life force energy?

Crystals (minerals) receive their life force from the sun and other planetary sources and when used for treatment purposes will emit powerful vibrations and frequencies, which will be effective in balancing and attuning the body, mind and spirit.

Grounding

Before carrying out *any* holistic treatment, it is important to ground yourself. Grounding means keeping both feet on the ground, physically and mentally. Grounding is a process by which a person or object is reconnected with the energy of the Earth and the physical plane. When performing any treatment it is important to 'be in the here and now' and not thinking about what you will have for dinner or that the car needs fuel on the way home. Before starting a treatment, you need to allow a little time; it only takes a minute or two to relax and to remove from your mind your own problems. They will still be there at the end of the treatment, but for the duration of the treatment your focus must be on your client, not yourself.

Sit or stand quietly so that your feet are firmly flat on the ground – preferably without shoes – and your back is straight. Let your body relax and your mind be calm. If the thoughts keep creeping in, imagine them

Tip

As a quick grounding exercise, become aware of your feet, wiggle your toes, and imagine that your shoes are weighted down!

inside clouds and let the clouds, with your thoughts inside them, float gently out of your mind. Be aware of your breathing – breathe right down into your abdominal area as this helps the grounding process. You may want to concentrate on the colour red, which is the colour of the base chakra, or the shape of a square, which is the shape of the base chakra. You may want to think about your adrenal glands, the glands associated with the base chakra, and imagine them calm and peaceful, not madly pumping out adrenaline to get through the day! Then concentrate on your feet, and imagine roots growing out of them into the ground. A drink of water is also helpful.

Choosing, storing, cleansing and energizing crystals

Choosing

Never buy crystals in a hurry. They will become very special to you and if you are to work well together, it must be the right crystal. Trying to work with crystals that are not right for you will produce poor results. It is said that you do not choose the crystal, but the crystal chooses you! It is not recommended that you buy crystals by mail order or from the Internet. It is so important for you to see, touch and feel the crystals you will be working with. You need to use your senses and following these guidelines will help you.

- Look
- Listen
- Touch
- Trust your intuition

First of all you may see a crystal that 'takes your eye'. This is a good start, but remember what happens when you are clothes shopping? You may see an item of clothing that you love, but when you try the garment on it may look terrible, be the wrong size or the wrong colour for you, or just not be you. Even though you love the garment you would be foolish to buy it as it would probably end up in the wardrobe and never be worn. It is the same when buying crystals. First you see the crystal, then you want to touch the crystal and take a closer look. Take it into the natural light, look deep into it and go with what you are feeling from within, not with what your brain is saying. Look right into the centre of the crystal – What do you *see*? What do you *feel*? What do you *hear*? You should trust your intuition when buying crystals. The most important thing of all is to *listen* to your heart and not your brain.

If you are looking at many crystals all at the same time, you may want to 'feel' by hovering one hand over them. This method may also enhance the intuitive process, as your hand will be picking up the vibrations of the crystals and conveying that information back to you. It is like the crystals are speaking to you through your hand. Carefully place your hand, palm down, about 10–15 cm (4 to 6 inches) above the crystals under consideration. Relax as deeply as possible, block out as much of what is going on around you as you can and note what sensations you can now feel. BELIEVE in what you feel. That tingling, feeling of heat, or cold, or strange sensation in your hand is not your imagination; you are picking up the energy of the crystals. What do you do if you 'feel' one crystal is for you, but like the look of another? Use your intuition – you could even ask the crystal 'Which crystal wants to help me with my work?' This may sound ridiculous at the moment, but when you start buying and working with crystals it will seem very natural. Remember you have small chakras in the palms of your hand. These small energy centres will help you resonate with the crystal that is right for you. Be open-minded and let your intuition go with the flow. Stay relaxed.

When choosing naturally pointed crystals such as clear quartz, amethyst, citrine or smoky quartz, try to choose those with undamaged points. One of the energy sources of the crystals is this main termination – the point. Any damage may affect the energy release of the crystal.

Storing

Crystals hate being left in cupboards or drawers or anywhere dark. Once you start working with your crystals they become part of you and want to be near you. The more they are around you, the more you will attune yourself to their vibrations, and the more you will become sensitive to them and, ultimately, to your surroundings.

When you are not working with them, leave them in a place where they can be seen, in a glass cabinet for example. An excellent place for them is on a windowsill where they will absorb the energy of the sun. A quartz cluster can be left in any room or office to absorb negative energies or an amethyst cluster can be placed near your computer to absorb negative electrical pulses.

Cleansing

It is important to clean crystals and gemstones after a therapy session because they will pick up and store negativity and thought patterns.

There are several ways of cleansing a crystal.

- You can bury it in the garden for 24–48 hours for Mother Earth to cleanse. (Unlike being kept in a dark drawer unused, the crystal came from deep within the Earth, and will be cleansed by the Earth, which will take in the negativity.) Rinse before use.
- You can wash crystals in water to which you have added sea salt.
- You can wash them under running water.
- You can wash them in water to which you have added a few drops of Bach Flower Remedies.
- You can use the element of fire by passing a crystal through the flame of a candle.
- You can place a new crystal on a large crystal cluster of quartz for a few days.
- You can put (male) crystals in the sunshine and allow the sun to cleanse them.
- You can put (female) crystals in the moonlight and allow the moon to cleanse them.

The choice is yours – but cleanse them you must. Crystals reflect light, life, colour and clarity, and because they vibrate at a low level they are sensitive and will pick up vibrations, frequencies, impurities and other imprints.

Today crystals are used abundantly in watches, clocks, computers, and medical and other specialized equipment because of their ability to work on a frequency, emitting and transmitting light. So with this understanding it is easy to see that they will pick up negativity. This is not only in the atmosphere: because they work on a thought vibration, they pick up thoughts also. Just think of the emotions a crystal may pick up just lying in a shop somewhere, being handled by people with all kinds of problems, both emotional and physical. If crystals are not cleansed regularly they will become dense and heavy with negativity. They may lose their lustre, their colour or even their powers.

 Interesting fact

Dr Edward Bach was an English doctor who concluded from studies of his patients that negative emotions could lead to physical illness. He was also convinced that flowers possessed healing properties that could be used to treat emotional problems and so restore health and harmony to the mind and body. During the 1930s Bach began to produce his remedies, which are made by infusing or boiling plant material in spring water. Bach Flower Remedies and other flower essences are today popular around the world, and are often taken for self-help during times of emotional crises or stress. Rescue Remedy is probably the best known of the Bach Flower remedies.

Energizing

Just as human beings need food for energy, crystals too need energizing or charging. As with cleansing, there are many ways of energizing crystals, but the most popular are as follows:

- sun (male crystals)
- moon (female crystals)
- thunderstorms
- streams
- breath.

Harnessing the power of the sun or moon, by leaving your crystals outside on a windowsill or somewhere safe, is a powerful way of energizing them. Thunderstorms that release huge amounts of energy are also an excellent way to energize crystals – but put them somewhere safe!

Charging crystals by streams can be a more gentle method of energizing crystals. They will need to be left for 24 hours so you will need to leave them in a safe place. Put them in a small container made of natural products such as a wooden bowl or a pouch tied with silk and lodge carefully in place. You would not want to lose them downstream.

It is also possible to use your own breath to energize crystals. To do this you need to ground yourself, still your mind as much as possible and concentrate on the crystal. Breathe on it and focus on removing any negative energy held within the crystal. When you feel you have accomplished this, breathe on it again, with the intent (*having the attention sharply focused*) of adding good healing energy to feed the crystal. This is a useful process when faced with a situation where the other methods are not available or when there is insufficient time for a full cleansing.

Male and female crystals

A crystal can be male, female or androgynous, and if she is female it can be quite damaging for her to be left in the sunlight for too long. A female crystal should be cleansed and energized by moonlight and a male crystal by sunlight. Generally speaking, a female crystal will be softer, smoother and more rounded than a male crystal, which tends to be phallic, angular, pointed or rough. Male stones tend to give out strong vibrations, whereas female stones tend to be more subtle in what they emit. A male crystal transmits energy and a female crystal is receptive by nature.

Taking amethyst as an example, this female stone will often fade dramatically if left out in the sun because the strength of direct sunlight drains this crystal of its subtle and feminine attributes. Amethysts love to be cleansed by moonlight. *Not sure what your crystal is? Ask it!!*

Here are some examples of male stones. These direct energy outwards and are good for sending healing energy, for projecting wishes, for confidence and for self-assurance, willpower, lasting success and luck.

Amber
Bloodstone
Carnelian
Citrine
Haematite
Quartz (clear)
Topaz

Here are some examples of female stones. They can be used for the relief of stress, for fertility, for love and development of the heart, for wisdom and understanding, for meditation enhancement, for spiritual aspirations, for psychic development and for intuitive work.

Amethyst

Calcite (blue or pink)

Lapis lazuli

Malachite

Moonstone

Celestite

Quartz (clear, rose, smoky)

Turquoise

Tourmaline (green)

You will notice that the quartz crystals can be male or female. You will know by its qualities – trust your intuition.

Recommendations for a basic set of crystals

Twenty crystals

Amber

Amber is said to promote stability, help combat feelings of insecurity and to attract treasures (especially antiques). Amber is the sun stone for those born under the sign of Taurus and is one of the oldest substances to be worn on the body. Amber pendants have been found at Northern European grave sites dating from 8000 BC. Amber is not a true crystal, being made of fossilized resin from a coniferous tree similar to our modern pine. Sometimes insects or plant material became trapped in the resin as it fell to the ground and were caught forever in the developing fossil. Unlike crystals, amber is warm to the touch and so is said to contain the power of the sun – it has been used in fire ceremonies across the world. It has antiseptic and disinfectant qualities and is used to purify body, mind and spirit as well as to cleanse rooms of accumulated negativity. In ancient times it was ground up and used as an antibiotic elixir.

Amethyst

Amethyst enhances energy and thought waves; it kindles the spiritual flame within each of us and stimulates the third eye (the brow chakra), thus sharpening the sixth sense. Amethyst has a gentle (female) but powerful energy and is an ideal starting stone for anyone wishing to meditate or work with crystals. It absorbs negativity and emits positively. Worn around the neck it will protect the wearer from radiation, including low-level EMFs (electromagnetic fields) caused by electrical equipment such as televisions, mobile phones, microwaves and electrical wiring. Amethyst is particularly effective in the treatment of ailments affecting the head, including mental disturbances, hearing problems, dizziness and headaches. It also energizes the glandular, circulatory, nervous and digestive systems.

Aventurine (green)

Aventurine is a variety of crystal (most commonly quartz or feldspar) that is speckled with other crystals. It is usually a green colour and so is used to treat heart conditions. (The colour of the heart chakra is green.) It also

Interesting fact

Amethysts and electrical equipment
Put amethyst upon a piece of electrical equipment and it will absorb the radiation from that equipment, preventing it spreading into the room. The amethyst may appear to have black speckles over it when you next look. This will be the negativity it has absorbed and will disappear once the stone has been cleansed. Simply leave out overnight in the moonlight – preferably a full moon. Weekly cleansing is sufficient.

helps increase motivation and adventurousness by connecting you to all of creation and reducing inner fears. It is generally known as the crystal of 'balance'.

Bloodstone

Bloodstone is a variety of quartz and, as its name suggests, it is used in the treatment of all blood disorders and circulatory problems, including haemorrhages and varicose veins. In ancient Egypt, the bloodstone was used to open doors both physically and spiritually. It can stop nosebleeds and improve memory by stimulating cerebral blood flow. During the thirteenth century, magicians wore bloodstones engraved with the figure of a bat to increase their power and to give them protection. Being red, bloodstone will help you stay grounded and give you energy.

Blue lace agate

A stone of peace and happiness, and a welcome friend in a stressful situation. This stone is at home on a work desk or in a difficult atmosphere, radiating calming energies and releasing blockages from the nervous system. It is also a wonderful for meditation and visualization.

Carnelian

Carnelian is a form of chalcedony and is red, orange or red-brown. As well as possessing all the properties of chalcedony, carnelian has been used since Egyptian times to quell anger, fear and hatred. It removes lethargy and depression, and stimulates inquisitiveness and curiosity. It has also been used in the treatment of neuralgia, gallstones, kidney stones and skin disorders.

Calcite (orange)

Calcite teaches that 'learning is remembering what we already know' by helping us to unlock genetic and spiritual memories. This 'unlocking' takes the form of spontaneous realizations and insights. When you work with calcite, you will find new ideas and thoughts coming into your mind and you will not be able to pinpoint their origin. Calcite also helps to stimulate past-life memories and enables you to integrate the lessons of those memories into the here and now.

Citrine

This yellow to golden-brown stone used to be called the merchant's stone, as it was said that placing a piece of it in a cash box would attract more customers to the vendor. It is connected to the sun and so has links with clear vision and enlightenment. Placed upon a table during a discussion or meeting, it improves understanding and communication and allows problems and their potential solutions to be viewed more easily. It also aids all digestive problems and helps the elimination of toxins from the body.

Fluorite

Coming in a huge variety of shades and colours, from purple, white and green, to magenta, red and black, fluorite opens the mind to spiritual awareness, connecting you to all life. It also purifies and cleanses. To make an elixir, place a piece of fluorite in a glass of spring water in the sunlight for an hour then drink the water. This helps the body to eliminate toxins and boosts the immune system.

Haematite

Haematite is rich in iron and as such is known as the stone of blood. It balances the mind, encouraging better mental control over the emotional and physical state. Its magnetic properties mean that it is a useful stone for grounding excess mental, emotional or physical energy. It can be used to treat blood conditions (such as anaemia) and leg cramps.

Lapis lazuli

The ancient Sumerians associated lapis lazuli with kings and deities. Many other cultures, including the Egyptians and Jews have considered it a royal stone. It is a crystal that strengthens the mind and body, protects against negativity and attracts wisdom and truth. An inspiration stone, lapis lazuli helps to bring ideas from the subconscious mind into the conscious mind, while allowing all sides of an issue to be seen.

Malachite

This crystal is said to be particularly good for the teeth and mouth. It is a beautiful and gentle stone and so is suitable for children and the elderly. It strengthens the physical body and calms the emotions, soothes inflammation and swellings, and can also be used in the treatment of infertility.

Moonstone

As its name suggests, the moonstone is connected to the power of the moon and so also to the emotions. It enhances and develops emotional sensitivity to others and is a good stone for lovers. It gently calms and soothes the nerves and is useful in the treatment of period pains, irregular menstruation and infertility.

Quartz (clear)

Clear quartz can be used for all purposes as it vibrates the clear white light which contains all other colours. Quartz is abundant and widely used throughout the world. It was once believed to be frozen water as many of our ancestors saw its qualities as being similar to those of ice, and this was how it developed its long association with purity. It is a crystal of protection and is worn by many people both to attract positive energies and to repel negative ones. As well as 'clear crystal', quartz is also called 'rock crystal' and 'quartz crystal'.

Quartz (rose)

Sometimes known as the 'love stone', rose quartz facilitates the release of anger, resentment and other negative emotions, teaching you not only how to love others, but how to love yourself also. It is a stone of creativity and so is good for all artists, musicians, writers and therapists. Although the colour of the heart chakra is green and any green gemstone or crystal can be used with it, it is often the rose quartz that is placed upon this chakra to create harmony and balance in this area.

Sodalite (blue)

Sodalite is a consciousness-opening stone, bringing clarity and wisdom. A good brain balancer, it assists in mastering the ego and removing selfish behaviour and reactionary responses to other people's negative energies.

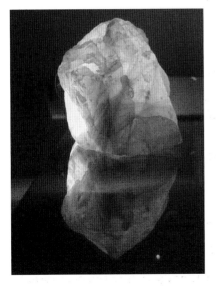

Rose quartz

It helps to regulate the endocrine system and is also said to be particularly helpful for insomnia if placed under a pillow at night.

Tiger's eye

Yellow stones represent the sun, fire and strength. Tiger's eyes are considered very lucky and are said to stimulate intuition and enhance awareness of any potential danger. The stone promotes a deeper understanding of our own inner resources. As a meditation stone, it is especially useful when trying to come to an important decision. Tiger's eye can be used to promote attention to detail and a willingness to listen to others' points of view.

Tourmaline

Tourmaline promotes co-operation and balance between the left and right sides of the brain. It allows you to see, not only your life's dream, but the steps you need to take to bring that dream to reality. It has long been regarded as a powerfully protective stone and is said to warn of dangers on the physical plane. Multicoloured tourmaline is particularly prized, as it is said to fill your life with rich colours and magic!

Interesting fact

All stones and rocks contain crystals, so any stone can be called a crystal. Some cultures hold all stones in high regard, whether they are the beautifully coloured crystals used in crystal therapy or the basalt rocks and stones used in stone therapy. What most people call crystals are in fact gem stones.

Types of crystal

Clear quartz crystals – single terminators

Clear quartz can be used for all purposes as it vibrates the clear white light which contains all other colours. The six sides of the quartz represent the six chakras with the termination being the crown chakra.

Clear quartz crystals – double terminated crystal

This is a crystal with a terminator (point) at each end. The energy within it travels in both directions and so helps to integrate the physical with the spiritual. These specialized crystals have the capacity to draw in as well as emanate out energy from either end. They have polarity and cleanse themselves. Wearing a double terminated crystal around the neck or by holding in each hand a double terminated crystal for even five minutes creates a protective energy and will calm and relax you into a state of mental and emotional stability. They are ideal to place between two chakras to bring into balance and unity the two and open the flow of energy.

Health & Safety

Don't wave crystals around. Remember – they are objects of power. They emit, transduce and transmute energy and in some respects can be likened to a laser, a laser for higher psychic levels of energetic vibration. Because of this, no terminated (pointed) crystal should be waved around in the presence of other people or animals. Remember that we have auric layers surrounding us which can be very sensitive to higher levels of energy.

Laser wand crystal

A long and slender crystal with a single termination or point. It is an amplifier and tuner of energies and so primarily is used to focus healing energies, although it can also be used as an aid in meditation also. It is said that laser wands carry the knowledge of ancient civilizations and have a profound and intimate relationship with both outer space and the depths of inner earth, serving to create a bridge between these worlds.

Channelling crystals

Channelling crystals (also known as transmitter crystals) have seven sides. They are used as a tool in personal meditation practices to gain inner clarity and to channel the light of wisdom into the mind and into daily affairs. They

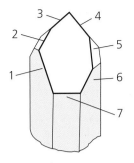

Rose quartz channelling crystal

can be used when specific answers are needed or when you want to gain information about a particular matter. The intention of channelling crystals is to teach personal empowerment by enabling one to channel all the different facets and all the various rays that exist within each person.

Phantom crystal

This is a crystal that holds one or more 'phantom' crystals within itself. The phantoms either appear as distinct crystals or as shadows within the crystal, rather like the growth lines on the rings of a tree. A phantom crystal is said to have known many lifetimes and can therefore help you connect with a past life or genetic memories.

Clusters

Clusters are formations of single terminated crystals that share a common base. These clusters gather negative energy and replace it with white light creating harmony and peace. They purify and recharge healing stones. They are very useful in distance healing when laying pictures of friends and family upon them.

Self-treatment

Getting to know your crystals

Select seven crystals to which you are attracted and which you feel you want to work with on yourself. As with all therapies, you need to know what a treatment feels like before you can recommend it to others. Using a simple visualization technique you will feel, touch and listen to each of your selected crystals individually before using them, all together, over the chakra areas of your body, in a whole self-treatment. The selected crystals below have been chosen in relationship to their colour and associated chakras.

> **Haematite** for the base chakra – haematite is shiny on the outside but when rubbed on a porcelain tile, used for testing crystals, it streaks red.
>
> **Carnelian** for the sacral chakra – as carnelian is orange which is the colour associated with this chakra
>
> **Citrine** for the solar plexus chakra – as citrine is yellow, the colour associated with this chakra.
>
> **Rose quartz** for the heart chakra – although rose quartz is pink, it can be used on the heart chakra as it is the crystal representing love.
>
> **Blue lace agate** for the throat chakra – as the colour for this crystal is pale blue, which is the colour associated with this chakra.
>
> **Sodalite** for the brow chakra – as sodalite is dark blue and dark blue or indigo is associated with the brow chakra.
>
> **Amethyst** for the crown chakra as amethyst is violet, which is the colour associated with the crown chakra.

Tip

Do not worry if when you first start using your crystals you think that nothing is happening. It will be! It just takes time to become attuned into your crystals. Be patient!

Getting to know individual crystals

This exercise will take approximately 40 minutes if all the stones are used. If you do not have time for a single session, then working through the stones one or two at a time is acceptable.

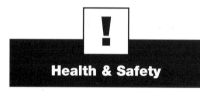

- Sit somewhere comfortable and warm, preferably with your back straight – on the floor or in straight-backed chair.
- Play some soothing music of your choice and pick up one crystal (start with haematite).
- Look at the crystal carefully, turn it over and study the size, colour, shape and everything about it. Now close your eyes and do absolutely nothing but visualize this stone. Turn it over in your hands. Give yourself time to respond. Just sit quietly and imagine you are looking at the stone with your eyes open – although of course they will be closed and you will be imagining/visualizing the stone.
- For a minute or two just do nothing – What do you feel? What do you hear?
- Think of the stone's qualities – haematite, for example, balances the mind, encouraging better mental control over the emotional and physical state. Its magnetic properties mean that it is a useful stone for grounding excess mental, emotional or physical energy.
- After four or five minutes, or whenever you 'feel' it is time, open your eyes, and *write down your findings immediately*, before going on to the next crystal.

Continue to work through the crystals, one at a time, in exactly the same way – the next will be carnelian, followed by citrine, moving up the chakras. Do not worry if you do not feel anything – you will in time – just relax and focus your mind on the crystal in your hand.

IMPORTANT: at the end of your session return to the haematite for a few minutes, to ground you before leaving the session. An alternative treatment would be to start with amethyst (crown chakra), moving down the chakras becoming more grounded as you do so.

Chakra balancing

You will be using the crystals used in the above exercise, plus two green aventurine crystals. Do not attempt this in the same session as the individual crystal exercise. This is a basic chakra balance and will give you an idea of what a chakra balance feels like, although it is not the same as having the treatment carried out for you. Prepare the room ready for a treatment – no telephones, disturbances, etc. Have the crystals ready for placing on your body, on the floor within easy reach. Here is an alternative list of crystals you may use, chosen from your basic set.

Bloodstone – used to open doors both physically and spiritually; a good red crystal to use for the base chakra.

Calcite (orange) – teaches that 'learning is remembering what we already know' by helping to unlock genetic and spiritual memories; a good orange crystal for the sacral chakra.

Citrine – yellow to golden-brown in colour this connected to the sun and so has links with clear vision and enlightenment; a good choice for the solar plexus chakra.

Green aventurine – used as a balancing crystal, this stone also helps increase motivation and adventurousness by connecting you to all of creation and reducing inner fears; a good choice for the heart chakra.

Blue lace agate – a crystal of peace and happiness, radiating calming energies and releasing blockages from the nervous system; an excellent choice for the throat chakra.

Sodalite – sodalite is a consciousness-opening crystal bringing clarity and wisdom; a perfect choice for the third eye (brow) chakra.

Amethyst – amethyst is used to enhance energy and thought waves, and has a gentle but powerful energy; a good choice for using with the crown chakra.

When you are ready:

- Place the base chakra stone (haematite or bloodstone) just below your feet and the amethyst just above your head. Lie down between them.
- Place the carnelian on the sacral chakra, just below the navel.
- Place the citrine on the solar plexus, just below the breast bone.
- Place the rose quartz on the heart chakra which is between the breasts.
- Place the blue lace agate in the indentation at the throat.
- Place the sodalite on the forehead just above the eyebrow.

Stones should be in a straight line along the centre of the body.

- Take two green aventurine crystals and gently hold one in each hand, resting them in the palm.
- Try to relax with the crystals placed upon you. Don't tense up trying to stop them falling or moving. As you relax, let any feelings wash over you. Do not try to feel what is happening, just note anything that happens or any feelings or sensations that come into your mind. If a stone should fall off, then let it be. It may mean that it should not be there or that its work is complete. After about 20 minutes take the crystals off, starting at the top and working down.
- Sit up slowly and check how you feel.
- Write down your results even if you did not feel anything.

Chakra balancing a client

Having worked upon yourself, now it is time to try a balancing treatment on a colleague. The whole treatment will take about half an hour. It is very easy, as at this stage you as the therapist do very little – the crystals are working for you; your role is merely to put them in the right places.

Prepare your working space. You can ask the relevant questions to ascertain which chakra needs working on the most (see Chapter 3, p.30). Remember that this is not a healing session, but a chakra balancing.

- Lie the client either on the floor or on a couch – they remain fully clothed, but shoes may be removed and tight belts and collars loosened. Have a blanket ready in case the client gets cold, as is often the case when people totally relax.
- The first crystal to place is the base chakra (bloodstone or haematite or another suitable crystal). Place either at the feet, on the couch or floor, or on the body. As it can be difficult to place because of the shape of the body and the nature of the clothing, place it as low on the trunk as possible, maintaining the client's dignity at all times.
- Next, place the amethyst at the top of the head. If you are using a terminated stone (one with a point), make sure the terminated end is pointing towards the client's head.
- Next place the other crystals on the body from the sacral upwards.
- Finally, place a piece of aventurine in each of the client's hands.
- Now move away from them and keep quiet. Do not encourage talking – encourage silence and relaxation. If they want to talk

Tip

Don't use the phrases 'crystal healing' or 'crystal healer'. This implies cure. You cannot and never must promise a cure. You are merely a channel – a channel for the healing rays of light from the crystal to the client.

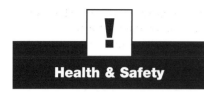

As with essential oils, more does not equate to better. Do not feel that putting more crystals on or around the body will make a better treatment. It does not. You may get great results with one small crystal. Remember – *less is often more*. Clients can suffer from a 'crystal crisis', which is the same as a 'healing crisis' in other therapies.

about what is happening to them that is fine. Just listen and respond with interest and empathy, encouraging quietness all the time. Suitable music may be played.

- Leave the client in peace for 20 minutes, but do not leave the room.
- Approach the client quietly and remove the crystals, starting with the crown and working down the chakras. Take the aventurine from their hands and replace with haematite to hold for a few minutes to ground the client before leaving.
- Obtain any feedback you can from them and write that down as soon as possible.

That is all there is to it. Keep the crystals you have used on this client away from the client as he or she prepares to leave. Do not let the client touch the stones you have just used as they may absorb back all the negative energy the stones have taken away! As soon as possible clean the crystals before re-using. As you progress through your training, sessions will become more complex. Once you start to read the energies of the chakras with your hands, or a pendulum (see Chapter 17, p.380), you can decide to use more or less of the crystals or combine the action of the clear quartz with the chakra stones to enhance their action.

Don't forget to make the connection that the chakras are all connected to different glands of the body (see Chapter 3, p.30).

Using crystals with other therapies

The use of crystals with other therapies can increase the effectiveness of those therapies. There are hundreds of combinations you could use. Start simply with one or two crystals; as you get more confident in their use, you may want to increase them in number or size. Given below are three examples each for using crystals with reflexology, aromatherapy and Indian head massage. List your own ideas for future use.

Reflexology

- With the client either sitting up or lying down, reflexology could be enhanced simply by the client holding one small aventurine stone in each hand. As the crystals of balance, this would enhance any holistic treatment you performed.
- If you knew the client was having infertility problems, you could place malachite over the client's sacral chakra. The key word for the sacral chakra is reproduction and the associated glands are the ovaries in women and the testes in men. Malachite is renowned for strengthening and balancing the reproductive system, and as such would enhance the treatment.
- Blue lace agate could be placed over the client's throat chakra if you knew the client was having communication problems.

Aromatherapy

- As with reflexology above, if the client is lying down, you can place any crystal on a chakra for a balancing or healing treatment that is appropriate to that client. Crystals can be placed above the blanket over the client, or placed on the floor beneath the client.

For example, you could place a rose quartz crystal over the heart chakra if the client was having any emotional problems.

- Each crystal has its own healing properties linked to its own chemical structure and vibration, but there are also properties shared by all crystals of a particular colour. Having decided which chakra is out of balance (see the chakra questionnaire on the companion website, www.thomsonlearning.co.uk/hairandbeauty/beckmann) you could then choose an appropriate essential oil of the same colour. For example, the colour orange relieves menstrual cramps, gas and draws out boils. It depresses the parathyroid and stimulates the thyroid, which in turn normalizes the metabolism. Orange crystals include amber, carnelian, citrine, smoky quartz and topaz. The client could hold these in their hands whilst the treatment was in progress, and you could choose essential oils of the same colour – orange essential oils include neroli, petitgrain and patchouli. By following this colour/chakra choice of oils, your choice of crystal will be correct – it is just a different way of selection than you are probably used to.

Indian head massage

- The client is seated for this treatment, so holding two small aventurine stones lightly in the palms of their hands will greatly enhance the effect.
- Placing any grounding stone on the floor by the client's feet will serve to keep the client grounded throughout the treatment.
- Offer a glass of water with a difference. Make an *elixir* especially for the client before the treatment commences. Place a piece of fluorite in a glass of spring water for the duration of the treatment and let the client drink the water at the end. This helps the body to eliminate toxins and boosts the immune system.

Specific after care advice for crystal therapy

In addition to the usual after care instructions given after all holistic therapies, you need to make sure that the person you have been working on is well grounded before leaving the salon. Do not underestimate the power of the crystals, and do not allow clients to leave if they are feeling 'spacey'. Encourage them to get up slowly. Give them a glass of water. If they appear a bit vague, give them a piece of haematite to hold for a minute or two to help earth/ground them or get them to touch the ground with their hands or stamp their feet. When you feel they are safe they can go but discourage them from driving immediately.

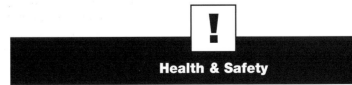

Health & Safety

Only use the crystals when your intuition says that it is right to do so. Don't use them just because someone wants to 'have a go'. If it doesn't feel right, don't do it. You can always say you don't feel up to it or the stones do not feel right. It is your prerogative to say 'No'. Listen to your inner self, to that little voice.

Knowledge review

1   Name four of the many cultures that held the highest respect for crystals and who used them effectively for power, influence and healing.

2   What are crystalline minerals?

3   What is a crystal?

4   How do crystals obtain their life force energy?

5   What is grounding?

6   What senses should be used when choosing crystals?

7   Where should crystals be stored when not in use?

8   There are many ways to cleanse crystals – name four.

9   Name three ways of energizing crystals.

10   What are the qualities of female crystals – give two examples.

11   What are the qualities of male crystals – give two examples.

12   What crystal is generally known as 'the crystal of balance'?

13   If amber is not a crystal then what is it?

14   Which crystal will absorb the radiation from equipment, stopping it spreading into the room?

15   Which crystal is known as the 'love' stone?

16   Which crystal is known to be a good brain balancer?

17   Which crystal may be beneficial in the treatment of infertility?

18   What is a double terminated crystal?

19   What is a cluster, and how could you use one?

20   What after care advice is specific to crystal therapy?

Colour therapy

Learning objectives

This chapter covers the following:

- **a brief history of colour therapy**
- **the electromagnetic spectrum**
- **how colour therapy works**
- **consultation for colour therapy**
- **colour therapy treatments**
- **ascertaining colour needs**
- **colour in our environment**
- **colours used in colour therapy**
- **contra indications to colour therapy**
- **specific after care advice**

Colour therapy is the use of the vibrational frequency of the seven colours of the spectrum to correct imbalance or disharmony in the human body. It can be used for balancing energies or as a preventative to avoid possible problems. Colour therapy can also be a catalyst for the body's healing process. However, to be able to treat a person with colour, the therapist must be able to ascertain the colour required in order to balance the colour energies. Several ways of doing this will be explained below.

The impact of colour on mood is widely recognized and colour therapy is being incorporated into holistic treatments more than ever before. Some aromatherapists select essential oils by their colour as well as their therapeutic values. Colour reflexology is gaining recognition and as many treatments now incorporate working with the chakras, therapists are using colour therapy already.

A brief history of colour therapy

The earliest association of colours with symbolic meanings arose from the close relationship between prehistoric humans and nature. Green was the colour of growth; blue represented the sky and heavenly peace. Cultural differences developed however: red, the colour of blood, spelled disaster for the ancient Celts, while the Chinese associated it with the sun, money and prosperity. In ancient Egypt temples were built where colour healing took place.

In these temples sunlight shone through coloured gems such as rubies and sapphires onto people for healing. The Egyptians influenced the Greek schools of Pythagoras and Plato, and according to Gimbel (1994) the Chinese have always diagnosed illness by reading the 'colour' of pulses. The *Nei Ching*, a medical text compiled almost 2000 years ago, also records colour diagnosis. In the West, healing with colour remained largely a folk tradition based on superstition until the nineteenth century, when discoveries were made about the light spectrum and electromagnetic waves. In the mediaeval cathedrals and churches of the West stained glass windows were widely used. It was thought that the light shining through these windows generated an atmosphere suitable for prayer and meditation.

The rainbow

For centuries rainbows created a challenge for the scientists and philosophers of the day searching for an explanation of exactly how they occurred. Originally it was believed that colours were the result of the differing mixtures of light and darkness. Pythagoras, Plato and Aristotle developed some of the early theories about light and colour. Pythagoras (582–507 BC) believed that objects themselves gave off particles that made them visible. Plato (427–347 BC) thought that the eye emitted light, which bounced off objects, and gave information on shape, size and colour. Aristotle (384–322 BC) studied how light travels, and his contribution was that light travels in waves rather than in particles. For the next 2000 years the controversy of particles versus waves continued.

It was Sir Isaac Newton (1642–1727) who in 1665 discovered that sunlight, although it appears to be white, is really a blend of colours. Newton was a mathematician and philosopher and he discovered that when he passed sunlight through a prism, the light was refracted, thereby producing the colour spectrum.

Through Newton's findings it can be concluded that a rainbow is created when the sun's rays are refracted through droplets of rain. Normally a rainbow appears as a single phenomenon, but if the raindrops are large enough for some of the sunlight to be reflected twice inside the raindrop, a second rainbow will appear. The second rainbow will appear above the first but its colours are always fainter and in reverse order.

Newton identified seven colours in the rainbow but colour therapists usually use eight or nine, including magenta and turquoise. Magenta can be seen very clearly when looking through a prism, but turquoise, being a mixture of blue and green, cannot be seen.

The electromagnetic spectrum

The universe is permeated with energy. During the birth, existence and death of stars, galaxies and other astronomical bodies, immense amounts of energy are produced. Cosmic rays and radiation, X-rays, ultra violet rays, visible light, infra red rays, microwaves and radio waves are collectively referred to as the electromagnetic spectrum and contain electromagnetic energy. The various forms of electromagnetic energy have two features in common:

- electromagnetic energy travels at the speed of light
- this energy has both an electrical and magnetic component.

For most purposes electromagnetic energy can be considered as travelling in waves. The distance between successive waves is called the *wavelength* and the number of times a wave oscillates in one second is called the *frequency*. The basic rule to remember is the longer the wavelength of the energy, the lower the frequency.

The electromagnetic spectrum includes energies from cosmic rays to radio waves. Energies are graded according to wavelength and measured in nanometres (nm): one nanometre equals one millionth of a millimetre. The spectrum of visible light falls between 760 nm at the red end and 380 nm at the violet end of the colour spectrum.

The sun's rays contain a whole spectrum of electromagnetic radiation that forms visible white or 'full-spectrum' light. The brain perceives these different wavelengths as different colours. When light is passed through a prism or refracted as a rainbow, the different colours (waves) of the spectrum can be identified.

As well as having its own wavelength, each colour has a certain frequency, the rate at which its wave vibrates. As cells and organs in the body also have vibrational frequencies, therapists can use colours to correct vibrational imbalances in the body and create a state of harmony. When colour is broken down into different wavelengths, we experience different colours. It is like holding a prism. Our eyes translate the energy of light into the nervous impulses, which the brain then interprets as colour. Those energies outside our conscious colour vision are not visible to us but we are still sensitive to them. Light and the constituent colours do have a strong effect on both mind and body and can have an effect on our physical, mental and emotional states.

Interesting fact

If you have ever had a cat on your bed at night, you may have noticed that, just as you are about to fall asleep, the cat begins to purr. This is because as you become very relaxed, your body's electromagnetic energy changes, emitting a pale blue light that is visible to cats. The cats find this colour particularly attractive and it makes them feel safe. They purr with pleasure!

How colour therapy works

To understand how colour therapy works, you must be aware of the following:

- the different vibrational frequency of colour
- the different subtle bodies of human beings which vibrate at different frequencies and which relate to colour vibrations
- the understanding that the chakras are the connection between the subtle (non-physical) body and physical body
- once the colour vibration has been transformed into accessible energy by the chakras this life-force energy is relayed through the meridian system in the body via the various organs (see Chapter 3, p.30).

The main uses for colour therapy

Colour therapy can be used to treat the following:

- emotional and behavioural problems
- stress-related conditions
- depression, insomnia

- fatigue and chronic fatigue syndrome
- headaches
- arthritis
- skin conditions
- menstrual problems.

It can also be used as part of

- relaxation therapy.

Consultation for colour therapy

Specific questions for a consultation

As with all treatments, a consultation must be undertaken before treatment whereby you need to note all the usual details (see Chapter 5, p.134). For colour therapy the consultation may also include the chakra questionnaire on the website (www.thomsonlearning.co.uk/beckmann) which would indicate which chakras needed balancing, and therefore the colours you need to work with. Additionally, you can ask general colour-type questions and make your own deductions as to the answers you are given.

What is your favourite colour?

What is your least favourite colour?

Describe the colour scheme of your home. Did you choose these colours? If you could redecorate, what colours would you choose?

Are there any colours you may avoid – why?

The reason for trying to identify both the positive and negative colours is an attempt to associate and correlate the psychological reasons. Both positive and negative associations can create an imbalance in the client's day-to-day colour exposure. A much-needed colour could possibly be avoided because of negative concentrations. The aim is to regain an equal acceptance of all colours.

If someone avoids the colour violet/purple at all costs, for example, could indicate someone who lacks self-respect and self-esteem and who may in fact need to work with this colour.

If someone is always wearing black, then a change to navy blue could make all the difference to how they feel generally – blue is a calming and grounding colour that makes you feel safe, and such a change could bring about big alterations in how someone feels.

You may have to use your counselling skills to find out why someone is averse to particular colours – but don't get in too deep, they really may just simply not like it.

Colour therapy treatments

Visualization and meditation

These techniques are described in Chapter 15, pp.350 and 352.

Colour breathing

The purpose of colour breathing is, firstly, to heighten the awareness of colour, and secondly to encourage a balance of all the seven main chakra colours for well-being.

Self-treatment

This treatment can be carried out lying down or standing. Be relaxed, whether lying or standing, with feet slightly apart and arms by the side, palms turned to the front. Relax the shoulders and concentrate on your breathing, consciously relaxing all of your body from the top of your head to the tips of your toes. Breathe in deeply through the nose, hold for a few moments, then breathe out through the month. As you breathe out, imagine expelling all the stress, negativity and toxins from your body. This should last a minimum of five minutes.

When completely relaxed, start to breathe in 'red' from the earth. Imagine it rising up through your whole body, from the feet upwards, giving you strength and courage. With each inward breath, the red rises further and further up the body. The first breath may take the red to the ankles, with the next in-breath the red may get to the knees, and with the next the red may reach the upper thigh. Depending on how much you are concentrating, and how deeply you are breathing, will affect how slowly or quickly your whole body is filled with red. Remember to breathe in slowly and deeply through the nose and out through the mouth. With each out-breath, breathe out all the stress, negativity and toxins from the body.

When the body is full of red, take a deep breath, and on the out breath, breathe all the red out – imagine it leaving your body through your feet, the same way that it entered. You will then start the whole process over again, but this time using orange, and the next time yellow. These first three colours are absorbed from the earth, so the colours rise up from your feet to your head, before being expelled.

The next colour to move onto is green, the heart chakra colour. This colour is absorbed horizontally through the heart. As you breathe in, imagine the colour entering your heart, and staying in this heart area. Take as many in-breaths as is necessary to completely fill the chest cavity with a beautiful green. When it is full, take a deep breath and breathe the green out. It will leave through your back.

You will then breathe in blue, indigo and finally violet. These three colours come from the sky and will be breathed in through the top of your head, and once the body is full, right down to the feet, it will then be expelled back out of the top of your head, back to the sky.

Concentrate on each colour totally. It will get easier the more you do it.

Client treatment

You can do the same self-treatment for a client. The client will be lying on the couch, eyes closed, with maybe an eye-sized beanbag over the eyes. With this light weight over the eyes, it is sometimes easier for the client to relax and only be aware of your voice and the colours she or he is thinking of. You can either talk the client through the above exercise 'live', or you could pre-tape it and play it. By preparing a tape recording, you can listen to it yourself, and actually do the exercise as if you were the client. This is an excellent way to 'test' the tape, as you can tell if you are going through the exercise too quickly. You can make the tape last 20 or 30 minutes. Wherever the colour is, when you move onto the next colour, the client will breathe out all of the previous colour and start the next. You still need to remember treatment time – or you could be there for hours. You could give the client the tape to practise with at home. At the end of the session, the client will sit up gently and be offered a glass of water. Ask for feedback and make a note of it on the record card. How did the client feel? Did they experience the colours? Explain the purpose of the exercise – by doing the exercise daily, colour awareness develops, balancing and enhancing the body's energies.

Colour Me Beautiful

The Colour Me Beautiful technique correlates colour and skin tone and designates a person as a spring, summer, winter or autumn person. Although a valid system of working with colour, it unfortunately correlates with skin colour and is not a therapeutic system. However, in enhancing the image of woman and men, it does contribute to a positive self-esteem.

Material and swatches

Using coloured scarves or swatches is another way of working with colour. When working with this technique, the material should be natural, like cotton or silk. The scarves or swatches of material are placed over the part of the body which needs colour. The following are examples of how to use scarves and swatches as part of a treatment.

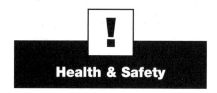

Health & Safety

Some therapists use candles in treatment rooms. While these are visually attractive and help to set the scene, they are nonetheless a fire hazard. Do not use candles when using coloured swatches.

- Use a piece of full-length blue material in either cotton or silk. Lie underneath this in a warm, light room for 20 minutes. For this exercise the material needs to be either against the skin or placed over white clothing. A blue woollen blanket over a white sheet would be very beneficial. This practice counteracts stress and insomnia.

- For a sore throat, use a blue silk, cotton or woollen scarf. Wrap this around your neck until your throat starts to heal. Remember that blue is the colour of the throat chakra. Wearing a scarf of this colour will also improve communication.

- If you suffer from tired or sore eyes, especially if this is caused through working with a VDU screen, place a piece of thick indigo cotton over your eyes and relax for 15 minutes. Remember that indigo is the colour of the third eye chakra, making it a good choice for this area.

- Sometimes therapists use two colours in a treatment. For depression a therapist might use orange silk for 20 minutes, followed by blue, its complementary colour, for 10 minutes.

Once the deficient colour has been identified, coloured silks may be draped over the body or worn on the body to treat symptoms.

Illumination therapy

A computer-controlled colour-therapy machine directs coloured light at the patient as he or she sits or lies in a darkened room. The main treatment colour, for example orange, is alternated with its complementary colour, in this case indigo, and each dose is precisely timed. The light is directed on to a specific part of the body through a 'quartz-tipped crystal torch', or is diffused as the client sits under the light source. Different hues are selected according to their vibrational frequencies and their particular effects on internal organs. The practitioner often uses both the main colour and its complementary opposite alternately in treatment. If you are being treated with violet for example, you will usually also be exposed to yellow. This is said to ensure a healthy balance of colour in the body. Sessions are usually about an hour long, and a course of treatment may last several weeks, depending upon the condition. Companies offering these light machines usually include specialized training in colour therapy also.

Aura-Soma

Described by its creator as 'non-intrusive, self-selective soul therapy' Aura-Soma is a form of colour therapy. It was developed, or 'envisaged', in 1984 by Vicky Wall, a UK chiropodist who allegedly developed extrasensory powers after losing her sight. The therapy is mainly available in the UK, although there are a small number of practitioners working in the USA and Australia. The client is presented with a selection of over 90 specially prepared 'balance' bottles, then asked to choose four. Each contains two coloured liquids: a mixture of essential oils on a layer of spring water containing herbal extracts. The colours the client chooses are said to provide insights into their physical and emotional condition. The four bottles are shaken and the mixtures applied to the skin daily for as long as necessary; this allows the colours to enter the body and rebalance disturbed chakras. There is no standard length of treatment or number of sessions, and the therapy is used primarily for long-standing emotional problems and stress.

Aura energy or reading

The chakras into which different coloured light streams play an important part in colour therapy. Related to the chakras is a person's 'aura', a subtle body consisting of multicoloured layers which surround every individual. Although invisible to most people, some therapists can see auras. They will read the colours of the aura to determine the patient's state of health, then visualize healing colours to counteract negative or dull colours in the aura. Sometimes the aura may appear to have a hole in it, so the therapist would help the client through a visualization to assist in repairing the hole.

Interesting fact

White light
The most healing colour is daylight, because it contains the full spectrum of the visible range of light – in other words, all the colours. If in doubt as to which colour to use, choose a 'white' light.

Tip

When working with colour therapy, work in natural daylight as much as possible, to enable clients to receive the full impact of the colour being used.

Ascertaining colour needs

How does one go about ascertaining the required colour needed to balance the colour energies?

Muscle testing

Muscle testing, also known as kinesiology, is a means of testing weaknesses in the body by means of testing certain muscles. The client holds up each of the colours of the spectrum in turn, at eye level, with their left hand. The right hand is held horizontal to the body. As each colour is looked at, the therapist applies gentle downward pressure to the client's right arm. If there is no resistance to this pressure it indicates that the client needs the colour he or she is holding. Kinesiology can also be used for allergy testing and to test for general body weakness. See if you can get your tutor to arrange a demonstration for you by a qualified therapist. As with all therapies, it is not something you can do yourself without training.

Dowsing with a pendulum

A pendulum can be used as a method of diagnosis when choosing:

- colour
- crystals
- essential oils.

When used in a therapeutic situation, dowsing is performed with a pendulum on a length of string. By relaxing the mind and quietly focusing inwards, the therapist is able to contact their intuition and receive answers 'Yes', or 'No' through the movement of the pendulum. The movement of the pendulum can be in a clockwise or anticlockwise direction, or from side to side or forwards and back. Before working with a pendulum, the therapist must learn the specific response of his or her pendulum to a 'Yes' or 'No'. It is very personal and the therapist must feel confident using the pendulum. Always keep your pendulum for your own use only.

A pendulum can be used to ascertain your client's needs as to which colour is deficient and needs to be worked with. List the eight predominant colours (see below) on a piece of paper, leaving plenty of space between each, or have a colour chart of the eight colours in a vertical column. Start with magenta and 'ask' each colour if it is needed for your client, carefully noting the direction of the pendulum before moving on to the next colour.

Buying a pendulum

If you decide to buy a pendulum, do not go into the shop with any predestined ideas of what you want. As with buying crystals, you will be working with this pendulum and you need to make sure you are compatible! Look at the choice of pendulums and see if any immediately take your eye. Take the pendulum and hold it approximately 3 inches above the palm of your hand. To establish your 'Yes' and 'No' with a pendulum, keep it very still, then ask 'What is my Yes?' Allow time for the pendulum to start its movement. Remember the result. Before the pendulum stops moving ask 'What is my No?' Let the pendulum give its own direction. Do this several times, with different pendulums. You will know which one you will be able to work with well. Of course you do not have to buy one. A wedding band or any ring tied onto a piece of string will work just as well. Always ascertain the 'Yes' and 'No' before you begin working with any pendulum.

Chakra questionnaire

Use the questionnaire given on the companion website, www.thomsonlearning.co.uk/hairandbeauty/beckmann, to establish which chakras need balancing and use the appropriate coloured scarves or drapes accordingly.

Interesting fact

The link between colour and sound was familiar to the Druids who, at the winter solstice, retreated to their caves for three days. On the third day each cave was flooded with light and sound that seemed to have no source. By chanting the Druids produced the full spectrum of harmonic overtones, which created a state of awareness that 'let in' the full spectrum of light (Gimbel, 1994).

Colour in our environment

Colour is used in our environment in many ways: examples include décor, clothing and food. Colour therapy can be used in different ways including visualization and meditation (see Chapter 15, pp.350, 352) and colour breathing can be used as an easy exercise and an introduction to meditation and visualization. These three methods can be used in relation to décor, clothing and food or used for general balancing work. When we think about colour and light in the environment – in other words the colours we live with in our homes, the clothes we wear and the foods we eat – we are dealing with a very important influence on daily life, well-being and, ultimately, on health.

Clothing

Colour can be absorbed into our bodily systems through the clothes we wear. This is particularly so if it is a natural fibre such as cotton, wool, linen or silk, which acts as a filter through which light passes. The more sensitive we are to the vibrational energies of colour, the more we are able to discern the colour we require at any one time. We have all experienced being drawn to a colour on a certain day. When we are drawn towards a colour, it is indicative of our needs for the energy of the colour on that particular day. When our need is satisfied, we no longer feel attracted to it. Although we are influenced by fashion to a certain extent, try not to wear the same colours every day. A balance is needed. If there are colours that you think don't suit you, then use these colours as accessories, or even as underwear or socks.

Décor

The colour of light and the colour in decoration must be used in conjunction with each other if interior decoration is to be successful. The interior decoration of your home should reflect your own personality and nurture your inner needs. Important factors that influence the colour scheme of a room include:

- the functions of the room – if you are to relax in the room, do not use red, orange or yellow but instead choose colours from the blue end of the spectrum
- your personal needs and preferences
- the physical attributes of the room – take into consideration the size and shape, the number of windows, the direction in which the room faces and the hours of sunlight the room receives.

Generally, warm colours would be used to stimulate activity in a room and cool colours would be used to produce a calming effect.

Turquoise, for example, is a good colour for the kitchen as it promotes a calming effect. But use bright colours with it to promote alertness and highlight health and safety matters in the kitchen. Keep bedrooms in relaxing blues or greens, and colour studies and workrooms in reds, russets or browns which are more stimulating. Greens and peachy oranges create a peaceful place to digest food and enjoy company.

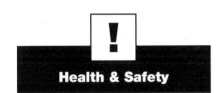

Health & Safety

Bright colours should be used for kitchens. Kitchens are dangerous places so use colours that help to keep your mind focused and bright colours so you can see what you are doing.

Food

Eating food of different colours adds another dimension to colour healing. The natural colour of foods is a way of getting colour vibrations into our systems. Be aware of the additives added to food to enhance the colour – these are chemically based and toxic to our bodies. When preparing food, attempt to include as many colours as possible in the meal and concentrate on natural sources of foodstuffs.

Colours used in colour therapy

There are eight predominant colours in colour therapy:

- red
- orange

- yellow
- green
- turquoise
- blue
- violet
- magenta.

Interesting fact

It is interesting to note that all colours have their own spectrum, which ranges from a very deep to a very pale colour. The bright translucent shades of a colour reveal its positive aspects, while the dark, dingy shade reveals its negative side.

Beneficial and detrimental attributes and effects of each colour

Like many things in life we take colour for granted. Colour dominates our senses. We tend to use colour to describe our physical health, moods and attitudes. For example we often refer to 'feeling blue', being 'green with envy', having a 'golden opportunity', being 'red' or 'purple with rage' or 'being in the pink'. Colours can have both beneficial and detrimental attributes, so the consultation stage, as always, is important to ascertain which colour is suitable for your client's needs at the time of treatment. You may also decide to use the complementary colour for a lesser time, to balance the treatment.

Red

Red is the colour of dynamic and expressive energy. We use phrases such as 'like a red rag to a bull' and 'seeing red', and these are linked to the anger and rage aspect of this colour. Red is a very stimulating and exciting colour and an amplifier of emotions. To use red properly, in a healthy way, we should use it to assist our expression, not to fuel our aggression. Red is the symbol of life, strength and vitality, and is regarded as the great energizer. Like the glowing coals of a fire, red is a warming energy and this makes it useful in the treatment of any illness where there is coldness or a lack of movement in the body, such as arthritis, rheumatism, lumbago, sciatica and any stiffening of the muscles and joints. It increases red blood cell production, improves sluggish menstruation and stimulates the autonomic nervous system. Red is also linked to sexual and reproductive energy and will therefore help with problems of impotence, frigidity and conception.

Red crystals include: agate, carnelian, garnet, ruby, spinel.

Red foods include: tomatoes, radishes, red peppers, beetroot, cherries, raspberries, red plums, red apples.

Orange

Orange is less dynamic and less aggressive than red, but is still considered an active and stimulating colour. Orange contains a mixture of intellectual and female reproductive energy – the energy of creation. It stimulates the digestion, allowing us to absorb nutrients from food, and knowledge from experiences (mental digestion). Orange is the colour of joy and happiness and enables us to create a balance between the physical and mental bodies. It gives freedom to thoughts and feelings and disperses heaviness, allowing the body natural and joyful movements. On a physical level orange has the ability to bring about change in the biochemical structure, which helps in dispersing depression. A warming colour, orange also helps to increase oxygen levels within the body by stimulating the lungs. Orange can relieve menstrual cramps, release gas, draw out boils and bring abscesses to a head. It depresses the parathyroid and stimulates the thyroid, which in turn improves milk production in nursing mothers.

Orange crystals include: amber, carnelian, citrine, smoky quartz, topaz.

Orange foods include: carrots, pumpkins, orange peppers, oranges, tangerines, apricots, mangoes, clementines, orange melons.

Yellow

Yellow is the colour of intellect and intelligence, and therefore stimulates mental activity. It is an excellent colour to have in a place of study. Yellow has the highest reflectivity of all colours, and appears to radiate outwards. It works directly upon balancing the mind and so is particularly useful in the treatment of mental problems and illnesses. When used in counselling it assists in releasing deep-seated problems, helps to reinforce self-confidence and stimulates courage. Yellow strengthens and improves the lymphatic system and energizes the liver, gall bladder, eyes and ears. It also helps to loosen arthritic lime deposits by encouraging the body to dissolve uric and lactic acid crystals, which cause rheumatism and gout. The yellow rays carry positive magnetic currents and these vibrations strengthen the nerves including motor nerves in the physical body, thus generating energy in the muscles. It is traditional in many cultures to take yellow flowers to a sick person to stimulate healing. Holding a yellow crystal or wearing something yellow is very helpful when you are feeling mentally drained or are looking for mental stimulation.

Yellow crystals include: citrine, topaz, yellow zircon.

Yellow foods include: sweetcorn, yellow peppers, marrow, winter squash, golden plums, pineapple, grapefruit, honeydew melons, lemons.

Green

Green is the colour of intuition and wisdom. It is the point of balance between the hot and warming red, orange and yellow colours and the cooler blue, indigo and violet colours. It is known as the colour of duality, being midway in the colour spectrum, and is composed of yellow, the last of the warm colours and blue, the first of the cold colours. It is the colour of nature and harmony and is linked to the heart, because true healing from the heart is balanced and non-judgmental, neither hot nor cold. Green helps to restore balance in the mind and body. Next time you feel stressed, try taking a walk in a park or in the countryside and you will soon understand the balancing and soothing power of this colour. Green also stimulates the pituitary gland and aids cell growth and regeneration, making it a good colour to help in healing open sores, cuts, bruises and scars. It helps to dissolve blood clots and heal infections. Green brings integration and therefore balance between left and right brain functioning. Therefore it is a good colour for schools, colleges and offices.

Green crystals include: emerald, jade, moss agate, peridot, tourmaline.

Green foods include: green peppers, spinach, cabbage, lettuce, peas, beans, green apples, kiwi fruit, green lentils.

 Interesting fact

Turquoise
Turquoise is not normally considered a spectrum colour, but many colour therapists use turquoise as it is the colour of the thymus chakra, which is situated midway between the heart chakra and the throat chakra.

Turquoise

Turquoise is not normally considered a spectrum colour because it is a combination of blue and green. In colour therapy this gentle soothing colour is used to boost the immune system, hence its association with the thymus. The human immune system depends on the strength of the lymphatic system in combating inflammation and as turquoise has a strengthening effect on the immune system, it is used for infections, inflammations and septic conditions in the body.

Turquoise crystals include: turquoise.

Turquoise foods include: eating blue and green foods together will have a 'turquoise' food effect.

Blue

Blue is a cool, calming colour. It radiates to form a protective capsule around an individual, helping them to feel happy and safe. It grounds flighty energy and calms over-excitement. Because of its downward energy (it calms down and grounds), blue has become linked with excesses of 'downward' energy – for example, 'feeling blue' and 'having the blues'. This colour aids sleep, quells fevers and helps with infections, inflammations, mental depression, irritation, itches and burns. It is also associated with the throat, especially in connection with speech and song. Blue is a very purifying colour and it is said that well water, stored in a blue glass bottle, will never go off. Many vibrational therapists keep their essences in blue bottles, and aromatherapy oils and other products can also be bought in blue bottles. Blue is a colour which symbolizes inspiration, devotion, peace and tranquillity and thus is a good colour to use during meditation and in places of healing. Because it is a colour which slows things down, it gives an impression of expansion and creates a feeling of space.

Blue crystals include: aquamarine, blue lace agate, celestite, sapphire.

Blue foods include: grapes, blueberries, blue plums.

Violet

Violet is the colour of creativity, inspiration, transformation and spirituality. It inspires healing through art, music, colour, crystals, aromatic oils, movement and sound. It is a consciousness-raising colour sometimes emitted by shamans. It is good for headaches, and for promoting peaceful sleep and dreams. It has also been used as a slimming aid. This is the seventh colour belonging to the visible part of the electromagnetic spectrum. It vibrates at the shortest wavelengths and therefore emits the highest energy. In the electromagnetic spectrum it lies next to ultra violet, a radiation not visible to the human eye. The colour violet is a uniting colour – it unites the person with their higher self, it balances the masculine and feminine energies, connects the conscious and subconscious and tends to restore. This colour pertains to spirituality, self-respect and dignity. It assists higher states of consciousness and this leads into the realm of spiritual awareness. In colour therapy treatments, violet is frequently needed by individuals who have no respect for their own thoughts, feelings or physical body. These persons often lack self-respect and self-esteem and are unable to accept, appreciate or love themselves.

Violet crystals include: amethyst, fluorite, sugilite.

Violet foods include: aubergine, purple grapes, plums, purple broccoli.

Magenta

This is a combination of red and violet. On a physical, emotional and mental level, magenta is the colour of 'letting go', so as to allow change to take place. It assists in letting go of old thought patterns born out of conditioning, which could have originated in childhood and/or adulthood. What occurs when conditioning happens is that the person becomes rigid and static and is no longer able to grow and evolve. Many people find it difficult to let go and flow with the tide of life. Change causes feelings of insecurity and uncertainty. Letting go and having faith in the future often implies letting go of a 'comfort zone' and trusting your intuition, and this can also be very unsettling for the personality. On the emotional level, magenta signifies letting go of feelings which are no longer relevant or stopping living in the past. In order to move on, we must learn to emotionally let go of the past, but this is not easy for many people. Clients who are in a transition phase in life will benefit being treated with magenta colour. When magenta fades to a pale pink, it becomes the colour of

Complementary colours

Violet	Yellow
Indigo	Orange
Blue	Red
Green	Magenta
Yellow	Violet
Orange	Indigo
Red	Blue
Magenta	Green

Interesting fact

Magenta
Magenta is the eighth colour and is not part of the visible spectrum, but is a combination of red (base chakra) and violet (crown chakra), thus combining the energies of those two colours. That is to say, magenta helps us to use our earthly experience and grounding together with intense spiritual awareness. It can help us both to release past conditioning and to move forward.

spiritual love and this can mainly be used on the emotional aspect of a person. If someone is suffering the loss of love, treating with this colour is beneficial. Do bear in mind that magenta is the complementary colour of green, the great balancing colour.

Magenta crystals include: dark rubies, garnets.

Magenta foods include: strawberries, cherries, red-pink watermelon.

Any crystal, essential oil, natural fibre clothing or food without chemicals that emits one of the above colours will possess all the therapeutic properties of that colour.

Complementary colours

When using a light box (see Illumination therapy above, p.378), therapists may use a complementary colour in addition to the main colour needed for the therapy. Complementary colours are the colours 'opposite' each other on the colour wheel (see the table above). Although 'opposite' each other, they are used together in colour therapy to give balance. We need the balance of the electric/cool colours and the magnetic/warm colours for our well-being and smooth functioning of the body.

The colour most needed would be used for 20 minutes and the complementary colour for 10 minutes – to give balance.

Contra indications to colour therapy

There are few contra indications to colour therapy, but care must be taken with anyone suffering from severe emotional disturbance, a psychological disorder or a physical illness that is being treated medically, and religious and/or other strongly held beliefs must be taken into consideration before offering treatment. Don't underestimate the value of colour therapy – colour can have dramatic effects on some people.

Specific after care advice

After care advice for colour therapy may include eating different coloured foods or wearing a specific colour on specific occasions. After care may include visualization exercises, colour breathing or meditation. Drinking plenty of water and balancing colour in the client's life are also recommended.

Knowledge review

1 With what do the Chinese associate the colour red?

2 Who discovered that when sunlight passed through a prism, the light was refracted, thereby producing the colour spectrum?

3 Name six main uses of colour therapy.

4 What is the purpose of colour breathing?

5 How can colour be taken into the body via clothes?

6 What important factors should be taken into consideration when deciding a colour scheme for a room?

7 What is kinesiology? How is it used in colour therapy?

8 What is the most healing light colour?

9 How can using a pendulum be a method of diagnosis for colour therapy?

10 Which colour is known as the great energizer?

11 Which colour is used as a balance between the warm colours and the cool colours, is the colour of nature and harmony and is linked to the heart?

12 Which colour is described as having 'downward energy' – that is, it calms down, grounds and aids sleep?

13 Why do many therapists keep their products in blue bottles?

14 What is the complementary colour to violet?

15 If a client were ready to 'let go', so allowing change to take place, what colour might you recommend for use in treatment?

16 What specific contra indications are related to colour therapy?

17 What specific after care advice could you offer for colour therapy?

18 What is the difference between a wavelength and a frequency?

19 What connects the subtle (non-physical) body and the physical body?

20 Turquoise is not a colour of the visible light spectrum so why do colour therapists use turquoise?

Thermal auricular therapy

18

Learning objectives

This chapter covers the following:

- **a history of ear candling**
- **contra indications and contra actions to ear candling**
- **the manufacture and composition of ear candles**
- **how ear candles actually work**
- **the benefits and effects of ear candling**
- **ear candling treatment**
- **after care advice**
- **essential anatomy and physiology of the ear**
- **medical terms explained**

Thermal auricular therapy, also known as ear candling, is a centuries-old method of bringing an enhanced state of health to the ear, nose, throat and sinuses of the body. It is a gentle, non-invasive and relaxing experience carried out using hollow tubes known as ear candles. Ear candling also loosens earwax and the client generally. Not only is the treatment beneficial for the upper respiratory tract, but also for the circulatory and lymphatic systems, making it a whole body treatment. Ear candling has captured the imagination of many through its amazing effects and its simplicity.

A history of ear candling

There is very little clear evidence of the history of ear candling. We do know that it was used by the Egyptians, Essenes, Mayans and Tibetans over 3000 years ago. It is believed that the history of ear candles (or ear cones as they are sometimes referred to) began in ancient Egypt and spread throughout the Orient and into Europe. There is evidence that the Greeks and Romans used ear candles, but the best evidence comes from the Native American Hopi Indians of northeastern Arizona. It is thought that these Indians used the candles for spiritual cleansing purposes before meditation or before entering into a trance state. These civilizations did not have ear candles as we know them today. It is thought they used hollow twigs or glazed clay with a double helix carved inside to create the spiral of smoke and that they used herbs and incense while performing the ritual.

Ear candling today is mostly used for its physical benefits, such as healing ear, nose, throat, respiratory and sinus problems, but feedback from clients suggests many psychological and subtle benefits also.

Contra indications and contra actions to ear candling

Contra indications

Despite being an extremely safe and effective treatment, when practising ear candling professionally, there may be certain conditions presented by the client which contra indicate treatment:

- any recent head or neck injury
- grommets*
- infections in the area
- perforated eardrum*
- high or low blood pressure
- circulatory disorders
- dysfunction of the nervous system
- epilepsy
- eczema
- treatment of children without express permission of parent or guardian.

*See Medical terms explained, p.396, for more details.

Contra actions

Clients may feel light-headed after a treatment and ears may 'ache' for a short time while afterwards. As with most other holistic treatment, clients may sometimes experience a healing crisis.

The manufacture and composition of candles

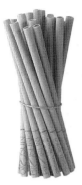

Ear candles

Ear candles are completely natural. There are many varieties on the market but they are all basically made in the same way. The candles are hollow and consist of an organic linen interior which is coated with a wax exterior. The wax should be beeswax, but some manufacturers use paraffin wax, producing an inferior product which should be avoided for this treatment. Candles are approximately 12 inches long. Manufacturers also use different herbs and/or essential oils, which are embedded into the beeswax and are released when the candle is burned. As many as three or four 'active' ingredients are added to the beeswax. The following are some examples of the active ingredients used.

- *Chamomile* – as an anti-inflammatory, anti-spasmodic sedative.
- *Sage* – as a carminative, astringent and circulatory stimulant which relaxes peripheral blood vessels.
- *St John's Wort* – as a restorative tonic for the nervous system and an analgesic.
- *Frankincense and cedar* – producing an oriental and ceremonial fragrance; recommended for spiritual opening.
- *Orange and lemon* – producing a mild and fruity fragrance; recommended for relaxed awareness.
- *Patchouli and bergamot* – producing an exotic and stimulating fragrance; recommended for female strength.

Tip

Keep candles in a dry cool place – preferably in a tin. Never leave in a retail area of a shop or car seat where sunlight and heat will distort the candles.

There are dozens of different candles on the market. Buy from a reputable supplier and check with your insurance provider that you have the necessary cover for the candles you are using. There are many companies selling ear candles over the Internet. Don't be tempted by the price, as many appear to be very inexpensive. Many of these ear candles are home-made efforts and are not safe. Remember you are dealing with a naked flame, so every precaution must be taken that you are using a safe product.

How do ear candles actually work?

The healing properties of ear candles are based on two physical actions of the candle. Firstly, the chimney effect inside the ear candle and the vibration of the rising air column serve to gently massage the eardrum and promote secretion in the frontal and paranasal sinuses. This has an immediate subjective effect of regulating ear pressure. Users often describe a soothing, light sensation in the ear/head area. Secondly, the locally applied warmth stimulates vascularization, invigorates the immune system and reinforces the flow of lymph.

The otoscope and its use in treatments

An otoscope is a medical instrument, which is placed in the ear enabling you to inspect the ear before treatment. Otoscopes have a magnified lens and a bright light. Whilst ear candling does not *remove* earwax, it can soften it, which can lead to it falling out either later on the same day of treatment or at any time over the next 24 hours. Using an otoscope is a

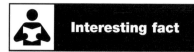

Interesting fact

In Germany, physicians are taught the art of ear candling.

useful diagnostic tool to see into the ears both before and after treatment; information should be recorded on the client's record card. Otoscopes come with removable end funnels, which must be sterilized between use, and these are placed into the ear canal. A bright light is shone down the ear canal and you will be able to see extremely clearly the condition of the ear. You will be able to identify a normal healthy ear, grommets, ear infections, swimmer's ear, hard impacted wax and soft wax, and you will be able to see all the hairs in the ear, as the magnification is so strong.

The benefits and effects of ear candling

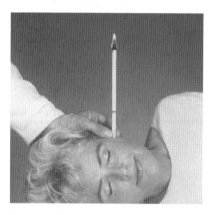

Ear candling treatment

Ear candling works on physical, psychological and subtle levels and the techniques used represent a cleansing programme for the whole body not just the ears.

Physical benefits

- Improves blood flow to the head and neck, increasing distribution of oxygen and nutrients to nourish the tissues and encourage healing.
- Stimulates and improves lymphatic drainage to the head and neck thus helping to eliminate waste material from the body.
- Is effective for tinnitus.
- Revitalizes the whole body.
- Relieves sinus congestion, colds, flu, sore throats, earache, lymphatic congestion, swollen glands, snoring, allergy symptoms, hearing difficulties (most forms), and pain or pressure when flying, scuba diving or other elevation change discomfort.

Psychological and subtle benefits

- Creates a 'balanced' feeling.
- Helps clearer thinking by increasing alertness and concentration.
- Re-balances the energy flow to the body.
- Releases stagnant energy.
- Revitalizes the whole body.
- Aura cleansing.
- Spiritual opening and emotional cleansing.

Ear candling treatment

Preparation for the treatment

Have everything you need to hand before the client arrives. You will need:

- two candles
- small bowl of water – to extinguish the candle after use
- lighter

- towel to cover client's shoulders
- pillow
- soft music
- otoscope (not essential).

Clients have a choice of position. They can either lie on their front with their head to one side, changing position halfway through. Alternatively, they may be more comfortable lying on their side, and turning over halfway through the treatment. The treatment should be performed on a treatment couch, but in the absence of a couch it can also be performed on the floor, or somewhere safe. Do not treat on a bed or anywhere where there is inflammable material. A pillow placed under the client's head will keep the spine straight. The client must be comfortable as once the candle is lit, they will be unable to move for the next 15 minutes whilst the candle is burning. When the client is comfortable, place a towel over their shoulder to protect their clothes from any falling ash.

Tip

Don't stare at the flame as it may make you sleepy. You are monitoring a naked flame, and therefore you must keep alert throughout the treatment.

The treatment

The treatment may vary slightly depending upon which make of candle you are using. As with all products, always read the directions provided by the manufacturer. Some ear candles need to be used with a paper plate either waxed or covered in foil; others can be placed directly into the ear.

BioSun – Hopi ear candles

These candles are placed directly in the ear.

Tip

A lighter is used as it can be used with one hand, leaving the other hand free to support the candle.

1 Check ears with otoscope if using one and record findings on client record card. To insert the candle, pull the client's ear back, opening up the ear canal and insert the candle before letting go of the ear. Ask the client if the candle feels comfortable. You do not need to 'push' the candle in, just place it in far enough so that it feels comfortable and the client's ear has sealed around the candle. The candle must be upright.

2 Only when the candle is in place correctly do you light the top of the candle with a lighter, and leave to burn down to the red safety mark. The burning candle will produce a black ash. This may fall onto the back of your hand, but will not burn you. When the candle reaches the red safety mark, remove from the client's ear and extinguish it in the bowl of water. The ear candles will burn for approximately 12 minutes each.

Tip

Bring your treatment chair close to the couch and make yourself comfortable – once the candle is alight, you want to make as little movement as possible.

3 Always treat both ears. Repeat treatment on the other ear for balancing, then extinguish the candle safely. When the treatment is finished, the client is asked to lie on their back for the facial massage.

4 Performing a lymphatic drainage facial massage (see below) completes the treatment.

5 If using an otoscope, check ears again and record findings.

6 On completion, ask the client to sit up slowly and always offer a glass of water.

Lymphatic facial massage

When the ear candling is over, an efficient and effective ending to the treatment is a lymphatic drainage facial massage, which will further assist in draining the sinuses and increases the circulation of the blood and lymph. This should last approximately five minutes. With the client lying on their back proceed as follows:

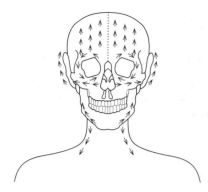

Facial lymphatic massage

1 Place your whole hand 'cupped' over the ears and hold for a slow count of 15.

2 Using middle fingers, gently massage temples, using no pressure and circular movements.

3 Anchor thumbs into scalp and using middle fingers, starting in between eyebrows, drain towards hairline ×3, continue working towards the temples from eyebrows to hairline. You should be able to complete three or four 'rows' of draining.

4 Using both middle fingers, starting over eyebrows, make one large circle, sweeping over eyebrow and under the eye, around the eye socket and ending up at the bridge of nose ×3. No pressure under the eye.

5 Place middle fingers at sides of nose and using a pumping action, work along the zygomatic bone ×3 – from nose towards ears.

6 In the same area, but this time using draining movements, slide your middle fingers from nose outwards under the zygomatic bone, draining to behind the ear ×3.

7 Using both hands together, drain under jaw line to behind ears ×3.

8 Gently but firmly, turn head onto one side and massage down the sternomastoid towards the main lymphatic ducts (just under collar bones) ×3.

9 Repeat for other side. Gently but firmly turn head to the left and massage down the sternomastoid towards the right lymphatic duct (just under the collar bones) ×3. Return head to centre.

10 Twiddle the ears. In auricular therapy, the lobe represents the head, so massage the lobe well before continuing up the ear, unravelling as you go. Continue two to three times up and down the ear.

11 To complete, as for step 1.

How does the treatment feel and does it hurt?
The treatment feels wonderful – warming, soothing, relaxing and very gentle. You may feel gentle warmth and a 'wave-like' sound in your ears. It does not hurt, and many clients fall asleep during the treatment.

The safety filter

It is not necessary to open the candles to look at the residue. The only residue there will be is a little of the beeswax lying above the filter. A filter is built into candles to make them safe. The filter makes sure that nothing drops down into the ear, and if nothing can drop down into the ear, then nothing can be sucked up into the filter either. Contrary to popular belief, the contents of the filter at the end of the treatment is not earwax. If the contents were scientifically examined, there may be a tiny amount of earwax under the filter, but the waxy substance above is from the candle itself. The earwax does get softened and loosened however, and many clients report that the wax simply falls out any time up to two or three days later.

Children and the elderly

The treatment is perfectly safe for children; however, for children under eight, use half a candle on each side. For safety reasons the candle is extinguished while the child changes position and a new candle used for the second ear. Never be tempted to share one candle between ears. This could cause cross infection and could also be dangerous.

The treatment is also excellent for the elderly, who regularly have problems with their ears.

Tip

To enhance your treatment you could make a blend of 5 ml almond oil with two drops chamomile and one drop of lavender essential oil and massage this behind the ear after the facial massage.

Interesting fact

Ear candling does not pull up earwax into the candle. The waxy residue found in the candle after use is from the candle itself.

Frequency of treatment

The time frames will be different for each person. Those who have severe problems may use candles up to three times a week, until symptoms improve. Following this, you may want to use the ear candles once a week, then once a month. For general maintenance once every four months is a good guide, usually with the change of season.

After care advice

Ear candling is a 'whole body' treatment where cleansing outcomes are expected. In order to aid the healing process and to get the most from their treatment, clients should be advised to take the following measures after treatment.

- Drink a glass of water immediately after the treatment and get up slowly from the couch, but only after first resting for at least five minutes.
- Keep ears out of water for 24 hours – when taking a shower, swimming or any water-based activity wear ear plugs.
- Keep out of cold winds and draughts – this includes driving with the window open.
- Reduce consumption of dairy products such as milk and cheese as these produce mucus.
- Cut down on tea, coffee and alcohol and stick to herbal teas or fresh juices.
- Avoid smoking.
- Rest as much as possible to allow the body to heal and do not tap into any sudden surges of fresh energy as they are there for healing purposes!
- Take a warm bath to help unwind.

Essential anatomy for ear candling

Anatomically, the ear is divided into three principal regions:

- the *external* or *outer ear* (pinna, external auditory canal and tympanic membrane)
- the *middle ear* (auditory or Eustachian tube, ossicles, oval and round windows)
- the *internal* or *inner ear* (bony labyrinth and membranous labyrinth); the internal ear contains the spiral organ (organ of Corti), the organ of hearing.

External (outer) ear

The external (outer) ear is structurally designed to collect sound waves and direct them inwards. It consists of the pinna, external auditory canal and tympanic membrane.

The pinna (auricle) is a flap of elastic cartilage shaped like the flared end of a trumpet and covered by thick skin. The rim of the pinna is called the helix, the inferior portion the lobule. The pinna is attached to the head by ligaments and muscles.

The external auditory canal is a curved tube about 2.5 cm (1 inch) in length that lies in the temporal bone. It leads from the pinna to the eardrum. The wall of the canal consists of bone lined with cartilage that is continuous with the cartilage of the pinna. The cartilage in the external auditory canal is covered with a thin, highly sensitive skin. Near the exterior opening, the canal contains a few hairs and specialized sebaceous glands called ceruminous (se-ROO-mi-nus) glands that secrete cerumen (earwax).

The combination of hairs and cerumen (se-ROO-min) helps to prevent dust and foreign objects from entering the ear. Usually cerumen dries up and falls out of the ear canal. Sometimes, however, it builds up in the canal and impairs hearing (impacted cerumen).

The tympanic membrane (eardrum) is a thin, semi-transparent partition of fibrous connective tissue between the external auditory canal and middle ear. Its external surface is concave and covered with skin. Its internal surface is convex and covered with a mucous membrane.

Middle ear

The middle ear (tympanic cavity) is a small, epithelial-lined, air-filled cavity hollowed out of the temporal bone. It is separated from the external ear by the eardrum and from the internal ear by a thin, bony partition that contains two small openings: the oval window and the round window.

The posterior wall of the middle ear communicates with the mastoid air cells of the temporal bone through a chamber called the tympanic antrum. This anatomical fact explains why a middle ear infection may spread to the temporal bone, causing mastoiditis, or even to the brain.

The anterior wall of the middle ear contains an opening that leads directly into the auditory tube (Eustachian tube). The auditory tube connects the middle ear with the nasopharynx of the throat. Through this passageway infections may travel from the throat and nose to the ear. The function of the tube is to equalize air pressure on both sides of the tympanic membrane. Abrupt changes in external or internal air pressure might otherwise cause the eardrum to rupture. During swallowing and yawning the tube opens to allow atmospheric air to enter or leave the middle ear until the internal pressure equals the external pressure. If the pressure is not relieved, intense pain, hearing impairment, tinnitus and vertigo could develop.

Any sudden pressure changes against the eardrum may be equalized by deliberately swallowing or pinching the nose closed, closing the mouth and gently forcing air from the lungs into the nasopharynx.

Extending across the middle ear are three exceedingly small bones called auditory ossicles. The bones, named for their shape, are the malleus, incus and stapes, commonly called the hammer, anvil and stirrup, respectively. They are connected by synovial joints. The 'handle' of the malleus is attached to the internal surface of the tympanic membrane. Its head articulates with the body of the incus. The incus is the intermediate bone in the series and articulates with the head of the stapes. The base or footplate of the stapes fits into a small opening in the thin bony partition between the middle and inner ear. The opening is called the oval window or fenestra vestibuli. Directly below the oval window is another opening, the round window or fenestra cochlea. This opening is enclosed by a membrane called the secondary tympanic membrane. Auditory ossicles are attached to the middle ear by means of ligaments.

In addition to the ligaments, there are also two skeletal muscles attached to the ossicles. The tensor tympani muscle draws the malleus medially, thus

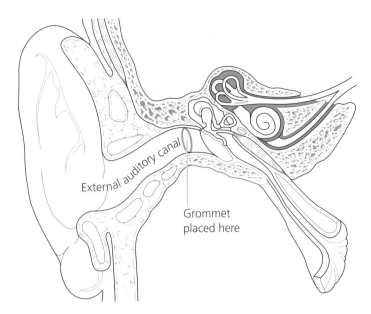

External auditory canal

Grommet
placed here

Position of grommet

limiting movement and increasing tension on the tympanic membrane to prevent damage to the inner ear when exposed to loud sounds. Since this response is slow it only protects the inner ear from prolonged loud noises, not brief ones, such as a gunshot.

The stapedium muscle is the smallest of all skeletal muscles. Its action is to draw the stapes posteriorly, thus preventing it from moving too much. Like the tensor tympani muscle, the stapedius muscle has a protective function in that it dampens (checks) large vibrations that result from loud noises. It is for this reason that paralysis of the stapedium muscle is associated with hyperacusia (acuteness in hearing).

Internal (inner) ear

The internal (inner) ear is also called the labyrinth (lab-I-RINTH) because of its complicated series of canals. Structurally, it consists of two main divisions: an outer bony labyrinth and an inner membranous labyrinth that fits into the bony labyrinth. The bony labyrinth is a series of cavities in the petrous portion of the temporal bone. It can be divided into three areas named on the basis of shape: these are the vestibule, cochlea and semi-circular canals. The bony labyrinth is lined with periosteum and contains a fluid called perilymph. This fluid, which is chemically similar to cerebrospinal fluid, surrounds the membranous labyrinth, a series of sacs and tubes laying inside and having the same general form as the bony labyrinth. The membranous labyrinth is lined with epithelium and contains a fluid called endolymph, which is chemically similar to intracellular fluid. The vestibule constitutes the oval central portion of the bony labyrinth. The membranous labyrinth is the vestibule consists of two sacs called the utricle (YOO-tri-kul = little bag) and saccule (SAK-yool). A small duct connects these sacs to each other.

Projecting upwards and posteriorly from the vestibule are the three bony semicircular canals. Each is arranged at approximately right angles to the other two. On the basis of their positions, they are called the *anterior*, *posterior* and *lateral canals*. The anterior and posterior semicircular canals are oriented vertically; the lateral is oriented horizontally. One end of each canal enlarges into a swelling called the ampulla (little jar). The portions of the membranous labyrinth that lie inside the bony semicircular canals are called the semicircular ducts.

Medical terms explained

Paranasal sinuses

Sinuses are not cranial or facial bones but cavities in certain cranial and facial bones near the nasal cavity. The paranasal sinuses are lined with mucous membranes that are continuous with the lining of the nasal cavity. Skull bones containing paranasal sinuses are the frontal, sphenoid, ethmoid and maxillae. Besides producing mucus, the paranasal sinuses lighten the skull bones and serve as resonant chambers for sound as we speak or sing.

Glue ear

The Eustachian tube usually keeps the middle ear full of air. If this tube becomes blocked, air cannot enter the middle ear. When this happens, the cells lining the middle ear begin to produce fluid. The fluid makes it harder for sound to pass through to the inner ear. It can be like listening to the world with both fingers stuck in your ears. Glue ear is temporary and can come and go.

Grommets

Grommets are tiny plastic tubes measuring about 2 mm in diameter that are put in the eardrum for people, usually children, suffering with glue ear. This is done during a short operation at hospital under general anaesthetic. The grommets are inserted after the fluid in the middle ear has been drained away. The grommets allow air to circulate in the middle ear and stop more fluid from building up. Grommets usually stay in until the eardrum has healed and pushed them out.

Vertigo

Vertigo is a sensation of spinning or movement in which the world is revolving or the person is revolving in space. Depending on its cause, vertigo may be classified as: (1) peripheral, which originates in the ear, has a sudden onset and lasts from minutes to hours; (2) central, which is caused by an abnormality of the central nervous system and may persist for more than three weeks; and (3) psychogenic, in which the cause is of a psychological origin.

Otitis media

Otitis media is an acute infection of the middle ear caused primarily by bacteria such as *Streptococcus pneumoniae* and *Haemophilus influenzae*. It is characterized by pain, malaise, fever and a reddening and outward bulging of the eardrum, which may rupture unless prompt treatment is given (this may involve draining pus from the middle ear). Abnormal function of the auditory (Eustachian) tube appears to be the most important mechanism in the pathogenesis of the middle ear disease. This allows bacteria from the nasopharynx, which are a primary cause of middle ear infection, to enter the middle ear.

Perforated eardrum

A perforated eardrum is a hole in the tympanic membrane that reduces sound transmission. The condition is characterized by acute pain initially, ringing or roaring in the affected ear, hearing impairment and sometimes dizziness. Causes of perforated eardrums include: ear syringing, compressed air, an explosion, scuba diving, trauma (skull fracture or from objects such as ear swabs), or acute middle ear infections. If the condition does not resolve itself, a surgical procedure called myringoplasty can be performed, in which a graft of skin, a vein or fascia is used to repair the perforation.

Tinnitus

Any noise (buzzing, ringing, etc.) in the ear. The many causes include a build up of wax (cerumen) in the ear; damage to the eardrum; diseases of the inner ear, such as otosclerosis and Menière's disease; adverse reactions to drugs such as aspirin and quinine; and abnormalities of the auditory nerve and its connections within the brain.

Knowledge review

1 Define thermal auricular therapy.

2 For what purpose did the Native American Hopi Indians use the candles?

3 State four active ingredients of ear candles.

4 What is an otoscope and why might you consider using one for an ear candling treatment?

5 State four physical benefits of an ear candling treatment.

6 State four psychological and subtle effects of an ear candling treatment.

7 How long do the candles burn for approximately?

8 How far down the candle do you burn?

9 What do you do with the candle when the burning is complete?

10 What is the benefit of the facial massage after an ear candling treatment?

11 Name two safety features ear candles may have.

12 Name four after care recommendations.

13 Name the three principal regions of the ear.

14 What are the individual names of the auditory ossicles?

15 Name the bones containing the paranasal sinuses.

16 What is vertigo?

17 Give four causes of a perforated eardrum.

18 Give four causes of the condition known as tinnitus.

19 What is the recommended frequency of ear candling treatments?

20 What are grommets?

19 Reiki

Learning objectives

This chapter covers the following:

- **what Reiki is**
- **intent**
- **the benefits and effects of Reiki**
- **Reiki precepts and principles**
- **understanding Reiki attunements**
- **contra indications and contra actions to Reiki treatments**
- **Reiki 'self-healing'**
- **how to give a Reiki treatment to others**
- **the meaning of the Reiki symbols**
- **using Reiki with other treatments**
- **causes of *dis*-harmony and *dis*-ease**

To become a Reiki I, II or III practitioner requires specialist training and attunements *in person* from a Reiki Master who has also received training and attunements from another Reiki Master. No book or Internet course can substitute for that direct personal initiation process.

The art of laying on of hands is as old as the hills. People have been doing it since the beginning of time. It is a natural instinct to put your hands on somebody who has been injured or is not well. Mothers are a prime example of this. When a child is hurt a mother will lay their hands on the injured spot instinctively. When we hurt ourselves, we instinctively rub or hold the injured spot for a few seconds. Human touch conveys healing, care and love.

What is Reiki?

Rei-Ki (pronounced Ray-key) is a system of natural healing involving the laying on of hands; it is said to be thousands of years old. Reiki assists us in balancing our physical, energy and emotional bodies, and those of our clients. It is believed that the technique was first used by Tibetan Buddhist monks and was rediscovered in the 1800s by Dr Mikao Usui, a Christian minister working in Japan. The Usui system of Reiki is a very simple but powerful healing technique that is easily given, and received, by anyone. The word healing is used in the sense of regaining harmony and wholeness, and Reiki addresses the whole person – physical, emotional, mental and spiritual. Reiki is unique in that the energy is drawn *through* the channel (the practitioner) by the recipient, as opposed to being directed *by* the practitioner.

Interesting fact

Other words for Ki
You may have come across the word Ki before and not realized it. Ki has been identified by all cultures and consequently has a variety of names. Other words representing Ki are Qi or Chi in Chinese, Prana in Sanskrit, and Mana in Hawaiian but they all mean the same thing – 'life force energy'.

Intent

Intention is very important in healing. The definition for intent is *having the attention sharply focused*. This means that you must concentrate on the client, the treatment, the hand positions, the chakras and the symbols, wholeheartedly. When we decide to work on someone we first *intend* to start channelling the Reiki energy through ourselves and into the client. It is our *intent* to be a pure vessel for the Reiki energy to flow through. We also *intend* that the person that we are healing accept this healing. However much you may want to heal somebody with Reiki, that person must want to be healed. Not everybody does! The whole aspect of intent can be quite complex, and your Reiki Master will go into this with you in much more detail. If the client has come to you for a Reiki treatment, then he or she will want to be healed. If, however, they have come to you for any other treatment, you cannot include any Reiki healing unless you have asked the client's express permission to do so at the consultation stage.

The benefits and effects of Reiki

Reiki energy is a unique form of energy and as such it is difficult to describe exactly the physiological effects of treatment. However, it is a powerful healing tool and its benefits are generally far reaching. Reiki is something that has to be experienced and is often impossible to describe clearly in words.

Reiki can help to:

- relieve pain(physical and emotional)
- accelerate natural healing

- aid the detoxification process of the body
- induce a state of deep relaxation
- calm the mind, body and spirit, restoring a feeling of peace
- dissolve energy blockages in the body
- generally improve health and well-being
- release stored emotions
- re-balance and amplify the body's energy
- release tension and negative stress
- focus the mind, helping to negate confusion and help solve problems.

Reiki precepts and principles

The two Reiki precepts

1   **The person must ask to be healed.**
    It is not considered ethical to give anyone healing unless they have requested it, or your have asked permission to give it. In asking to receive or agreeing to receive the person is putting forth a conscious decision to be come involved in the healing process.

2   **There must be an exchange of energy for the services.**
    The healing energy belongs to the Universe. However, there needs to be some exchange from the recipient to the person whose time and services are being rendered for the healing. If you offer the healing for nothing it is stating that the healing is of no value to you, thereby causing imbalances of energy exchange. An energy exchange therefore maintains the balance. Energy exchange can be anything from the concept of energy we call money, or a bunch of flowers or any exchange of services between the person being healed and the Reiki healer. Reiki healers offering services on a professional level should establish a fee.

The five Reiki principles

One of the things that makes Reiki unique compared to other healing practices is the Reiki principles. Whilst Reiki is not a religion, it remains true to Eastern philosophy. There are a number of variations of the Five Principles, but this list, as given by Mrs Takata on her audio tape *The History of Reiki as Told by Mrs Takata*, is probably the closest to the original.

1   Just for today – do not worry.
2   Just for today – do not anger.
3   Honour your parents, teachers and elders.
4   Earn your living honestly.
5   Show gratitude for every living thing.

Tip

Your Reiki will be enhanced by learning the Reiki principles and incorporating them into your life. Pass them on to your clients too.

These principles bear careful thought, and using them daily makes Reiki a way of life. They violate no one's religion or religious ethics. How these compassionate commandments are interpreted can vary according to the individual. For example, if you are angry about something that has occurred in your life, this Principle suggests that you do not to nurse your rage and resentment, or to hold on to it until it explodes. Taking one day at a time, expressing honest feelings and clearing the air without letting the anger smoulder unresolved, seems to be the essence of this Principle.

How would you interpret the other Reiki Principles?

Understanding Reiki attunements

Reiki is a powerful spiritual experience and consequently is not taught in the same way as other healing techniques. The ability to attune to the Reiki energy is passed from Master to student during an attunement process, which opens the crown, heart and palm chakras. This process also creates a special link between the Master and the student.

Reiki I – the First Degree – is usually taken over a two-day period, and the attunements are usually spread over these two days. Reiki I has a four-stage attunement process which has the effect of greatly opening the channels of the student to the energy. The first three attunements open the healing chakras and the fourth seals in the energy. This means that, once given, the ability to give Reiki is for life and will always be an ever-present ability, even if the energy is dormant for any length of time. Some Reiki Masters amalgamate the four attunements into one. This may be to save time or they may feel it is better received this way. However, by receiving four small attunements over the training sessions, students become accustomed to the attunement process and relax and enjoy each one more, thereby adding value and refinement to the process. Further attunements during a student's life, as when continuing their studies with Reiki II and Reiki III, produce a clearer channel and therefore an increase in the physical sensitivity and consciousness of the individual.

The attunements are a group concern, unless you are having one-to-one tuition. Students will be seated with the Reiki Master behind them. With their hands on their thighs and eyes closed, students wait in turn for their attunement. The larger the group, the longer this takes, so comfortable chairs are recommended. At the end of the attunement session there may be group feedback discussions on the experiences of the students during the attunement process, or one-to-one feedback with the Reiki Master. After the attunements, students would then perform a 'self-heal' treatment on themselves.

Reiki attunements begin a spiritual cleansing of the physical body as well as of the mind and emotions. It is usual for students to go through a release of emotional energy and to begin to see a refinement of their belief structures and feelings. Your Reiki Master should talk you through the attunement process before commencement.

The three degrees of the Usui system of Reiki

The Reiki healing system comprises three degrees: First Degree, Second Degree and Third Degree. Most students will go through a period of readjusting to the new energy even though they may not feel anything at the attunement. Reiki creates change! Old beliefs and attitudes will be lost and a new sense of 'being' is generally experienced. The consciousness is awakened and the newly initiated Reiki practitioner will find himself or herself with renewed enthusiasm and lust for life. The different degrees of Reiki are said to have been added to the Reiki system of healing by Dr Chujiro Hayashi.

It is recommended that a period of time is taken to adjust to these new energies. Some Masters offer First Degree Reiki (Reiki I) and Second Degree Reiki (Reiki II) over a single weekend teaching period. It is very difficult to assimilate such a vast readjustment to the system in this short time frame. Different students have different energies and abilities and usually the student 'feels' when the time is right to progress to the next degree. It is generally accepted that six months should elapse between Reiki I and Reiki II and one year between Reiki II and Reiki III.

First Degree Reiki (Reiki I)

In Reiki I you receive the appropriate attunements and learn a self-healing routine that you can administer on a daily basis. You will learn techniques and hand positions that can be incorporated into a meditation routine or used at any convenient time. Also taught on a Reiki I course are using Reiki with other therapies, treating plants and animals with Reiki, giving a Reiki treatment to someone else, group healing techniques and hand positions. Often the chakra system of energy is also taught on a Reiki I course.

Second Degree Reiki (Reiki II)

Reiki II is a more advanced application of the energy, concentrating more on the subtle, or aetheric, body rather than the physical. During this course students are initiated into the three sacred symbols of the degree, which increase the power of the energy and allow the practitioner to project the Reiki energy at a distance, effecting a powerful form of absent healing. Reiki II also helps the practitioner to focus the energy to remove and heal mental and emotional blocks in the client.

As a Reiki II practitioner you will have all the tools necessary to provide very effective healing for yourself, clients and friends, on all levels – physical, emotional and mental. You will be able to heal issues pertaining to the past or future and you will be able to give effective healing whether the other person or people are in your presence or not.

Third Degree Reiki (Reiki III)

Many practitioners, having experienced the universal energy and wonder of Reiki II, wish to progress to become Masters themselves. Master energy brings new powers, and also new responsibilities. As a Master Practitioner you will be able to pass on the power of Reiki through attunements, and teach classes, extending the energy to others. The word 'master' should not be considered in the same way as a spiritual master, but should be considered like a school master or a head master, who, by virtue of their training and commitment to a subject, have achieved a position that should be respected. Taking the Third Degree in Reiki should be a very important step in your life and students should feel absolutely confident in their Master, who should be available at all times to offer support and advice. Master classes are often conducted at sacred sites around the world such as Bali, Hawaii, Cyprus, Ayers Rock in Australia, Machu Picchu in Peru; Tenerife, the Great Pyramids in Egypt, and Glastonbury.

Contra indications and contra actions to Reiki treatments

Contra indications

There will be very few people to whom you cannot administer a Reiki treatment. However, as with all holistic and alternative therapies, there may be specific contra indications and Reiki is no exception. The following conditions are contra indicated to Reiki treatment:

- pacemakers
- epilepsy
- fractures and sprains

- severed limbs and digits
- recent operations
- identified acute or chronic medical disorders.

Conditions, which need special consideration, are as follows:

- *Pregnancy* – although pregnancy is not an illness, it is wise to avoid treating anyone during the first trimester. Provided that the pregnancy is uncomplicated, great benefits may be gained from Reiki during the later stages of pregnancy.
- *Babies and children* – a Reiki treatment can be invaluable to babies and children with either physical or emotional problems, and can help to bond the relationship between babies, children and their parents. If babies and/or children are treated, it is of paramount importance that you not only obtain parental or a guardian's permission to carry out the treatment, but also for ethical reasons, that the parent or guardian is present during the treatment. A Reiki treatment for a baby or child would be shorter in duration than that for an adult.

Contra actions

As with all other holistic and alternative treatments, some clients may experience a variety of symptoms after their treatment, whilst others experience nothing at all except stress relief and relaxation. However, a thoughtful therapist will identify the following contra actions to clients before they leave the salon so that they will not worry unnecessarily *should* any occur.

- a healing crisis
- somnolence
- weepiness
- laxative and diuretic effects
- emotional release
- increased energy flow.

Reiki self-healing

Tip

Reiki 'self-treatment' can be used whenever you feel stressed or anxious, or run down and exhausted. Your hands are placed against your body without pressure.

When you give a Reiki treatment, the practitioner will also receive the energy, and therefore receive healing at the same time. However, it is unlikely, especially in the beginning that you will be giving Reiki treatments every day, so it is recommended that you undertake a Reiki 'self-treatment' preferably on a daily basis. It is worth waking up a little earlier to ensure that time is available to give yourself this treatment.

After a few treatments the general beneficial effects on your health and ability to deal with issues in your life will be apparent and you will actively look forward to receiving the energy. If you don't have time or a complete self-treatment, you can place your hand or hands on yourself anywhere, anytime. Just placing your hand over your throat chakra for a couple of minutes for example will energize that chakra and may make it easier for you to say something difficult to somebody. You will read more about channelling energy to all organs, glands and associated chakras later in this chapter (see p.408). It is the client's choice to be healed or not.

Self-healing

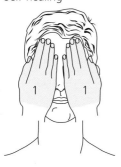

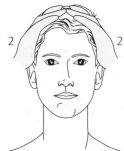

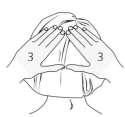

Head and face, 1–3

Procedure for a Reiki 'self-treatment'

Position 1 (head and face)
Hands cover the front of the face, with the tips of the fingers touching the hairline or top of the forehead. Hands are together and covering the nose. This first position balances the left and right sides of the brain and is wonderful for headaches and eyestrain. It also covers the brow or third eye chakra.

Position 2
The tips of the middle fingers are placed on the crown of the head. Allow the fingers and hands to rest gently on the head. This position covers the crown chakra.

Position 3
The heels of the hands are cupped under the occiput. The fingers extend straight upwards with the thumbs and index fingers touching. If this is awkward, the hands can be adjusted slightly into a more comfortable position, with one hand above the occiput ridge and the other below. This position also covers the crown and the third eye chakra.

Position 4 (front of body)
The left hand is placed at the neck and rests on the chest, with the right hand on the chest directly below. This is the position for the throat chakra, but because many people do not like to be touched around the throat area, we move down slightly and the heels of the hands should rest on the collar bone.

Position 5
Hands are placed across the centre of the chest, with the right hand on top. The hands are placed either gently on the body, or slightly away, about one inch, from the body. Never place your hands directly over a female's breasts. This is the position for the heart chakra.

Position 6
Left hand over the centre of the navel with the right hand placed above, but with hands touching. This position covers the solar plexus chakra.

Position 7
Hands pointed down. Thumbs and index fingers are touching. Fingertips touch the pubic bone. This position is covering the base or root chakra.

Position 8 (back of body)
Place hands over the waist area on the back of the body. The hands are equally spaced on either side of the spine.

Position 9
Hands pointed downward, with the heels of the hands at the waistline, middle fingertips pointing towards the spine.

How to give a Reiki treatment to others

Tip

The practitioner and the client will remain more grounded if they remove their shoes when performing and receiving Reiki treatments.

The treatment room

Set up your room so that you have the couch at the right height for you to sit or stand without having to bend or stretch. This will help you to perform your Reiki treatment without stressing your own body. The room should be decorated tastefully with soft colours. This helps both therapist and client to feel relaxed. Having a special treatment room or Reiki room is ideal but Reiki can be done anywhere, at any time, in classrooms, in client's homes, on trains or buses or in the street.

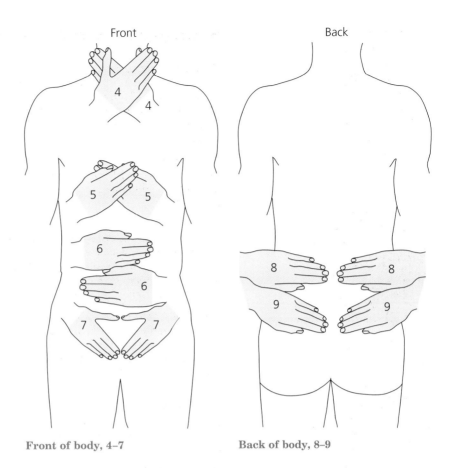

Front of body, 4–7   Back of body, 8–9

The client always keeps their clothes on during a treatment with the exception of the shoes, but it is recommended that tight garments, such as belts and ties, be loosened. The therapist should wear loose comfortable clothes. A blanket should be near to hand, as the client may feel cold after a treatment. Appropriate music may be played during the healing session. You may choose this but check with the client that it is to their liking too.

The treatment

Once attuned, the Reiki practitioner has only to place their hands on the subject and the healing energy will flow automatically. Reiki is an automatic process and will flow to the area that needs the most healing. Any attempt to force the process will result in a general lessening of the power available. Remember that the practitioner is a channel for the energy to be given, and not the source of the healing. This explains why treatments do not drain the giver, but actively replenish and charge Reiki practitioners.

As with all treatments, a consultation will precede the treatment. You need to know the client is suitable for treatment, by checking any contra indications they may have and finding out the client's expectations of the treatment. You need relevant information concerning the client's lifestyle, physical and emotional state, which will be recorded on the client's consultation form. The client needs to be fully and accurately informed of the concepts of Reiki and informed regarding possible contra actions resulting from treatment.

Interesting fact

Energy will go where it is needed in the body – the therapist does not need to direct it.

Tip

It is very important that you ground yourself and surround yourself with white light before you heal, otherwise you may take on the client's energy in some way.

A full Reiki treatment will normally last for about an hour during which time the energy will communicate to the higher self of the recipient. The practitioner ideally should attempt to allow the flow for about 3–4 minutes in each of the hand positions. The best results are achieved when the practitioner is calm and relaxed, becoming at one with the energy. Depending on the relative sensitivity of the individual, Reiki will begin to allow the practitioner to use their intuition as to where, and for how long, they place their hands on areas of the body. This produces a wonderfully flowing procedure with the energy fields of the practitioner and client joining to produce balance, harmony and understanding.

It is important that practitioners do not become too reliant on results, and trust that the recipient is receiving the required amount of Reiki energy to restore harmony. Remember that you cannot make a mistake in the application of the energy, and that you are not responsible for the results. Reiki I works on a physical level – when you touch, you heal, and when you take your hands away, it stops. Reiki can never cause harm and, has a beneficial effect on most causes of *dis*-ease.

If the client wants to talk to the practitioner, the flow of energy will not be stopped; however it is best if conversation is kept to a minimum. Usually the Reiki energy relaxes the recipient so efficiently that this invariably ceases to be an issue once treatment commences.

Leave sufficient time at the end of the treatment to give after care advice, for feedback from the client, and time for the client to gather their thoughts and return to the present.

Reiki treatment routine – seated chair position

A Reiki treatment can be given with the recipient seated in a chair. Shoes can be removed before commencing the treatment. The seated chair position usually takes approximately 45 minutes of actual hands-on work. Prepare the working area by dimming the lights, making the room warm and playing some suitable music if possible. There are ten positions for this treatment and each position should last between 4 and 5 minutes. In time you will know intuitively when to move to the next position.

Position 1
Standing behind the client, place your hands on the client's shoulders.

Position 2
Standing to the side of the client, place your right hand on the client's forehead, with the left hand behind the client's head, over the occiput.

Position 3
Standing behind the client, place your hands over the front chest area. Thumbs and index finger tips should be touching.

Position 4
Right hand in front of the client and left hand placed on the client's back. This is at the heart chakra level and the hands are placed very gently – hardly touching at the front.

Position 5
As for position 4 but hands are lowered so that right hand is over the solar plexus chakra and left hand is corresponding at the back of the client.

Position 6
The right hand holds the client's hand gently while the left hand is placed on the client's shoulder.

Seated positions

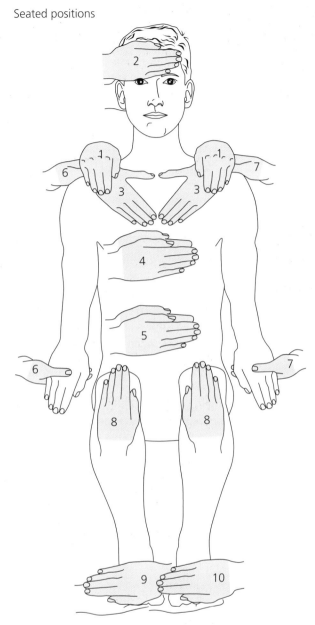

Seated, 1–10

Position 7
The right hand is placed on the client's shoulder while the left hand gently holds the client's hand.

Position 8
Kneeling in front of the client, place your hands on the client's knees.

Position 9
Still kneeling, your right hand is placed on the top of the right foot, and the left hand beneath the sole of the right foot.

Position 10
Still kneeling, your right hand is placed on the top of the left foot, and the left hand beneath the sole of the left foot.

As with all treatments, offer the client a glass of water at the end of the treatment and give the after care advice.

Tip
Burning sage 'smudge' sticks after a treatment cleanses the treatment room of any negative energies.

Front

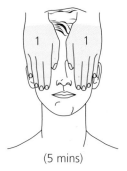

(5 mins)

Hand positions

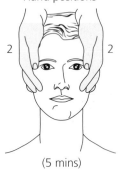

(5 mins)

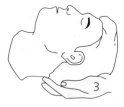

(5 mins)

Hands/face, 1–3

Reiki full body treatment routine

A full body Reiki treatment will last approximately 60 minutes. The major hand positions will be left for between 3 and 5 minutes on each position, whilst the minor hand positions of the lower limbs are left on for approximately 30 seconds each. You may want to leave about an hour and a half in total for a complete treatment to include the consultation and after care processes. Be aware of your own movements. Be as still as possible, gliding from one position to another, and as with all Reiki treatments make every possible attempt to have no interruptions. Remember that all the hand positions are placed over the main chakras, organs and glands of the body.

Position 1

As the first four positions may take up to 20 minutes, you will need to be sitting comfortably behind the client. Place your hands over the client's eyes, gently 'cupping' your hands so they are not placed directly over the eyes. A tissue may be placed over the eyes without covering the nose if you wish. The heels of the hands are placed at the top of the forehead (hairline). The hands are always held gently over the body, but especially so with the face and head. Hold the position for 3–5 minutes. This first position balances the left and right sides of the brain. Discourage talking for at least the time it takes to complete the head positions.

Position 2

Slide your hands so they are covering the cheeks, with your little fingers placed just beside the ears. Hold the position for 3–5 minutes. Where position 1 covered the third eye chakra, position 2 reaches both crown and third eye chakras.

Position 3

Gently slide your hands under the client's head. Fingertips are touching the lower edge of the occipital bones with hands together. This position reaches the crown and third eye chakra, as with position 2. Hold the position for 3–5 minutes.

Position 4

Still sitting comfortably, place your hands over the client's upper chest with the thumbs and index fingers touching. This position is the throat chakra position, but as so many people panic when hands are placed directly over their throat, place your hands over the client's collar bone. Hold the position for 3–5 minutes.

Position 5

Standing, sitting or kneeling (on a cushion), on your client's right-hand side, place your right hand under the breast line and left hand immediately under the right hand. Hold the position for 3–5 minutes.

Position 6

With both hands in the same position as for 5 above, move them over so that the heels of your hands are on the mid-line of the body. Hold the position for 3–5 minutes.

Position 7

Moving down the body, position 7 has the right hand at the outside of the client with the left hand in the centre as shown in the figure. Hold the position for 3–5 minutes.

Position 8

Position 8 differs between male and female clients. The right hand is pointed downwards whilst the left hand is pointed slightly upwards. Check the figure for positions. Remember to maintain the client's modesty at all times and hold the position for 3–5 minutes.

Position 9

The next five moves (positions 9–13 inclusive) are performed for only 30 seconds each. With these moves you are working down the front of the legs,

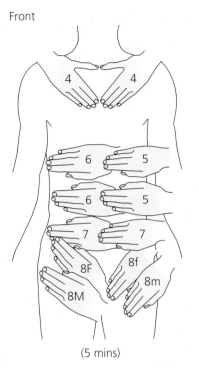

Front

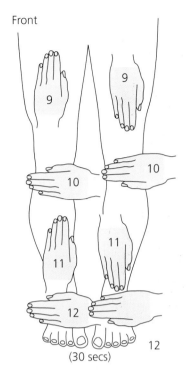

Front

(5 mins)

Front of body, 4–8

(30 secs)

Legs, 9–12

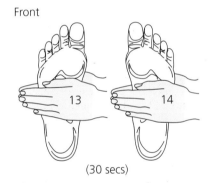

Front

(30 secs)

Feet, 13–14

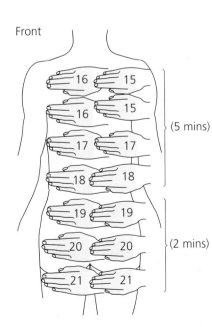

Front

(5 mins)

(2 mins)

Back of body, 15–21

finishing with the client's feet. Always keep your right hand closest to you. Position 9 is performed with your right hand placed on the client's thigh with fingers pointing downwards and the left hand on the other leg, with fingers pointing upwards. Hold the position for 30 seconds.

Position 10
Your hands are placed over the client's knees, your right hand closest to you.

Position 11
With your hands on the client's shins, right hand closest to you, fingers pointing down, left hand on the other leg and pointing upwards. Hold the position for 30 seconds.

Position 12
One hand on each of the client's upper feet and with the right hand closest to you. Hold the position for 30 seconds.

Position 13
Starting with the client's right foot – the one furthest away from you – sandwich their foot between your hands. Hold the position for 30 seconds.

Position 14
Repeat for other foot.

Ask the client to turn over so you can work on the back of the body.

Position 15
You are now going to move back to the client's body again, and start working on the back area. With hands together and thumbs touching, hands are held over the scapula area of the back. Hold position for 3–5 minutes.

Position 16
Slide hands over to other side of body and repeat, holding for 3–5 minutes.

Position 17
Moving down one hand's width, align the hands with your right hand nearest to you. Hold for 3–5 minutes.

Back

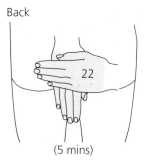

(5 mins)

Glutes, 22

Back

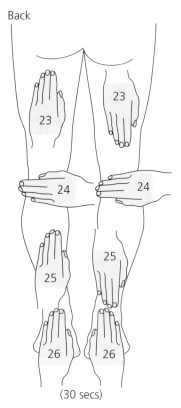

(30 secs)

Back of legs, 23–26

Tip

Sitting or standing still for 3–5 minutes with your hands gently resting on somebody can seem like a long time. Visualizing the colour and key words of the chakras when working over these areas will help keep you focused during those minutes.

Position 18
Repeat similar movement at waist level and hold for 3–5 minutes.

Position 19
Move hands to sacral chakra position and hold for 3–5 minutes.

Position 20
Keep moving hands down the body. This time you are over the gluteal area of body, the area that also represents the base (root) chakra. Still using gentle pressure, hold for 3–5 minutes.

Position 21
Move hands down to top of thigh and hold for a further 3–5 minutes. You may be standing, sitting or kneeling at this stage. Try not to move around too much in between moves – just *glide* into each new position.

Position 22
Right hand over coccyx with fingers pointing towards feet and left hand over right hand – hold this position for 3–5 minutes. The base (root) chakra is being worked in this position.

Position 23
Positions 23–26 inclusive are held for 30 seconds each, working down the backs of the legs as we did on the fronts of the legs. In position 23 your right hand is closest to you with fingers pointing downwards, with your left hand on other leg with fingers pointing upwards.

Position 24
Hands placed over the backs of the client's knees, right hand nearest to you.

Position 25
Right hand nearest to you and pointing downwards and left hand on client's other leg with fingers pointing upwards. Hands placed over the client's gastrocnemius muscle.

Position 26
The last position is the placing of your hands over the soles of the client's feet. Hold for 30 seconds.

If doing a whole body treatment, you may want to skip the feet positions 13 and 14 on the front of the body and choose to do the feet positions at the end of the session for a longer time. Although the front and backs of legs and the feet positions are held for only 30 seconds, they are extremely important. For the first half-hour or more the person receiving the healing has been lying quietly. He or she may appear to be asleep or just totally relaxed. The hand positions on the legs and feet begin to bring the client back to Earth – this helps to 'ground' the client. The backs of the legs and the final foot positions are extremely important for the same reason. In the last position the therapist's hands are placed on the soles of the feet, as this is where the Earth or grounding chakra is located. You may feel streams of energy moving through the feet. This position integrates the healing and completes it. The receiver of the healing will be far from grounded when they get up from the session but they will be functioning – without the feet positions they would not be grounded at all.

Group healing sessions

You will probably only be treating one client at a time in a clinic situation, but in a classroom situation or at a Reiki healers' meeting, group healing can take place. One member of the class will lie on the couch and the others will take up various positions around the couch. Look at the positions shown in the figures on p.411 for suggestions as to where to stand. The practitioners can either maintain their positions which is preferable as there is less movement within the room itself, or the therapists can move around the couch, changing their positions. Leave enough time so everyone takes a turn on the couch. You can adjust the treatment time accordingly – the more therapists the less the treatment time. For example, a 20-minute session (10 minutes on the front and 10 minutes on the back) will be long enough with four practitioners working on one person. Remember you can't over treat or do anything wrong. The Reiki energy will direct itself to where it is needed.

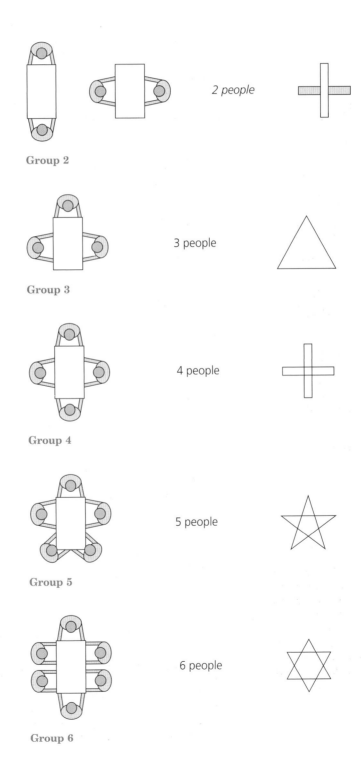

Group 2   *2 people*

Group 3   3 people

Group 4   4 people

Group 5   5 people

Group 6   6 people

The meaning of the Reiki symbols

In Reiki II, you will learn how to use the first three Reiki symbols. Only a Reiki Master can teach these, and usually only after the student has had about six months' experience using Reiki I. The symbols are visualized by the Reiki practitioner in violet, silver, white or gold light, and when learning them, are usually drawn in the air using the index and middle fingers of the dominant hand. The thumb and ring finger should also be joined which creates an energy circuit.

Symbol 1 – The Power Symbol

The Power Symbol is always referred to as the 'First Symbol' or 'Power Symbol', and these are the phrases to use when talking about the symbols to non-Reiki attuned persons. You will learn the sacred name of the symbol in your classes and this can be used when speaking with other attuned Reiki practitioners.

The meaning of the Power Symbol is to 'set right'. It also means, 'The Key to unlock the Power within', or 'The Light Switch'. It represents a powerful universal symbol. The Power Symbol is the only symbol that can be used independently of the other symbols as it works on the principles of radionics, where lines or objects create a force by their being. The 'power' in the Power Symbol is therefore between the lines, not the lines themselves. The Power Symbol needs to be invoked three times for best results. The main purpose of the Power Symbol is to increase the power of the Reiki given during the attunement process used in Reiki I. Further uses are as follows:

- empowerment
- clearance of negative energy
- sealing
- protection.

Symbol 2 – The Mental/Emotional Symbol

This symbol is referred to as the 'Second Symbol' or the 'Mental/Emotional Symbol'. As it implies, the symbol is used for all healing which involves mental or emotional issues. The symbol balances both hemispheres of the brain, bringing calmness and clarity and relieving shock. As with the Power Symbol above, you will learn the sacred word for this symbol in your class work.

All areas of emotional or mental imbalance can be dealt with effectively using this symbol. This would include nervousness, anger or sadness, as well balancing temporary or longer-term conditions. The major uses of this symbol are:

- relieving conditions that have a mental or emotional basis
- countering addictions
- improving the memory
- enhancing affirmations
- creating harmony in relationships.

Symbol 3 – The Distant Symbol

The Distant Symbol is based on Japanese script. It is made up of 21 lines that form to make one symbol, which you will learn from your Reiki Master in your classes. There are five individual words within the Distant Symbol, but when joined together the whole symbol brings the meaning of Wholeness, Completion and Enlightenment.

When learning the symbols, it is important to learn them exactly as taught by your Reiki Master. The slightest change to the strokes radically alters the meaning, which means that while the intent remains strong the symbols are having an altogether different effect on the energy body. Many say that the symbols work even through they are different, and that will and intent is very powerful and will produce an effect. However, whilst this is true, if something is worth doing, it is worth doing well, so learn the symbols exactly as taught.

Tip

Learn the symbols by visualizing them. As you become more experienced you can visualize them in the palms of your hands as you hold the hand positions.

Using Reiki with other treatments

Reiki not only complements other therapies and disciplines but actively increases the amount of healing power normally available. At First Degree level, Reiki will add a great deal of power to any hands on healing, especially aromatherapy and reflexology.

Crystal healers too will find that crystals store the Reiki energy and this can then be used to enhance the quality of the crystal's power for healing. Crystals should be 'charged' (after cleansing) by being held in both hands and allowing the Reiki to flow through for 5–10 minutes. Further infusions of Reiki energy are necessary to maintain the crystal as a Reiki conductor.

There are a couple of disciplines, which require a different use of the Reiki energy. In shiatsu for instance, where diagnostics are undertaken by pressing areas of the abdomen, Reiki will begin to heal areas of disharmony, thereby giving a false and confusing diagnosis. In this case the practitioner needs to actively close down the Reiki channel by force of will during the time needed to perform the diagnosis; this completed, the Reiki can be allowed to flow freely again.

With homeopathic remedies, many contain an element of poison that creates the energy to provide the basis for the healing. According to some homeopaths, Reiki applied directly to the remedy will try to produce harmony by neutralizing the poison, thereby making the remedy ineffective. It is better therefore to perform Reiki either before or after the remedy is ingested.

Holding aromatherapy oils in the hands and applying Reiki can purify the oils, if you are not sure of their source. This will overcome effects of pollution during growth, or mishandling during extraction.

Reiki and Indian head massage can be practised together easily, and often an Indian head massage treatment will end with balancing the chakras and a few minutes of Reiki. Remember to ask at the consultation stage if giving the Reiki is acceptable to the client.

Causes of *dis*-harmony and *dis*-ease

Have you ever thought why it is that some people are always suffering with their backs, or their knees, or with headaches or digestive disorders or constantly have sore throats, while other people go through life apparently symptom-free? What causes *dis*-harmony and *dis*-ease in some people and not in others? As our minds and bodies are not separate entities, a connection can be made of all our physical weaknesses to our mental state. Physical symptoms therefore may be brought about by emotional factors. For example, it is said that tinnitus is an 'emotional problem'. Someone who does not want to hear something has turned noise in upon him- or herself so that they will *not* hear it. Look at these other examples and see if you can identify any, either in yourself, or in family and friends. When someone next says to you 'I've got butterflies in my stomach', look for a possible emotional connection too.

Head

Our head is the place where we put everything that is going on in our lives; it is the control centre for the body. Too much analysing results in headaches or migraines, or a general imbalance in the physical, emotional, mental or spiritual level. It can be a repository for confusion and unexpressed emotion. Remaining 'level headed' and 'keeping your head above water' are expressions we may use when we are overwhelmed or have taken on too much.

Eyes

Eyes relate to our inner seeing and feeling. To the need to be seen by others, or not seeing their needs. Not seeing what is plainly in front of our eyes, or what is ahead. The eyes are also connected to the sinus and link to unshed tears.

Ears

Hearing others, being heard by others or blocking out what we don't or didn't want to hear (tinnitus). Also related to high blood pressure, balance and clarity.

Throat

Dis-harmony in the throat by becoming 'choked up' may mean the inability to express to others how we really feel. Difficulty in speaking the truth; throat blockages or sore throats caused by not saying what needs to be said, talking too much, feeling gagged.

Neck

The link between our intellectual and physical processes. A 'stiff-necked' view, or inability to put your 'neck on the line'. Rigidity in thinking. Also related to shoulders carrying burdens and responsibilities.

Intestinal tract/abdomen

Blockages, constipation, unable to let go of the past or old feelings. Holding in anger. Diarrhoea or colitis is letting go of the past without dealing with the issues. The abdomen can be the storage area for anger or unresolved issues. Lack of 'gut feeling', indecision, 'no guts'.

Liver

Anger stored over long periods of time and/or long-term insecurity may affect the effectiveness of the liver. If the liver is not detoxifying efficiently this may show up as eczema or psoriasis.

Gall bladder

Anger that has turned to bitterness may result in gall bladder problems.

Stomach

Being unable to digest aspects from the past, such as old ideas or social conditioning, may result in stomach conditions. Difficulty in having to 'stomach' issues. Ulcers show the eating away of the gut, whilst 'butterflies in the stomach' represent anxiety about the future. Fear of change, or of possible disapproval.

Pancreas

Losing the sweetness of life. Lack of spark or the 'spice of life'.

Spleen

Unfinished business, especially within relationships. The need to 'vent one's spleen'. Sometimes related to the death of someone or something close, e.g. person, lifestyle, job, etc.

Ovaries or testicles, uterus

Deep sexual issues such as abuse. Guilt to do with miscarriage or abortion. Anger about sexuality.

Bladder

Stored issues that need to be expressed.

Prostate

Sexual guilt, anger with women, helplessness with birth or sexual issues, and powerlessness.

Hips

Body's physical support system. Stored problems or anger or fear result in excess of fat making a barrier to the world. Being too vulnerable or unprotected in life results in thinness. The inability to deal with a changing environment.

Knees

The body's shock absorbers. The need for support for emotional or practical issues, and inflexibility in dealing with 'the rough ground' of life.

Ankles

Difficulty in being able to react to rapidly changing circumstances. Lack of understanding or trying to analyse things not relevant to our progression.

Feet

Lack of grounding in life. Unable to 'take a stand', to 'stand up' for ourselves. Unable to 'stand something' any more. Difficulty in setting standards for the self.

Shoulders

Burdens and responsibilities and the inability to 'shoulder' those burdens. Tension, and a difficulty in dealing with or carrying the things we need in life. Feeling that the 'whole world' is on our shoulders.

Upper back

Too much giving and little receiving. Creating a 'rod for one's back'. Repressed feelings of another's ingratitude or guilt may cause upper back problems, or just something getting one's 'back up'.

Adrenals/kidneys

Shock, trauma, stress and fear all may produce weakness in this area. An inability to deal with fear or uncertainty in life. Overstretching of the nervous system.

Lower back

Lower back problems may indicate that someone is uncomfortable with life, or the stress of life itself. Just doing too much may cause problems in this area.

Coccyx

Connected to the survival instinct. Sometimes indicates fear of success in life.

Knowledge review

1 What is Reiki?

2 Give a definition of the word Reiki.

3 What do the words Chi, Prana and Mana mean?

4 What are the Two Reiki Precepts?

5 How many Reiki Principles are there? Name them.

6 What is your understanding of the Reiki attunement process?

7 How many 'degrees' of the Reiki system are there?

8 There are six specific contra indications to a Reiki treatment – what are they?

9 There are six specific contra actions to a Reiki treatment – what are they?

10 How often should newly qualified practitioners practice the Reiki 'self-treatment'?

11 When can you use the Reiki 'self-treatment'?

12 Are clothes removed for a Reiki treatment?

13 All Reiki hand positions are placed over the main chakras, organs and glands of the body. How many main chakras are there?

14 How many Reiki symbols are there in Reiki II?

15 What is the meaning of the Mental/Emotional Symbol?

16 What may be a cause of dis-harmony in somebody who suffers from upper back problems?

20

Hot stone massage

Learning Objectives

This chapter covers the following:

- **brief history of stone therapy**
- **basalt stones**
- **the benefits and effects of heated basalt stones**
- **marine stones**
- **the benefits and effects of cold marine stones**
- **standard set of stones**
- **care of the stones**
- **contra indications and Contra actions to stone therapy**
- **the importance of grounding**
- **preparation for massage**
- **back massage treatment using hot and cold stones**
- **specific after care advice for hot stone massage**

Stone therapy has become one of the most sought after treatments in our industry. This grounding and unique form of massage, using hot and cold stones, is gaining great popularity among clients drawn to this cosseting, warming, earthy, and deeply balancing treatment. Stone massage incorporates the use of basalt stones, which are used after heating, and marine stones, which are kept refrigerated. Both hot and cold stones are then incorporated into a normal massage routine enabling the client to have the luxury of a spa treatment in the beauty salon or holistic clinic. As with all new treatments, there is a range of training now available. Some include simply incorporating the stones within a regular massage, some include working with meridians or the chakras while others include working with crystals as well as the stones. The choices are wide and varied, in cost and length of course, so shop around to get the best value in terms of product and training.

Brief history of stone therapy

By looking at ancient cultures and civilizations we can see that as humans we have used stones for thousands of years. Huge stones were used for building temples and pyramids from Egypt across the world to South America, smaller stones were used to build basic shelter for human beings and animals. For practical purposes smaller stones were heated and then used for heating living accommodation or for healing purposes by placing warm stones on areas with pain, and for sacred rituals.

No one really knows where the modern treatment of Hot Stone Therapy came from. Some say Arizona, and others say from the sweat lodges of New Zealand, but wherever it was, it is now one of the most sought after luxury treatments on offer in beauty salons and spas today.

Hot basalt stones

Basalt stones are spat out of hot lava from erupting volcanoes. Throughout the years the Basalt stones are exposed to a rigorous workout from all the seasons, with varying weather conditions metamorphosing the multi-colored stones (grey, green and black) to bundles of minerals and crystals. The stones need to be 'oiled' before use, to enable them to glide over the skin.

Benefits and effects of hot stones

Interesting fact

Basalt stones can be found all over the world, however, it is thought that stones originating from the least polluted areas carry the most benefits. Basalt stones from Hawaii and Peru are said to have great healing powers.

- The direct heat from the stones relaxes muscles, allowing manipulation of a greater intensity than with basic massage movements. This will help to alleviate minor aches and pains.
- The hot stones give additional warmth to the body by expanding blood vessels, a condition known as vaso-dilation. This will then make normal Swedish massage movements even more effective at increasing blood flow and eliminating waste.
- Lymphatic circulation is assisted by the general increase in circulation.
- As crystals carry energy, so too do stones and the energy of the stones promote a meditative and sedative effect, creating a state of quietude and calm within the client.

Conditions that would benefit from a hot stone massage

There are certain conditions where the application of heat speeds healing, and are therefore conditions that would benefit from a Hot Stone Massage – these conditions include:

- Muscular aches and pains, sprains and strains
- Fibromyalagia

 • Back pain

 • Stress, anxiety and tension

Cold marine stones

Cold marine stones originate from the sediment in ocean basins and are formed via plant life and coral reefs. These stones change into a green hue when cooled in a refrigerator and are smooth enough to use directly without lubricant.

Benefits and effects of marine stones

 • Cold stones are used where there is muscular injury or inflammation, and are used on specific areas.

 • Cold stones have the opposite effect of hot stones; they have a de-congesting effect as they constrict blood vessels – thereby reducing inflammation by cooling the area.

 • Cold flat small stones can also be used to cover the eyes to give a cooling and relaxing feeling for the client.

Standard set of stones

A standard set of stones would comprise of approximately 60 basalt stones and 10 marine stones divided as follows:

Basalt stones

 • 7 large flat stones – these can be used to place over chakra areas, or can be placed on a towel for the client to lie on, when you are performing massage to the front of the body.

 • 8 large stones for general massage – large areas like the back.

 • 25 medium sized stones for general massage – the back and backs of legs.

 • 12 small stones to massage arms and face.

 • 8 small flat toe/finger stones.

Marine stones

 • 2 medium sized flat marine stones – to be used over the eyes during a facial massage.

 • 4 small oval stones for facial work.

 • 4 medium stones for general massage work.

Care of the stones

As with crystals, the stones absorb negativity from the client and therefore must be cleansed thoroughly before use on another client. As you finish using the stones, they can be placed either back in the heater, or into a bowl ready to be taken to a sink for cleaning. At the end of each treatment the basalt stones should be immersed in an anti-bactericidal product and individually washed ensuring any massage oil and any residue from the skin is completely removed. Complete the cleaning by rinsing thoroughly under cold running water.

If you have several treatments during a day, you may not have time for this thorough cleaning in between clients. If this is the case, as you finish using each stone lay them on a large towel, which has been placed under the couch. When the client has left you can then pull out the towel with all the used stones on and use a spray of alcohol or anti bacterial product on both sides of the stones. Wipe each stone clean, ensuring all oil is removed, before returning to the heater bin. Be sure to do a thorough wash at the end of the day with the anti bacterial product and running water.

Although the cold marine stones do not need a medium to work over the skin, they will still pick up oil from the skin and therefore should be cleansed in exactly the same way.

Contra indications to stone therapy

Tip

Always have a bowl of cold water on your trolley. If the stones are too hot to use, you can reduce their heat very quickly by placing them in and immediately out of cold water.

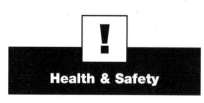

Always test the temperature of both hot and cold stones before use. If they are too hot or too cold for you, they will most certainly be too hot or too cold for your client.

Care must always be taken in checking for contra indications before commencing any treatment. This is particularly the case in hot stone massage, as there may be additional side effects due to heat or temperature changes. Page 137 of this book details a full list of both general contra indications and contra indications on specific areas. All these are relevant to Hot Stone massage.

Contra actions to stone therapy

Warm Stones

Care must be taken that the stones are at a temperature comfortable to hold in your hands. If they are too hot for you to hold, they will certainly be too hot to place on the client's skin. Even when the stones are at the right temperature, if an area is very congested, the rapid increase of blood flow may result in a contra action known as hyperemia – which is shown by the congested area becoming red. This redness usually returns to normal by the end of the treatment time.

Cold Stones

As with the warm stones, cold stones may also leave a red mark, or even freezer burns could be left on the skin if the cold stones were too cold before use. Ensure that the temperature is comfortable for you to hold, before placing on the client's skin.

The importance of grounding

As with all therapies, the importance of grounding yourself cannot be stressed enough. It is particularly important with stone massage. Stones have vibrational qualities and absorb negative energies from the client. You do not want these negative energies transferred to you, or the next client. Therefore at the commencement of the treatment perform a grounding exercise for yourself, to make you less sensitive and vulnerable to receiving these energies (see Grounding, p. 359).

Massage treatment

Preparation

The success of any treatment is in the preparation. Make sure you have everything ready before the client arrives for treatment.

- Ensure that the heating unit for the stones has been turned on in plenty of time to warm the stones before use – and that the stones are covered by water.
- Have a bowl of cold water easily accessible – to put the hot stones into should they be too hot to use. When put into cold water they will lose a lot of heat immediately and are ready for use.
- Have towels ready – hot towels heated in a heating cabinet will add luxury to the treatment.
- Have appropriate music ready.
- Put a large plastic bowl, lined with a large towel to reduce the noise level, ready to receive used stones under the couch. Alternatively, have a large towel under the couch ready to place used stones on for spraying in between clients if there is more than one treatment per day.

Order of treatment

You can incorporate the stones into your massage in any order you feel appropriate. There is no right or wrong way – just an appropriate way. For a full body massage, the following order is recommended.

- the back of the body
- the back of the legs
- the front of the legs
- the arms
- end with a facial massage using the cold marine stones.

Back massage treatment using hot and cold stones

The following sequence is recommended for a hot stone back massage.

1 Commence the massage by applying hot towels to the client's feet. This serves four purposes.

    (a) Cleanses the feet

    (b) Introduces heat to the massage

    (c) Makes the client feel comfortable and cosseted immediately

    (d) Grounds the client

After cleansing the feet, wrap up with a warm towel.

2 Take one large flat stone from the heater and place over the lower lumbar vertebrae of the client. This stone is then placed over a towel and wrapped up. Place your bottom hand over this towel where the stone is placed. Place your second hand horizontally flat across the back at mid thoracic level and mentally prepare for the massage. Now is a good time to do your grounding exercise. Don't be in a rush to get started – the client will be able to feel the warmth of the chakra stone and will be relaxed already. Take your time and focus on the massage ahead.

3 Apply appropriate massage oil to the client's back and effleurage for a minute or so. Take 8 medium stones from the heater and safely place 4 each side of the client's head – ready for use. Do not worry about leaving the client and breaking contact. Your chakra stone is in place, and this stone is keeping the contact for you. The unused stones will maintain their heat for a long time (20 minutes), but as soon as you start using them on a client's skin, they will lose their heat quite quickly – approximately 5 minutes for each side of the stone.

4 Continue with effleurage movements. Incorporate more heat into the massage by warming your hands on the stones. As your hands reach the client's shoulders, extend over the shoulder to pick up and hold, two stones from the top of the couch and feel their temperature for a second or two. Replace the stones on the towel above your client's head and continue massaging, from the shoulders back down to the sides of the client. The heat from the stones will now be felt on your hands and the client's back. Continue doing this (feeling the heat of the first two stones) and incorporating the heat to the client's back until the stones are a comfortable heat. At this stage, on the next upward stroke of effleurage, extend over the shoulders and take hold of the stones to continue with your effleurage movements down the back with the stones in your hands. The stones should fit comfortably in the palm of your hand, and become an extension of your hand.

5 The stones will start to lose their temperature as your massage progresses – the heat being transferred into the client. Continue massaging for five minutes with one side of the stone. When you feel the stone is losing its heat, turn the stone in your hand and continue with the warm side of the stone. Be imaginative with the stones. Turn them in your hands and whilst using the edge, work around the scapular areas with small circular movements each side of the spine area, and deep circular movements over the uncovered hip area. When the warmth has gone from the first stone, effleurage up the back and upon reaching the shoulders, extend over the shoulder replacing the used stones at the top of the clients head.

6   Continue your usual back massage using hands only and tapotement and petrissage movements.

7   After a couple of minutes, take the next hot stone and continue with effleurage movements as before, turning the stone when the heat has been transferred to the client.

8   Continue until all the stones have been used.

9   Place the used stones under the couch either in the bowl for thorough cleansing or on a towel for spraying.

10   If the massage were to continue, you would take 8 medium sized stones from the heater, and place them at the foot of the couch, or somewhere within easy reach and work on the backs of the legs – using 4 stones for each leg.

11   For a full body massage, the client would be turned over and you would work the front of the legs, the arms and complete the massage with a facial massage using cold stones.

This is just one example of many ways you can incorporate hot and cold stones into a body massage. Be imaginative when working with stones, and remember to use them as an extension of your hand. You will need a lot less pressure, as the stones are doing the work for you.

Large flat stones

There are two purposes for using the large flat stones.

- The first purpose is for grounding when used over the lower lumbar area (placed over a towel, and then covered). This area is close to the base chakra and the continued warm feeling the client receives during the massage will help to keep the client grounded.

- The second purpose of placing a large flat stone is to maintain contact when you leave the client to either put stones into the bowl under the couch, or to get new stones from the heater. The client will be able to feel the heat and weight of the stone.

Tip

Selecting and replacing stones from the heater and into the bowl or towel after use will be noisy. Be aware of this potential interruption to your client's massage and make every effort to maintain the tranquility of the room.

Specific after care advice for hot stone massage

After care advice following a hot stone massage is the same as for a body massage or any other holistic treatment: light diet, drink plenty of water; avoid alcohol, caffeine and other stimulants. However, after receiving such a warming massage, it is advisable for the client to remain warm and rest. If there is a rest area in the salon, the client should be encouraged to rest for 15–20 minutes before leaving the salon.

Knowledge review

1 Describe basalt stones.

2 Describe marine stones.

3 What is the main effect of the cold stones?

4 Why is it important to cleanse the stones thoroughly after each use?

5 Are hot stones recommended for use over varicose veins?

6 Why may an area remain red.

7 What could happen if the cold stones are too cold?

8 What would you do if the stones were too hot to use?

9 What do you do with the stones after use?

10 Why do you commence the massage by putting hot towels to the client's feet?

11 Is massage oil needed for a stone massage?

12 Do you use the hot stones immediately on the client's skin?

13 How long do the stones hold their heat once taken out of the heater?

14 What can you do to reduce the noise of the stones?

15 What are the purposes for using a large flat stone over the lower lumbar area?

16 Is there any specific after care advice for clients having received a hot stone massage?

Managing and marketing

21

Learning objectives

This chapter covers the following:

- **choosing premises**
- **business planning**
- **stock**
- **accounts and your accountant**
- **time management**
- **effective marketing**

Managing and marketing are absolutely crucial to your business. Effective management is as important as offering the right treatment to the right client. It doesn't matter how qualified or experienced you are, if your management and administration skills are poor and potential clients don't know that you exist, your practice cannot be successful. To be successful in running your own business, whether working from home, renting time in a clinic, buying an existing business, or leasing or buying premises, you *must* be business minded. If your working life is starting to work for somebody else, you will still need to be business minded. You need to 'manage' yourself and your client list. At the end of the day, you have chosen to become a therapist because you are a caring and hard-working person and love the type of work you have chosen. We all work, however, as a means to an end, and that end is an exchange of energy – in this case money! You have bills to pay and commitments to meet, and when it comes to running a business, or being an employee, managing and marketing should be at the top of your 'TO DO' list.

Choosing premises

If you have decided to work for someone else, work from home or go it alone by being self-employed, the most important decision you will have to make is *where* you will work from. Whichever option you choose, there are many advantages and disadvantages to consider. This will be the first of many important management decisions you will have to make.

Working for someone else

An excellent start to your working and business career is to work for somebody else. As well as gaining valuable experience whilst carrying out treatments on clients, you can observe the way the business is run and make notes for the future, when you may want to go it alone. As an employee you will work a set number of hours per week, which should be written in a contract of employment, and be paid either a set wage or a basic wage plus commission on treatments and retail sales. You will also receive holiday and possible sickness pay. Your income is guaranteed and you do not need to keep business accounts, as your employer will deduct the necessary National Insurance and income tax from your wages. You will be provided a room to work in and all the equipment and stock needed to carry out your treatments.

However, you still have managing and marketing skills to acquire. You will need to understand your contract of employment. If you are not offered one, ask for one! Always check your contract very carefully, and never sign without reading it thoroughly. If you are unsure about any aspect of it, ask for an explanation. You will need to be able to work out commission rates to check your wages, if this is the method by which you will be paid. You will need to run your client list smoothly by good time keeping, thereby using 'time management' skills, and you will need to look professional at all times, thereby 'marketing' yourself.

Most salons will have staff meetings during which you may be given an opportunity to express grievances – what is working well in the salon and areas that need improving – thereby sharing your ideas for improving the business. Employers cannot put problems right unless they are aware of them, so speak your mind. A successful business needs open communication channels between staff and employers. What would you do if this were your business? What would you not do? What would you do differently? Never think of your self as 'just' an employee – without the staff there would be no business, and all businesses are only as good as the staff they employ.

Partnerships

You may decide either at the outset or after a few years of work experience to join with a partner or colleague to make a partnership. Legal advice should be sought before the partnership begins in order to establish the basis on which the partners will act. It follows that it is vital to choose the right partner from the outset. The partnership will be required to keep detailed accounts, with all partners reporting their share of the profits on their tax return. All sorts of issues must be sorted out at the start of the partnership *before* anything is signed. Always go to a solicitor and have proper paperwork drawn up. This applies even to husband and wife partnerships! Many partnerships start with two people, however, there is no limit to how many partners there may be in a partnership. If a partnership of two had a very successful therapist working for them for a length of time who had proved his or her worth, it may be worth considering offering them a partnership position in the business. After two years the successful therapist may well be thinking of moving on, or even opening up a salon of their own, so it may make good sense to have a third partner in the business rather have them competing for business. You may be that successful therapist, and may be ready to take on more responsibility in the running of the salon. If you are, then ask for a meeting with the other partners to explore the chances of you becoming a partner – you don't always have to move on, there may be opportunities right under your nose – you just need to identify them.

Although starting out as friends, many partnerships end in disaster because of lack of communication skills. Each individual partner may think they are doing more than their share and carrying the other(s). It is very difficult to work exactly the same hours, put into the business exactly the same as each other or even to agree on important issues. One partner may want to re-invest profits into the business, the other partner may want an end-of-year bonus. Regular meetings are very important in all partnerships. You need to identify your individual skill areas, and to identify and rectify problems before they occur. Little problems only turn into bigger ones, so immediately you feel there may be a problem, no matter how small it is, get it out into the open and discuss it with your partner(s). Partnerships can be extremely rewarding nonetheless as you are never alone – there is always one or more people working towards the same goals.

Working from home

Many therapists start a practice from home. This offers a number of advantages. However, whilst working from home may suit you very well, do consider the disadvantages, especially to your security. You need to be strict with your timing when working from home. Some clients feel that because it's your home, their appointment is more of a social call than a business one. You don't want a one-hour appointment turning into a one-hour appointment plus an additional half-hour chat before the client leaves. If you have clients like this, then a good idea is to have a friend phone you 10–15 minutes after the client is meant to have left, thus giving you the perfect opportunity of showing her the door, should she be hanging around. You could even say that you are expecting an important phone call to hasten her departure. The table below lists the advantages and disadvantages of such a practice.

Going mobile

Being a mobile therapist can be a very rewarding experience; it can also be a very harrowing one! As with working from home there are many advantages and disadvantages to take into consideration.

Pros and cons of working from home

Advantages	Disadvantages
● No additional rent	● May not reflect professionalism
● No long-term commitments	● Disruption to other family members
● Home offers total privacy and anonymity for your clients	● Looks unprofessional if you have only a one-bathroom house (used by family)
● No additional heating costs	● Cats, dogs and all pets will need to be quiet and out of the way
● More flexible working hours	● There may be no waiting room facilities
● No lost travelling time or expenses	● Security – for yourself and your possessions
	● Sometimes difficult to get clients to leave – especially if no next appointment appears

As a mobile therapist, what you save by renting a room you lose on transport costs and time taken travelling to the client's home. All these factors should be taken into account when deciding your fee structure. Clients should be willing to pay a higher price for the convenience of having the service come to them. You could charge an additional amount for the travelling time and costs in your therapy fees – especially for minor treatments. An example could be 35 pence per mile from your home. This fee could be waived, or reduced, if the client has treatments over a set price, for example, reduced travel costs of 20 pence per mile for treatments over £50.00 and all travel costs waived for treatments over £75.00.

The following are some examples of calculating costs.

For a client who lives 12 miles from your home:

Cost of treatment	£20.00
Travel costs (24 miles at 35p per mile)	£8.40
Total cost	£28.40

You may think this a bit steep. However, remember the client's situation. They have benefited by not having to go into a salon, which would include savings of travel/fuel costs, parking costs and their time getting there and back. If they complain about the travel costs, then encourage them to have more than one treatment, which would benefit both of you.

Cost of treatments	£50.00
Travel discount (24 miles at 20p per mile)	£4.80
Total cost	£54.80
Cost of treatments	£75.00
Travel costs	None
Total cost of treatment	£75.00

Do not forget that it may take you half an hour to drive 12 miles there and another half an hour to drive back again. That is one hour when you are not working.

There is a huge misconception that mobile therapists should be cheap – quench this misconception now. You are doing the client a big favour going to them – they should respect your services and pay you accordingly for your time and effort.

When you are in a new area, take advantage and do a leaflet drop before or after treating your client. Or give the client a discount if she can recommend another client in the same area.

Your cancellation fee must be strictly adhered to when offering a mobile service. What would you do if you turned up at a client's home to find out she was out! You would leave a bill. Have black invoices in the car for such an event, as it is sure to happen at least once. The best policy is to phone any clients the day before to remind them of their appointment. Whilst you should not have to do this, it may just save you a useless journey.

The table above lists the advantages and disadvantages of being mobile.

Renting time in a clinic

Renting time in a clinic is becoming increasingly popular as more and more holistic centres open. Working in a clinic can be very advantageous if you don't want a full-time position as you can rent a session. A session is a morning, an afternoon or an evening slot or one or two whole days. As your client base increases, so you can increase the amount of time you rent. Often the more sessions you commit to, the cheaper the rent becomes. Try

Pros and cons of being mobile

Advantages	Disadvantages
• No additional rent • No long-term commitments • Client's own home offers total privacy and anonymity • No additional heating costs • Flexible working hours • No disruption to the family home	• Personal security – entering someone's home you do not know • Practising in a strange environment • Uncertainty regarding available facilities • Heavy work involved – carrying massage couches, equipment and products in and out of your car, up and down stairs, etc. • Wear and tear on your car • Additional transport costs • Lost time in travelling to and from each client

Pros and cons of renting time in a clinic

Advantages	Disadvantages
• Professional image • Personal safety will be improved • You may receive referrals from other fellow therapists who use the centre • There may be a receptionist to take your bookings • Availability of a waiting/changing room • No long-term commitments – rooms usually available on 3/6 month 'leases' • Shared advertising costs with other therapists • There should be wheelchair access • Networking with other therapists based there will reduce feelings of isolation • A quiet environment in which to work • Flexible working hours • No disruption to the family home	• Paying for the room –whether you have clients booked in or not • Inflexibility in working hours – you can only book clients in on specific days at specific times • You can never run over time – another therapist may be waiting for the next session • Travelling times and costs getting to and from the clinic

Tip

Check the small print of a contract carefully and have a solicitor look at it for you, if you are not absolutely sure what you are signing.

to meet the other therapists – so often therapists only know each other by sight/name/brochure. The more of the other therapists you know, the more networking and recommending you can do for each other. Be sure to find out the lock-up procedure if you are going to be the last one out. Again, and as with leasing premises, there will be some kind of documentation stating the rules of the tenancy. You may be asked to take the room for a three-month period and you may have to give three months' notice of leave.

The table above lists the advantages and disadvantages of renting time in a clinic.

Buying a salon with a client base

Like any other business, beauty salons come on the market as a going concern. A going concern is an established business with a clientele and usually has three years' accounts for you to inspect. A going concern is a business that is ready for you to take over and start trading immediately. You will need professional help when buying an existing business. You will need to see at least three years' accounting, to read the lease thoroughly and ask to see the existing and old appointment books. What exactly are you buying? Sometimes a price may seem unbelievably good until you read the small print. Sometimes stock is included and sometimes not, and often huge amounts are added for 'good will'. If stock is included you need to make absolutely sure it can be sold. Check all sell-by dates carefully too. If a quarter of the stock has passed its sell-by date and another quarter has only say three months on left on it, that leaves you in a strong position to refuse either the entire stock or do some serious negotiating. Your money would be better spent on new stock with two or more years on the sell-by dates, or just left in the bank as working capital. Never just accept what is being offered – always check and negotiate.

Whatever the deal, remember that there is no guarantee existing clients may stay with a new proprietor. They may see it as a good time to have a change of salon themselves. The advantages are that you are taking over an established business and that set procedures and systems should be in place. There should be no equipment to buy and the appointment book should be full of *genuine* appointments. There may be existing staff with clients of their own, and the goodwill can get you off to a flying start – but take care as the initial outlay can be very large. You need to ask some very important questions:

- Why is the business being sold?
- Do the existing clients know of the impending change of management?
- Is the equipment owned or leased? If leased, how much is outstanding on the lease and what options are available at the end of it? Leased equipment will have either an option to buy the equipment at the end of he leasing time, or to exchange for a more up-to-date piece of equipment. Has the equipment been maintained and serviced regularly?
- If you see a piece of expensive equipment that you really do not want, negotiate – you are the buyer so only buy what you want. Sellers will not jeopardize the sale of a business for the sake of one piece of equipment.
- Ask about existing product lines being offered in the salon – will you be able to take over accounts with these companies? Are there any outstanding invoices?
- If the practice is known by the (selling) therapist's name, will you be able to trade using that name even though they no longer work at the practice?
- Can you use the former owner's name in advertising and marketing?
- Is the former owner retiring or moving to another area? You would not want the existing owner to take all the existing clients that you are paying highly for if, for example, she had decided to sell the business and go mobile.

Website   @

For further information about the viability of leasing treatment rooms, go to the website available at: www.thomsonlearning.co.uk/beckmann

Business planning

The bank and the business plan

Financial matters are an important part of being in business and need careful consideration. Your bank manager will be only too pleased to listen to your proposals. Do not go to the bank without a detailed and well thought out business plan prepared. The purpose of a business plan is to help you set down on paper everything that is involved in your venture. It is not prepared to impress your bank manager, but as a point of reference for *you* to see how *your* business is doing on a weekly/monthly basis based according to your stated objectives. It is an essential document to draw upon whenever you discuss finances with bank managers, business partners, your accountant and anyone else interested in your welfare and plans for the future. Most banks will be only too pleased to provide you with a new business start-up pack, which will include all the paperwork you need for your business plan – all you need to do is to fill in the blanks. Most new business packs comes supplied with a CD-ROM, and as you complete the blank forms on screen, all the calculations are done for you. The business plan will also include an up-to-date CV detailing all your qualifications and experience to date. One of the most important documents to prepare, however, is the cash flow statement.

Cash flow

A profitable business can fail because of bad cash flow. All businesses need working capital, so make sure you're not under-financed. Most new businesses fail in the first two years because of poor cash flow. By operating on a no credit basis with customers, meanwhile getting 30 to 60 days' credit from suppliers, you can generate some working capital. This is achieved by selling stock before you have actually paid for it – the difference between what you owe for the stock, the wholesale price, and what you get for the stock, that is the retail price, will generate working capital. But make sure you pay all bills at the end of the 30 or 60 days agreed with the supplier. You can avoid problems if you do your estimates correctly at the outset and stick to your targets. A cash flow statement is a record of your monthly estimated income, which is set against your monthly expenditure. You usually have a good idea of what the expenditure is going to be, which would include items such as:

- rent
- your wages
- other staff wages and all national insurance
- heating and lighting
- insurance – premises and personal
- travelling and motor expenses
- telephone
- professional fees – accountants
- loan repayments
- advertising
- property maintenance
- tax provision.

When preparing a business plan, all the income figures are estimated at the outset and the bank will be only too quick to dampen your spirits regarding the amount of income you are anticipating. When you do start trading, your 'actual' income figures are inserted against the estimated ones, and the expenditure figures can be corrected to bring the cash flow statement up to date and make it accurate. If this is done religiously it will be easy to see how much you will have in the bank at any time in the future. If the figures do not work out on paper, the bank may be reluctant to help you with any sort of small business loan. Don't get in a panic if you see the bank position getting worse as the months pass in relation to your estimates. That is the whole point of a cash flow forecast – to 'forecast' the future position of the money in the bank at any one time. If it doesn't look good, you will have to increase income or reduce expenditure to get the figures right again. It may be that once you have really looked at the proposition you may decide not to go ahead. Be prepared for the bank to pull the cash flow to pieces – that is their job, so be one step ahead and put down very conservative income figures.

How much can you pay yourself?

Initially, you need to ask yourself here 'How much do I *need* to earn?' rather than 'How much do I *want* to earn?' It is important to set a realistic objective here. When you have worked out how much you need, this figure must be included in the cash flow forecast. Add together your monthly or weekly expenses, not forgetting rent, food, any car loans (although this may be transferable to the business), savings, bills and clothes. After the first year or two, you may be able to give yourself a rise to more than you actually *need*. Keep all personal finances totally separate from business finances.

In addition to the cash flow forecast, you will also need to produce a projected balance sheet/profit forecast. This will help you monitor your expected business performance month by month. Its main purpose is to show you how viable your business is likely to be. The more accurate the cash flow forecast is, the more accurate the profit and loss forecast will be.

Borrowing money

Having completed all the paperwork, you need to make some appointments with the small business manager of *several* banks and building societies. Banking is big business and there are many excellent deals for small businesses – shop around to get the best deal. It doesn't matter how small you think your business is, it is still business and the banks will be eager to take you on board as a new account. However, you will still have to sell your case, which is your business and yourself. This you should do with absolute confidence. Remember, it is the bank's job to lend you money and as long as they are certain that you are able to repay without problems they will be happy to do so. After all, that is how they make their living. If you want to borrow, say, £8000 for your initial start up costs, make absolutely sure you have included the repayments in your cash flow forecast – as if you already had the loan! – it is easy enough to work out the monthly repayment figures. Most banks will offer a range of services including business overdrafts, small business loans, property finance and business mortgages. They will, however, usually seek some security on larger loans. Don't forget to ask for your free banking – bank charges mount up considerably and most banks nowadays will give you the first year free of bank charges if you open a business account with them. Find out what special services each bank will offer you before you place your business with them. They may even offer preferential interest rates for a business starting up. Shop around and *do not* accept the first bank that offers you an account. Banks and building societies are very competitive these days and only too keen to offer you better terms than the one down the road.

Tip

When dealing with banks and bank managers, remember that you are the customer and they are providing a service. Don't let banks or bank managers intimidate you.

Stock

Stock and stock control will be another big part of your business, especially if you have your own salon. Stock needs to be 'turned around' quickly. In other words, you do not want to buy £1000 worth of cosmetics, make a pretty display and have them sitting there for a year collecting dust. If you don't sell the stock quickly, the cash would be better in the bank being used

Tip

As with the banks, shop around. Imagine the stock on the shelves could be money in the bank and never be persuaded by salespeople to buy more than you need – they are just trying to reach their targets too!

as working capital. Tying money up in stock may have a detrimental effect on working capital. As quickly as stock comes in you want it sold, ideally within a month or two, and the money back in the bank, along with any profit on sales; this will help keep the cash flow on target. Retail selling in any salon can make a huge difference to overall income and to overall profits. However, it can also have a detrimental effect on business if stock doesn't move. Take care choosing your product lines. Start with small companies, where there is no pressure on you to buy large quantities of stock you don't really need. You don't want to get tied into minimum orders and postage. Many companies will give you free postage if your order is over a certain amount – so be sure to check out all these things before committing to a product range. As stated earlier, they need you, as it is *you* selling *their* product.

Accounts and your accountant

You can save a lot of money by managing your own accounts to a certain degree and letting the accountant just complete them at the end of the year. Your accountant will also advise you on what you can claim on the business, As with banks and products, you need to shop around for an accountant. Word of mouth is always a good recommendation. Make sure that the accountant specializes in the setting up of small businesses and preferably has a basic grasp of your type of business. Ask for the basic scale of fees, which is usually assessed by the hour. Your accountant will advise you of the best period of time to choose as your accounting year, which need not coincide with the tax year. You pay tax on your taxable profits and your accountant will work out what you need to pay the Inland Revenue. Your taxable profits are your takings during the tax year. In addition, any money owed by you at the end of the accounting year plus any increase in the value of stock you own is taken into account and liable for tax.

Tip

A small business software product will keep you in control of your business. Internet banking also allows you to pay bills and transfer money, all without leaving the salon.

You can keep your books in excellent order with the help of many software packages on the market for the small business which, once set up and running, can show you the areas of your business that are doing well and the areas that are not doing so well. It is worth a few days out of the salon, going to either college or a training session with your bank, to learn how to use accounting software. Many banks recommend a small business accounting package and will also recommend someone who gives training with the product. Internet banking is quick and easy and there is absolutely no excuse in not knowing the exact position of your account. You need to know daily what has come into and gone out of your bank.

Time management

I often hear people say that reading time management books is a waste of time! Believe me it is not. There are some excellent time management books on the market, offering many different ideas of how to use your time wisely.

What is time management? Time management is learning how to use your working time effectively, thereby leaving enough time for leisure activities, family and friends. Time management is especially important for those working for themselves. As the business grows, so does the paperwork, with the result that we don't see our friends as often as we would like, family life may suffer and we have little time for relaxation and physical exercise. Time management skills will help you identify where your time goes and how to plan to use your time more efficiently. There are many techniques that are commonly used for managing time: making meetings more effective; delegating to other people, reducing interruptions, making more efficient appointments, dealing with the paperwork, the stock control and the filing. When running your own business, you need to keep on top of the paperwork. One hour a day, even if it means one less client a day, could save you five hours of paperwork on a Sunday!

Effective marketing

I often hear therapists say that they can't afford to advertise. The truth is that you can't afford *not* to advertise – clients need to know you exist, where you are and what you do. However, advertising alone is not 'marketing' but is just one part of the process. Marketing involves the six Ps:

- *Place*
- *Products*
- *Promotion*
- *Price*
- *People*
- *Persistence.*

Get any one of them wrong and you will lose business.

Product

The products you are offering not only include retail products but also your services. A full body massage, for example, is a product (service) that is 'for sale' in your establishment just the same as a jar of face cream is 'for sale'. But take care, as the more products/ services you offer, the more stock you will have to buy to perform those services. In the beginning it is very easy to offer too much too soon and end up spending all your money on expensive equipment and stock. You may have set your heart on using and supplying a top market product range, however, some product ranges may be out of the question for you at this early stage. Some of the larger companies will only provide their product if you take on the entire range – face, body and make-up. They may also insist that their product is the only one you can stock! This can not only be very expensive but you are allowing another company dictate to you how to run *your* company! Remember – they need you more than you need them; you are the customer and have many choices of products. If you do take on entire ranges at the outset, you then have the enormous task of selling all the retail products before their sell-by dates. This can be very stressful and can be described as a 'chicken and egg' situation. You need the stock to attract the clients, but you need the clients to sell the stock. Good advice is to get the clients first!

Decide what services/products you are going to offer and then shop around for a small but thorough range of products with a generous mark up and from a company that will provide free training and after sales support – after all, *you* are promoting *their* product!

Promotion

Promotion means promotional material to 'promote' your business. It includes: brochures, business cards, leaflets and handouts, pens and other such free merchandise. This is a vital part of the whole marketing process, but so many therapists get it wrong by trying to cut corners and doing it on the cheap! There are areas where you can save money and be prudent, but your salon brochure is not one of them.

Brochures

Your brochure is often the first impression a prospective client may have of your business – it *has* to be good. Collect as many brochures you can and study them all carefully. Compare them against each other. Which salon would you go to on the strength of these brochures alone? Ask yourself why you have chosen that particular salon – what caught your eye? the colour? the layout? the wording? the products/services offered? Whatever it was, you need to encapsulate that in your own brochure. Hand this collection of brochures to friends, family and colleagues, and ask them the same question – which salon would they choose on the strength of the brochure alone? Ask them why and make your evaluations. Use their comments wisely when designing your own brochure. What should you put in your brochure? Here is a list of essential details:

- **The name of the salon and your name**
  Take care to have a salon name that can be identified directly with your business. Whilst it is brave to have something completely different, the business name must reflect the activities of the actual business. Your individual name is also important in addition to the salon name. Make sure it can be identified if you are a male or female therapist – it could make all the difference to a client calling or not!

- **Contact details**
  Telephone numbers, e-mail address, website address – give as many options as possible for prospective clients to be able to contact you.

- **Address**
  Note the address of the salon in full – if a client cannot find you, they can ask directions.

- **Qualifications and professional bodies**
  In addition to adding qualification initials after your name, if room allows write out in full the qualifications and organizations you belong to. The general public are unaware of the initials of qualifications, and these often mean little to them; however, if they can read in detail of your achievements, they have much more of an understanding. Take the following as an example, imagining yourself as a member of the general public, and compare example A with example B.

  > *Example A*
  > A.N. Other
  > Dip Nut. FHT
  >
  > *Example B*
  > Angela N. Other
  > Diploma in Nutrition and Member of the Federation of Holistic Therapists

Example A does not give much away, however, example B is much more explicit. It may not be practicable to list all your qualifications but try to list the most important or the most relevant ones to your business. Another example appears below.

> *Example A*
> S. Le Quesne
> BANT
>
> *Example B*
> Suzanne Le Quesne
> British Association of Nutritional Therapists

Example A states what? A name which could be a male or female therapist and some initials many people have never heard of. Example B, however, lets prospective clients know that I am a female therapist and belong to a reputable organization. Some female clients only want to see female therapists so it is important to make this distinction. On the other hand, male therapists may be the first choice for many other clients. Take care if your name can belong to either sex.

- **Types of therapy you offer**
  A clear list of the services you offer is the main part of any brochure. A short description of treatments, and the *benefits* they offer, is important if space allows. Never assume clients will know what the various treatments are.
- **Opening hours**
  Make it quite clear on your brochure your opening hours, or session hours, whichever apply. Be flexible, but not too flexible – you have a life too!

Business cards

A business card is an absolute must for anyone in business, no matter how small that business may be. Although it may cost a little more, use both sides of the card. A blank reverse is wasting 50 per cent of the available space you have, but it will not *cost* you 50 per cent more to have the back printed on. Quality is of the utmost importance – use colour, symbols, and a clear typeface. Get a few different examples before finally deciding, and show them to friends, colleagues and family for valuable feedback.

Essential details to list on your business card are:

- salon and personal name
- qualifications and initials of any professional body
- your title (profession) – aromatherapist, holistic therapist, etc.
- telephone and other contact numbers
- e-mail address
- website address
- postal address.

The reverse of the card could include:

- details for recording appointments
- a list of services your business offers
- any cancellation rules (24 hours notice of cancellation, etc.).

Leaflets and handouts

Leaflets and/or handouts are a good way to get your business on the map yet so many therapist do not even consider it – the legwork usually puts people off! It is a very inexpensive way to let everybody know you exist. It is true that most 'junk mail' put through the letterbox does get thrown away. However, most people will glance at it first – just in case it may be of interest.

Leaflets can be printed on cheap paper, as most will go straight into the bin, however, you do have a valuable few seconds to get attention. Coloured paper gets more attention than white, but make sure the printing is clear and the message simple. A5 is big enough to be noticed and big enough to contain all the information needed for the purpose of the exercise. Consider including a discount voucher to be used by a certain date, upon presentation of the leaflet. Once designed, obtain feedback from friends, colleagues and family, then have a minimum of 1000 printed. At the time of writing, this should cost approximately £60. Ask the printers to guillotine them for you, as they will print 2 leaflets per 1 × A4 piece of paper.

The next stage is to get up very early one morning and start delivering. Depending on the location of your business you may want to start with the immediate area around your business and gradually work outwards. On the other hand, you may want to attract clients from different areas than your immediate location. However you do it, the return on your investment must be worked out. If you deliver 1000 leaflets to 1000 homes and other businesses, you can expect between 0.5 to 1 per cent return. This may sound too little for the work involved in delivering them, but between 5 and 10 clients is a good return, and even if they only have one treatment each, this will more than pay for the price of the leaflets. Of course, once they are in your salon, it is then up to you to get them to return again. One thing that is certain with this method is that you know every single household in a certain area knows you exist whether they need your services or not, unlike a newspaper advertisement, where the paper first has to be bought and the client then has to find and read your advertisement. Use different coloured paper for different areas to identify where clients are coming from.

Pens and other promotional ideas

You may at first think this is a cheap and nasty idea. However, if your business opens just when the new telephone directory has been delivered and you are not in it, it is an excellent way of giving people your contact details. There are all sorts of promotional freebies you can give to clients such as bookmarks, key fobs, pens, mouse mats – everyone loves a freebie and if it means more clients so much the better. Work out the cost to you and how many treatments you need to do to cover the cost. You can also hand these out at health fairs, lectures, anywhere in fact. People do not throw pens away!

Price and payment

You first need to do a survey of the competition to see what is being charged in your area. The biggest mistake a new business can make is to be too cheap. Clients will think your service lacks quality or that the therapists lack experience or that you are desperate for business. Too high on the other hand may be outside the affordability range for your particular area. There are many way of deciding your pricing structure. It is easier to come down in price, either by using special offers and promotions, than to go up in price when you realize you are too cheap. You need take into account your overheads – these will include:

- rent and council tax
- light, heat and telephone
- insurance and other professional fees
- products
- travelling/parking costs.

After calculating all the overheads, don't forget to add on your wages. There does need to be something left at the end of the week for you!

There are many different marketing strategies you can apply to your business:

- seasonal special offers – Easter, Christmas, summer, etc.
- introduce one/two new clients and receive a free treatment
- buy a course of treatments and get one/two free
- loyalty cards for treatments and products.

One strategy that works is that you choose a really popular treatment – a half-leg wax for example – at a *really* competitive price to get clients into the salon. Once in, clients will tend to have other treatments – 'While I'm here would you have time to do a . . .'. The objective is to get clients through the front door. It's then up to you. It is easy to get clients in once – the art of good business and good marketing is to get *repeat and regular* business. You will of course always get the clients who come for the cheap treatment only – that's life! You do, of course, put on an extra £1 here and there on other treatments to make up the shortfall on the really inexpensive treatment.

When it comes time for the client to pay their bill, you should be flexible with ways of payment. Cash is always the best, followed by personal cheque supported by the appropriate cheque guarantee card. However, many people these days only use plastic and it is highly recommended you look into having a credit card facility. Although it does cost you initially to set up, you can *lose* a lot of business by not accepting cards – especially retail selling at the end of a treatment.

Loyalty cards

Loyalty cards work in many different ways, and are offered by many businesses because they work. For example, some trendy coffee bars use them and each time you buy a coffee, a small card is stamped. After you purchase nine coffees, the tenth one is free. All that time of course card is in the client's purse as a constant reminder of that particular coffee shop. The same principle can work in a salon. After nine treatments, usually of the same value, the tenth is offered free of charge. With retail products, after say five products bought, the next one carries with it a discount. Or, rather than giving away cash incentives, you could offer say a complementary manicure, so your time is being given away but not your stock. There are many variables, but don't be half hearted if you introduce loyalty cards into the salon. You want clients who have not got one to hear you talking about them at the cash desk.

Always offer value for money. It is usually the little things that make the difference. Nice tableware and glassware in which to offer unusual herbal teas and caffeine-free coffee alternatives, as well as the usual tea and coffee. Up-to-date magazines, good quality daily newspapers to read either before or after treatments. A good selection of different music – not one CD playing for months at a time!

Concessions

You will from time to time be asked if you offer reduced rates for the unemployed, those on low incomes or who for one reason or another cannot afford to pay the fee requested by you. It is perfectly acceptable to say no. Although there are many genuine cases, often the clients that have the confidence to ask for reduced rates are the ones who can afford the full price the most! Some therapists offer a sliding scale of fees. However, this can become complicated and once clients know you do this you will get more and more enquiries for reduced treatments. You could offer say 10 per cent off for Monday mornings, Thursday afternoons, or times when you know your salon is not busy. However, these times can be busy, so be careful – you have bills like everyone else and you deserve to be paid for what you do, whenever that may be.

Cancellations

Have a cancellation policy right from the start of opening your business and *stick to it*. Less than 24 hours' notice of cancellation usually carries with it the full charge of the treatment. You may decide to charge half the treatment fee for less than 24 hours' notice – it is up to you. But don't forget you are running a business! There is nothing more frustrating after turning away appointments all morning to then receive a cancellation call five minutes before a client is due to come in. Of course if there is a genuine reason for calling at the last minute, an accident for example, you may be prepared to waive the cancellation fee. However, more often than not clients simply forget, or just can't be bothered. Some clients offer to pay anyway – say 'yes', and do not feel embarrassed – they have let you down, not the other way around. State your cancellation policy clearly in your brochure – it is much easier to waive a cancellation fee than to ask for one from a client who doesn't expect it.

Persistence

What do you do if your marketing strategies do not appear to be working? Keep trying, and trying again, because they will work in the end. Here are some other ideas.

- Have regular open days.
- Arrange a demonstration session of a particular treatment.
- Use an 'A' board outside your premises, if allowed, changing the information *regularly*.
- Put on special promotions for Christmas, Mother's Day, Easter, Summer, etc. You will need to work about six months in advance for these promotions – clients need to know as they are busy people too.
- Offer to write an article for your local newspaper – get your name in print as often as possible, become known.
- Do a talk for local social groups.
- Support a charity.
- Go on local radio – promote your services.
- If you have a window display, change it regularly and keep it clean – this is prime marketing space. Most companies will charge for posters, but if they know you have a shop front they will usually give them to you.

Knowledge review

1 How many people are needed to form a partnership?

2 Why should mobile therapists cost the same price as salons or higher?

3 Name three advantages of working in a clinic with other therapists.

4 Name three disadvantages of working from home.

5 What is a cash flow forecast?

6 How can you reduce the fees charged by your accountant?

7 What is time management?

8 Name six items of expenditure you need to include on a cash flow forecast.

9 What are the 6Ps of effective marketing?

10 What important facts must be on a business card?

11 How would you deal with cancellations?

12 What should you take into account when considering your pricing structure?

13 Why is it important not to be too cheap?

14 How do loyalty cards work?

15 List six different types of marketing promotions.

Glossary

abduction a movement away from the mid-line

acid mantle a protective layer on the surface of the epidermis

acne rosacea chronic skin disorder of the superficial capillaries of the nose and cheeks

acne vulgaris bacterial infection of overactive sebaceous glands

actin protein filament found in muscle cell

active transport substances use carrier proteins to carry out active transport

acute disorder or symptoms that come on suddenly and usually last for a short duration

Addison's disease disease caused by hyperfunctioning of the adrenal cortex

adduction movement towards the mid-line (*add*ing)

adenoid mass of lymphatic tissue at the rear of the nasal cavity

adipose tissue fat cells

adrenalin hormone/neurotransmitter that prepares the body for activity

adrenocorticotrophic hormone (ACTH) hormone secreted by the pituitary gland; regulates the cortex and adrenal glands

AIDS (acquired immune deficiency syndrome) full-blown viral disease interfering with the immune system

albinism total absence of melanin

aldosterone hormone regulating water balance

aliphatic compound molecule comprising straight chains of carbon atoms

allergen substance that stimulates an allergy

allergy inappropriate response (hypersensitivity) by the immune system to an allergen

alopecia baldness, loss or thinning of the hair

amenorrhoea absence of menstruation

anaesthesia loss of sensation

anagen active growth stage of the hair

analgesic pain relieving

anaphrodisiac agent that reduces sexual desire

androgen hormone regulating development and maintenance of secondary sexual characteristics

angioma tiny, red, raised area of skin

anion negatively charged ion

ankylosing spondylitis inflammatory disease of the joints between the vertebra

anterior front of the body

antibody (immunoglobin) protein that is produced in response to a specific antigen

anti-depressant agent that is uplifting/mood enhancer

anti-diuretic hormone hormone secreted by the pituitary gland; regulates water balance

antigen foreign substance to the body that causes antibodies to be to be produced

anti-histamine a chemical that blocks the effect of histamine

anti-inflammatory reduces the symptoms and signs of inflammation

anti-microbial agent that resists and destroys micro-organisms

anti-oxidant substance that protects against free radical damage

anti-rheumatic prevents or reduces the symptoms of rheumatism

antiseptic destroys and inhibits the development of micro-organisms

anti-spasmodic reduces muscle spasm, cramp

anti-toxic reduces the effects of toxins

anti-viral fights viral infections

anxiety unpleasant emotional state

aorta blood vessel carrying blood from the heart to the body

aperitive stimulates appetite

aphrodisiac agent that increases sexual desire

apocrine gland type of sweat gland

appendicular skeleton comprises the shoulder girdle, arms, hands, pelvic girdle, legs and feet

appendix small projection from the caecum

agranulocytes type of white blood cell

aromatic compounds carbon atoms joined together in a ring

arthritis inflammatory disease of the joints

associated neurone found in the brain and spinal cord; links sensory and motor neurones

asthma recurrent attacks of breathlessness and wheezing caused by inflammation of the bronchi

astringent substance that causes the tissue to dry and shrink by reducing the ability to absorb water

atherosclerosis degenerative disorder caused by a build up of fatty deposits in the arteries restricting blood flow

atom smallest particle of matter

atomic number number of protons an atom has

ATP (adenosine triphosphate) molecule in which heat is stored for energy

atrophy wasting away

auto-immune disorder when the immune system produces antibodies against itself rather than an invading micro-organism

axial skeleton comprises skull, spine and thorax

Ayurvedic Ayurveda is the world's oldest recorded healing system dating back nearly 4000 years; the book of *Ayur Veda* translates as the art of life and is a sacred book written around 1800 BC and includes massage amongst its hygienic principles

bacteria a single celled micro-organism

bactericidal agent which kills bacteria

balsamic fragrant substance which softens phlegm

basal metabolic rate metabolic rate when at complete rest

basophils white blood cells involved in allergic and inflammatory reactions

benign growth slow-growing growth confined to an area and which does not spread around the body

blood pressure force which the blood exerts on the arterial blood vessels

B-lymphocytes lymphocyte cells that produce antibodies and neutralize antigens

boil bacterial infection of the hair follicle

bonding attraction between molecules that hold them together

bromhidrosis unpleasant body odour

bronchitis inflammation of the bronchi

bruise discoloured area caused by blood leaking from damaged blood vessels

bunion displacement of the big toe joint

bursa fluid-filled sac between the bone and tendon

bursitis inflammation of the bursa

callus area of thickened skin

cancellous bone spongy bone tissue

cancer generic term for unrestrained cellular growth causing malignant tumours

Candida albicans naturally occurring yeast, mould

capillaries small blood vessels linking arterioles with venules

capsular ligament tough fibrous tissue surrounding a joint and holding the bones in place

capsulitis inflammation of the capsule of a joint

carbuncle multi-headed boil

carcinoma malignant tumour occurring in the epithelial tissue

carminative substance which causes expulsion of gases from the intestine

carpal tunnel syndrome pressure on the median nerve of the hand causing tingling or pain in the hand

cartilage firm, flexible and tough connective tissue

catagen period of change in the stages of hair growth

cation positively charged ion

cellulite dimpled, lumpy, fatty tissue

central nervous system brain and spinal cord

cephalic associated with the head

cerebrospinal fluid (CSF) fluid that protects the brain

cerebrum largest part of the brain, centre for learning voluntary movement and sensory perception

chemical reaction process by which different combinations of elements are created or destroyed

chloasma (melasma) area of darkened pigmentation

cholagogue agent that facilities the movement of bile from the biliary ducts

choleretic agent which increases bile secretion

chronic disorder or symptom/s that are persistent over a period of time

chyme soup-like mixture of liquid created as part of the digestive process in the stomach

cicatrisant aid to healing and the formation of scar tissue

circumduction circular movement of a joint (360°)

coeliac disease abnormal immune reaction to the protein gluten

co-enzyme small organic molecule that associates closely with certain enzymes; many B vitamins form an integral part of co-enzymes

cognition action or faculty of knowing, perceiving, conceiving as opposed to emotion and volition

colitis chronic inflammatory disease of the colon and rectum

comedone plug of sebum blocking a pore

compact bone hard bone tissue

compounds stable interaction between elements

conjunctivitis allergy or bacterial infection of the mucous membranes of the eye

connective tissue diverse group of tissues that support and protect the organs and hold body parts together

cordial stimulant and tonic

corn callus on a toe

covalent bonding bond with shared electrons

Crohn's disease inflammatory disease of the gastrointestinal tract

Cushing's syndrome disease caused by hypersecretions of glucocorticoids

cystitis bladder inflammation

cytophylactic agent which is cell-regenerating and protects other cells

cytoplasm contents of the living cell other than the nucleus

debility condition of weakness, general state of depression

deodorant substance which destroys odour

depression persistent low state of emotion

depurative substance which assists to purify the blood and internal organs

dermis deeper layer of the skin under the epidermis

desquamation the process of shedding dead skin cells, naturally or assisted

diabetes mellitus insufficient insulin in the body causing high blood glucose levels

diaphysis the shaft of a long bone

diastolic blood pressure pressure exerted in the arteries when the heart is at rest between contractions

diffusion random movement of molecules in a solute from an area of high concentration to an area of low concentration to a more dilute solution, through a permeable membrane

digestive chemical that stimulates the digestion

dipole negative or positive areas in a molecule

disease deviation from a normal state of health

distal furthest from the point of attachment of a limb

diuretic increases flow of urine

diverticular pouches of intestine which protrude externally into the abdomen

dorsal upper surface

dorsiflexion top of the foot moved upwards

dysmenorrhoea painful menstruation

eccrine gland type of sweat gland

eczema dry irritated skin disorder; not contagious

electron negatively charged particle

element substance with only one type of atom

embolism fragment of material blocking an artery

emmenagogue substance that affects the reproductive organs and assists menstrual flow

emulsifier substance added to products in industry to stabilize the ingredients and stop them separating

endometriosis endometrial tissue migrating outside the uterus but which continues to respond to the sex hormones

endoplasmic reticulum membranous canals in cytoplasm of cell involved in transportation of materials through the cell

enzyme catalyst that promotes or regulates a chemical reaction

ephilide freckle – small patches of concentrated pigmentation

epidermis upper layer of the skin

epilepsy recurrent seizures or temporary alteration of the electrical activity of the brain

epiphyses the ends of a long bone

epithelial tissue tissue from which glands, external layer of the skin are formed; also lines the hollow organs, blood vessels and orifices

erythema reddening of the skin caused by vasodilation

erythrocytes red blood corpuscles (cells)

euphoric agent that exaggerates the feeling of wellbeing

eversion movement to turn the sole of the foot outwards

excretion removal of waste from the body

expectorant removes excess mucus

expiration breathing out – exhalation

extension straightening or movement backwards from the mid line

facilitated diffusion uses a specific carrier protein, which temporarily binds to large molecules

fascia connective tissue covering a muscle

febrifugal reduces fever

flexion bending a move forwards from the mid line

follicle stimulating hormone (FSH) hormone secreted by the pituitary gland; causes growth of the Graafian follicle and stimulates production of spermatozoa

folliculitis bacterial infection of one of more hair follicle

fracture break in a bone

free radicals a molecule with an unpaired electron in its outer sheath is known as a free radical, resulting in these molecules becoming unstable; free radicals then damage healthy cells in an attempt to make themselves stable, i.e. 'paired' again

functional group distinctive part of a compound

fungi fungi are simple parasites and include yeast and moulds

fungicidal prevents or treats fungal infections

genito-urinary linked to reproductive and urinary systems

glucagon hormone that counter the effect of insulin, i.e. reduces the level of glucose in the blood

glucocorticoids hormone produced in the adrenal; has a variety of effects essential for life

glycolysis series of metabolic pathways which release energy by converting glucose into lactic acid or pyruvic acid

golgi body protein manufacture site in a cell

gout metabolic disorder causing attacks of arthritis

Graafian follicle formed in the ovary; usually only one follicle matures each menstrual cycle and releases an ovum

granulocytes type of white blood cell

growth hormone hormone secreted by the pituitary gland

haemorrhage bleeding or loss of blood

Haversian system arrangement of support cells in bone tissue

hay fever seasonal inflammation of the mucus membranes lining the nose, caused by an allergy to pollen

heart attack blood supply to the heart is obstructed causing an area of tissue to die; may be fatal

heparin chemical that prevents coagulation of plasma

hepatic associated with the liver

hepatitis inflammation of the liver

Herpes simplex contagious viral infection of the skin

Herpes zoster infection of one or more of the nerve pathways by the chicken pox virus

hirsutism abnormal growth of excess hair in a male growth pattern

histamine substance that causes vasodilation, bronchiolar constriction and increased permeability of the blood vessels

HIV (human immunodeficiency virus) retro virus that infects T-lymphocytes and causes defects in immunity

Hodgkin's disease progressive malignant disease of the lymph nodes

homeostasis an automated self-regulation to maintain a relatively constant internal environment within the body

homeostatic agent that regulates homeostasis

hormone chemical messenger

hyaline cartilage special clear cartilage covering the ends of bones in synovial joints

hydrogen bonds oxygen or nitrogen molecules with a small negative charge, and the hydrogen atom with a small positive charge

hydroxyl group structure with 1 hydrogen bonded to 1 oxygen atom

hyperaemic excessive quantity of blood in tissues

hyperhidrosis excessive perspiration

hypertension high blood pressure

hypertensors substance that increases blood pressure

hyperthyroidism overactive thyroid

hypertrichosis abnormal growth of excess hair in a general distribution

hypnotic agent which causes sleep

hypodermis *see subcutaneous layer*

hypomenorrhoea scanty menstruation

hypotension low blood pressure

hypotensors substance that lowers blood pressure

hypothalamus portion of the brain that with the pituitary gland regulates the autonomic nervous system, emotional response, body temperature, water balance and appetite

hypothyroidism underactive thyroid

ileum part of the small intestine

immune-stimulant stimulates protection against disease

impetigo contagious bacterial skin infection

inferior below

inorganic compound compound which does not contain any carbon molecules

insertion moveable attachment of a muscle

inspiration breathing in – inhalation

insulin hormone influencing the level of glucose in the blood

interstitial cell stimulating hormone hormone secreted by the pituitary gland; stimulates the testes to produce testosterone

inversion movement to turn the sole of the foot inwards

involuntary muscle *see smooth muscle*

ionic bonding attraction of atoms held by an oppositely charged atoms creating a crystal lattice

ions atoms with a negative or positive charge

irritable bowel syndrome (IBS) change in bowel habits with no cause

ischaemic heart disease reduced blood supply to the heart causing damage to the tissues

isomer compounds with the same chemical formula but different structure

isoprene unit structure comprising of 5 carbon atoms

isotopes variation of the number of neutrons occurring among elements

joint where two bones meet

keratin fibrous protein found in the skin, hair and nails

keratinization process by which cells change from living with a nucleus to dead, flat cells

keratinocyte cells of epidermis, secrete keratin

lateral away from the mid line of the body

lateral flexion sideways bend

laxative agent which causes a mild action of the bowels

lentigines flat, discoloured area of skin larger than a freckle

leukaemia type of cancer affecting the white blood cells

leukocytes white blood corpuscles

ligament tough connective tissue holding bones together at a joint

limbic system group of structures in the brain which includes the hypothalamus and hippocampus

London force momentary attraction between oppositely charged molecules

lunula visible part of the nail matrix

lupus erythmatosus auto-immune disorder when the body attacks its own connective tissue

luteinizing hormone (LH) hormone secreted by the pituitary gland; works with FSH to produce ovum

lymph fluid that bathes the tissues contains mainly water and a high concentration of lymphocytes

lymphocytes type of white blood cell involved in immunity

macromolecule molecule with a large structure

macule area of skin darker or lighter than that which surrounds it

matrix living part of the nail

ME (myalgic encephalitis) chronic fatigue or post-viral syndrome causing several debilitating symptoms

medial towards/closest to the mid line of the body

melanin pigmentation found in the epidermis

melanocyte cell that produces melanin

meninges membranes and connective tissue which cover, protect and nourish the brain

menopause the end of the fertile years in a female

menorrhagia heavy menstruation

menstrual cycle series of events which occur regularly in females

metabolic pathways series of chemical reactions

metabolism collective term for all the chemical processes that take place within the body

metasthetic spreading, transforming, transferring energies

migraine severe headache accompanied by visual disturbances, nausea and/or vomiting

milia firm, pearly white, contained spot

mitochondria powerhouse of the cell, site of cellular respiration

mitosis simple cell division where a new cell is created as an exact replica of the original cell

mole skin blemish; flat, raised, pigmented or unpigmented area of skin

molecule two or more atoms

monocytes phagocytic white blood cells

motor nerve conveys impulse from the nerve centre to a muscle or gland

motor point junction between a nerve and muscle, where the nerve enters the muscles

multiple sclerosis progressive disease of the nervous system which destroys the protective covering of the nerve fibres

muscle fatigue overuse of muscle; waste products build up in the muscle tissue

muscle tone incomplete contraction of some of the muscle fibres

myocardial infarction heart attack

myofibrils threads that make up a muscle fibre responsible for contraction of the muscle

myosin protein filament found in muscle cell

nail bed area on which the nail plate lies

nail plate visible portion of the nail

nervine associated with the nerves

neurone specialized nerve cell

neutron uncharged particle in an atom

neutrophils white blood cell; protects against pathogens

noradrenaline counters the effect of adrenalin

nucleolus located in the nucleus of the cell, contains DNA; initiates cell division

nucleus control centre of the cell containing cell DNA or core of an atom containing protons and neutrons

oedema abnormal accumulation of fluid in the tissues; medical oedema is a result of a serious systemic disease

oestrogen hormone that controls the development and function of the female sex organs

olfactory bulb region that receives nerve fibres from the olfactory region of the nose

olfactory epithelium mucous membranes in the nasal cavity

oligomenorrhoea irregular menstruation

onychomycosis fungal infection of the nail

organ group of tissues performing a specific function

organic compound compound containing carbon

origin fixed attachment of a muscle

oscillator something that moves to and fro between two points, e.g. a pendulum

osmosis movement of water molecules from a weak or dilute solution to a more concentrated solution through a semi-permeable membrane

osteoarthritis non-inflammatory disease causing restriction and pain in the joints

osteoporosis reduction in bone tissue making it brittle and easily fractured

oxytocin hormone secreted by the pituitary gland; stimulates the uterus to contract and triggers the release of breast milk

pacemaker electrical device fitted to maintain a regular heart beat

palmar relating to the hand

papillary layer upper layer of the dermis next to the epidermis

parasite organism that lives in or on another living organism

parasiticidal substance that combats parasites

parasympathetic nervous system inhibits the effect of the sympathetic nervous system and prepares the body for inactivity

parathormone hormone controlling excretions of phosphate and calcium

Parkinson's disease neurological disorder caused by the degeneration of the nerve cells in the substantia nigra

paronychia bacterial infection at the base of a nail

pathogen any type of micro-organism that causes disease

peripheral nervous system nervous system outside of the brain and spinal cord

pH scale the 'pH' stands for potential of hydrogen; a standard scale devised to measure the hydrogen ion concentration

phagocytosis action of phagocytes to engulf and ingest micro-organisms and other cells

Pityriasis simplex dandruff – increased activity in the skin cells of the scalp

plantar sole of the foot

plantar flexion sole of the foot moved downwards (toe pointed)

plasma blood with cells removed

platelets *see thrombocytes*

polar covalent bond bond with both a negative and a positive end

polymers smaller molecules joined in long chains

posterior back of the body

pre-menstrual syndrome (PMS) sometimes referred to as pre-menstrual tension (PMT); a collection of emotional and physical symptoms related to the fluctuation in the hormones oestrogen and progesterone

progesterone hormone which prepares and maintains the uterus for pregnancy

pronation palm of the hand turned downwards

prone lying face down

protons positively charged particle in an atom

proximal nearest to the point of attachment of a limb

psoriasis skin disorder caused by overproduction of skin cells; not contagious

puberty development of the secondary sexual characteristics stimulated by the gonadotrophic hormones

pulmonary associated with the lungs

pulmonary artery blood vessel carrying blood from the heart to the lungs

pulmonary vein blood vessel carrying blood from the lungs to the heart

pulse rate wave of pressure which passes along the arteries indicating the pumping action of the heart

reflex action involuntary automatic responses to an external or internal stimulus

refracted when a substance, e.g. water, air, or glass, deflects at a certain angle when it enters obliquely from another medium of different density

reticular layer layer of the dermis next to the subcutaneous layer

rheumatism pain and stiffness in both the muscle and joints

rheumatoid arthritis auto-immune inflammatory disease of the joints

rotation movement of a bone around an axis (180°)

rubefacient increased blood circulation, causing redness to the skin

sarcoma malignant tumour occurring in connective tissue

scabies contagious parasitic mite

sciatica pressure on the sciatic nerve causing numbness or pain

sebaceous gland gland which secretes sebum

seborrhoea excessively oily skin

sebum waxy substance secreted from the sebaceous gland

sedative agent that temporarily reduces functional activity and excitement

sensory nerve responsible for relaying sensation to the brain or spinal cord

serotonin chemical which causes vasoconstriction

skeletal muscle muscle under conscious control

smooth muscle muscle not under conscious control

solute substance that is dissolved in a liquid (solvent) to form a solution

solution liquid in which one or more substances are dissolved

solvent liquid that dissolves another substance (solute) to form a solution without a chemical change in either

spider naevus capillaries evident in a spider shape

sprain tear or overstretch of a ligament

staphylococci type of bacteria, which group together to form small clusters

stimulant agent that causes temporary increased functional activity or excitement

stomachic digestive aid, tonic

strain tear or overstretch of muscle fibres

stratum corneum top layer of the epidermis

stratum germinatum lowest layer of the epidermis

stratum granulosum middle layer of the epidermis

stratum lucidum 2nd layer of the epidermis

stratum spinosum 4th layer of the epidermis

streptococci type of bacteria, formed in chains

striated muscle *see skeletal muscle*

stroke interruption of the blood supply to the brain

subcutaneous layer also called hypodermis; lower layer of the skin which insulates and protects the underlying organs

sudiferous gland collective name for the sweat glands

sudorific agent which causes sweating

superior above

supine lying on the back (supine – spine side), face up

supination palm of the hand turned upwards

sympathetic nervous system prepares the body for vigorous activity

synapse junction between two neurones

synaptic cleft narrow gap separating synapses

synovial joint fully moveable joint

systolic blood pressure pressure exerted in the arteries during ventricular contraction

telangiectasia increase in the size of the small blood vessels beneath the surface of the skin

telogen period of rest in the stages of hair growth

tendons specialized connective tissue that attaches the ends of muscle to bone or skin

testosterone hormone producing male sexual characteristics

thalamus relay centre in the brain for transmitting nerve impulses between the spinal cord and the cerebrum

thoracic duct vessel that drains lymph from the legs, pelvic and abdominal cavities, left half of the head, neck, thorax and left arm

thorax protective cavity of the chest

thrombocytes platelets – small fragments in the blood involved in the clotting process

thrombophlebitis inflammation of part of a vein

thrombosis blood clot

thrush yeast infection of the mucus membrane

thymosin hormone produced in the thymus

thymus endocrine gland located in the chest

thyroid stimulating hormone (TSH) hormone secreted by the pituitary gland; stimulates the thyroid

thyroxin hormone regulating metabolism

tinea parasitic fungal infection

tissue group of cells which work together, performing a similar function

tissue fluid lymph

T-lymphocytes lymphocytes that combat antigens

tonic substance that tones or braces an organ or part of the body

tumour abnormal excessive growth of tissues

urethritis inflammation of the urethra

uterine relating to the uterus

urticaria allergic reaction

valency number of bonds an atom can make

varicose vein enlarged and distended vein

veins blood vessels carrying blood to the heart (excepting the pulmonary vein)

vena cava blood vessel carrying blood from the body to the heart

venules small veins

verruca small, localized, viral infection of the upper epidermis on the foot

virus the smallest known type of infectious agent

vitiligo area of skin lacking pigmentation

voluntary muscle *see skeletal muscle*

vulnerary substance that assists wound healing

wart small, localized, viral infection of the upper epidermis

Appendix 1: First aid box

Area of concern	Action
Burns and scalds	*Burns* are caused by dry heat – flames, e.g. oven. *Scalds* are caused by wet heat – steam, boiling water, fat, e.g. autoclave. *Dealing with burns* ● Cool the burnt area by either placing under running water (running tap or shower) or immerse in cold water (bowl, bucket, bath) for *at least* 10 minutes. ● If water is not available use any cold, harmless fluid, e.g. milk. ● Remove tight clothing and jewellery carefully. Never try to remove anything which has adhered to the skin. ● Protect injury by placing a sterile dressing large enough to cover the whole area. Alternatively, if appropriate, use a clean polythene bag. *Facts* ● Burns are classified by the area covered and the depth into the body. Burns larger than 2.5 square cm must have medical treatment. ● There are three levels of burns: superficial, severe and deep. ● Blisters form because of tissue damage and serum leaks into the burnt area. Never burst blisters as this will increase the risk of infection.
Chest pains – angina	● Sit the casualty down. ● Ask the casualty if they have medication for the condition, e.g. tablets or a puffer. ● The symptoms should ease within a few minutes. If the pain persists or returns it may be a heart attack.
Cuts and grazes	*Aim:* to clean and dress the wound. ● Protect the wound with clean piece of gauze or paper tissue. ● Wash hands and collect first aid equipment. ● If the wound is dirty gently rinse under running water until clean. Clean around the wound with gauze swabs or antiseptic wipes, working outwards. ● If present, carefully remove any loose or foreign material. ● Dry around the wound area and place an adhesive dressing over the area. Never use anything fluffy or cotton wool.
Diabetes	If sugar levels are not controlled they will either: ● drop below normal resulting in *hypoglycaemia* ● build up in the bloodstream resulting in *hyperglycaemia*. Symptoms of hypoglycaemia include: ● prolonged, low blood sugar levels with resulting unconsciousness and diabetic coma ● weakness, faintness, feelings of hunger ● pale skin, cold and clammy ● strong pounding pulse, palpitations

Area of concern	Action
	• muscle tremors • shallow breathing • as brain function is affected the casualty may begin to act strangely. To treat the attack sugar levels need to be raised quickly: • if conscious give sugary drinks – honey, chocolate or other sweet food • let the casualty rest and get medical assistance. Symptoms of hyperglycaemia include: • dry skin and rapid pulse • faint smell of acetone on the breath • laboured breathing. Seek urgent medical assistance. Most suffers of diabetes mellitus will have this type of attack and many carry kits to monitor their blood sugar levels. If the casualty falls unconscious call for urgent medical assistance and monitor breathing and response every 10 minutes.
Epileptic seizures	Minor seizures may pass unnoticed and the person may appear to be daydreaming.
Fainting	Fainting is a short-term loss of consciousness. Casualty may feel weak, giddy and sick. Skin may become pale (grey) and pulse slow down. • If possible lie casualty down on the floor. • Raise feet above level of heart. • Alternatively, sit casualty down and place their head between their knees. • Loosen clothing. • Make sure there is plenty of fresh air. • If casualty loses consciousness, place in the recovery position (on their side, upper leg bent up and pulled forward to rest on the floor, lower leg straight; upper arm forward in front of the body on the floor to support the body and stop it rolling).
Heart attack	Symptoms are like those described for chest pains/angina except they do not ease when the casualty rests, and even occur during rest. In addition there may be: • tightness in the chest • discomfort high in the abdomen, which can radiate down the left arm • shortness of breath • feeling of faintness or giddiness • ashen-looking skin • blueness at the lips • rapid, weak or irregular pulse • sudden collapse. To treat the condition heed the following: • Do not move the casualty. • Make the casualty as comfortable as possible. Put them in a half-sitting position, head and shoulders well supported and knees bent. Do not lie them flat. • Dial 999 and state that you have a suspected heart attack casualty. • Monitor breathing and pulse. • If the casualty has medication help them to take it. If fully conscious give them an aspirin (300 mg) to chew. • Be prepared to resuscitate.

Area of concern	*Action*
Leg cramps	Cramp is caused when there is a sudden tightening or contraction of a muscle or group of muscles. Stretching the affected muscle(s) can normally relieve the condition. Cramp may be as a result of: ● heavy sweating (due to heat, exercise) ● a chemical build up in the muscles after strenuous activity ● pregnancy (common occurrence). To relieve symptoms if persistent, sip a glass of water containing quarter of a teaspoon of salt. Eating a banana may also help.
Major seizures	There is very little you can do apart from remain calm and clear the space around the casualty to prevent injury. Do not restrain them. Once the seizure is over (no longer than five minutes) the casualty may appear confused and sleepy. Place in the recovery position.
Nosebleeds	● Sit the person down and get them to lean forward, this will stop blood going down the throat. ● Put on a pair of disposable gloves and pinch the base of the bone half way up the nose to encourage the blood to clot. ● Advise the casualty to spit out any excess fluid as swallowing may disturb the clotting process, and to avoid blowing their nose for some time afterwards to give the damaged capillaries times to heal.
Poisoning	A poison is any substance which when taken in the body in a sufficient quantity has the potential to cause temporary or permanent damage. Poisons can be swallowed, inhaled, absorbed through the skin, injected or splashed into the eye. If conscious ● do not make the casualty sick (if casualty has been sick keep a sample) ● rush to hospital ● take poison (e.g. tablets, essential oil) if known with you ● if mouth has been burnt by a corrosive substance give casualty sips of cold water or milk.
Resuscitation sequence	First check for a response (talk into both ears). If there is no response call for help. ● **AIRWAY**: Check for breathing; tilt the head back to open the airway. If patient is breathing, place in recovery position. ● **BREATHE:** Check that the mouth is clear and remove any obstructions. Tilt the head back, pinch the nostrils closed and give two breaths of mouth-to-mouth ventilation. ● **CIRCULATION**: Check the pulse rate for up to 10 seconds. If there is a pulse continue artificial ventilation. If there is no pulse begin CPR (if you know how) – alternate 15 chest compressions with 2 breaths of artificial ventilation.
Sensitivity	If you are in doubt as to the level of sensation in an area there are two quick tests you can perform: ● *To check for pain sensitivity* – (client should not be able to see you) randomly place the pointed end of an orange wood stick and the flat (hoof) end without damaging the skin and ask the client to distinguish between the two sensations. ● *To check for tactile sensitivity* – place randomly a very cold and a hot piece of damp cotton wool onto the skin and ask the client to say which is which (you can obtain special sealed tubes that the water can be placed in for performing this test).

Area of concern	Action
Serious wounds	• Apply direct pressure over the wound, preferably over a clean pad. • Pressure may need to maintained for up to 10 minutes. • Raise and support the injured part. It should be above heart or chest level. • Place a sterile dressing over the wound. The dressings should extend over the wound. Secure firmly with a bandage. • Refer to a casualty department or GP.
Sprains and swelling	Sprains are caused in joints when the ligaments that hold the bones in place become overextended or torn (acronym *R-I-C-E*). • *R*est the injured part. • Apply *I*ce or a cold compress (a bag of frozen peas works well) to reduce the swelling. • *C*ompress the injury. • *E*levate the injured part.
Unconsciousness	This condition may develop suddenly or slowly. Common causes include: • head/brain injury • lack of oxygen to the brain, e.g. loss of blood, heart failure, strokes • shock • lack of oxygen entering the lungs (asphyxia/suffocation) • poisoning • imbalance of heat (hypothermia, heat stroke, heat exhaustion) • certain medical conditions such as epilepsy and diabetes.

Appendix 2: Muscles table

Muscle	Position	Origin	Insertion	Action
Occipitalis	base of cranium	epicrananial aponeurosis	skin of eyebrows and bridge of nose	moves scalp backwards
Frontalis	frontal bone over forehead		skin of eyebrows and bridge of nose	moves scalp forwards raises eyebrows creates horizontal wrinkles
Temporalis	side of cranium	temporal fossa	coronoid process and rami of mandible	closes jaw muscle of mastication
Orbicularis oculi	encircles eye	an elliptical muscle, 3 points within the front of the orbit on the frontal, lacrimal and maxilla bones	fibres form an ellipse	closes eye tight partial contraction creates crows feet around eyes
Corrugator	inner edge of each eyebrows	frontal bone, supercillary ridge	skin of eyebrow	wrinkles forehead creates vertical lines on forehead
Buccinator	cheek, opposite to 3rd molar	maxillae above and mandible below	skin into angle/sides of the mouth	holds teeth against cheek when eating blows air out when cheeks have been filled (trumpeting) smiling
Risorius	sides of mouth	parotid fascia over masseter	angle of the mouth	draws mouth sideways (sardonic expression)
Orbicularis oris	encircles mouth (lips)	maxilla above and mandible below	surrounds orifice of the mouth	closes the lips compresses and protrudes the lips works with other muscles to produce speech
Masseter	side of face	under surface of zygomatic arch	inferior angle and lower part (ramus) of mandible	closes jaw muscle of mastication
Zygomatic major	zygomatic bone/cheek	zygomatic bone	into corner of the mouth	raises corner of mouth (smiling) minor raises upper lip
Mentalis	chin	incisive fossa of mandible	skin of lower lip	wrinkles skin of chin protrudes lower lip
Procerus	lies over nasal bone	fascia of lower part of nasal bone and upper part of cartilage	into the skin of the brow and forehead	depresses the wider part of the eyebrow producing wrinkles over bridge of the nose

Muscle	Position	Origin	Insertion	Action
Dilator naris (alar naris)	sides of nostrils	maxilla at sides of nose	skin over margin of nostrils	expands /dilates nostrils
Nasalis	over front of nose	maxilla at side of nose	over bridge of nose to meet muscles of the other side	compresses nose causing it to wrinkle dilates nostrils
Levator palbebrae	upper eyelid	inside of sphenoid bone and in front of orbital foramen	spreads out over surface of skin of upper eyelid	raises upper eyelid
Levator labii superioris	runs upwards from upper lip	lower margin of orbit, maxilla and zygomatic bone	skin of nose, upper lip	lifts upper lip assists in opening the mouth
Depressor labii inferioris	runs downwards from lower lip	inner part of mandible	skin of lower lip	draws down the lower lip assists in opening the mouth
Levator anguli oris (caninus)	runs upwards from corners of mouth	canine fossa of mandible	angle of mouth	lifts the corners of mouth
Depressor anguli oris (triangularis)	runs downwards from corners of mouth	outer part of mandible	angle of mouth	lifts the skin of the chin turns the lower lip outwards (sadness)
Digastric	deep muscle located under the chin (double chin)	two parts joined by a tendon, held in place by a fibrous loop from the hyoid bone *posterior*: mastoid process *anterior*: digastric fossa on inner aspect of base of mandible	as for origin	moves the bones involved with swallowing (i.e. elevates hyoid bone. depresses mandible)
Sternocleidomastoid	sides of neck	sternum and clavicle	temporal bone, mastoid process	flexes head (prayer muscle) one muscle alone rotates head towards opposite side
Platysma	front of chin and neck	fascia of upper part of deltoid and pectoralis major	lower border of mandible, blends with orbicularis oris and skin around corners of the mouth	draws corners of mouth down (pouting)

MUSCLES OF THE ARM

Biceps
Position: front of upper arm
Origin: short head – scapula carocoid process; long head – tubercle of scapula
Insertion: tubercles, proximal end of radius
Action: supinates forearm flexion forearm at elbow

Brachialis
Position: crosses the front of the elbow joint
Origin: lower 1/2 of anterior surface of humerus
Insertion: front of coronoid process of ulna
Action: flexion of elbow in pronation and supination

Brachioradialis
Position: crosses elbow joint on radial side
Origin: lateral supracondylar ridge of humerus
Insertion: styloid process of radius
Action: flexion of forearm at elbow

Flexors of the forearm

Flexor carpi radialis
Position: front of forearm
Origin: medial epicondyle of humerus
Insertion: base of 2nd metacarpal
Action: flexes hand at wrist abducts hand

Palmaris longus
Position: front of forearm
Origin: medial epicondyle of humerus
Insertion: palmar aponeurosis
Action: flexes hand at wrist

Flexor carpi ulnaris
Position: front of forearm
Origin: dual; medial epicondyle of humerus, posterior border of ulna
Insertion: pisiform, hamate, base of 5th metacarpal
Action: flexes wrist adducts wrist

Extensors of the forearm

Extensor carpi radialis longus
Position: covering back of forearm
Origin: supracondylar ridge of humerus
Insertion: posterior of base of 2nd metacarpal
Action: extends hand at wrist abduction of hand at wrist

Extensor carpi ulnaris
Position: covering back of forearm
Origin: dual; lateral epicondyle of humerus, posterior aspect of ulna
Insertion: base of 5th metacarpal
Action: extends and adducts hand at wrist

Extensor carpi radialis brevis
Position: inner side of forearm
Origin: dual; lateral epicondyle of humerus, radial ligament of elbow joint
Insertion: dorsal surface base of 2nd and 3rd metacarpals
Action: extends and abducts hand at wrist

Pronator teres
Position: elbow – forearm
Origin: dual; medial epicondyle of humerus, coronoid process of ulna
Insertion: middle of lateral aspect of radius
Action: pronates forearm flexes forearm at elbow

Triceps
Position: back of arm
Origin: 3 heads; long head – infra glenoid tubercle of scapula; lateral head – upper 1/2 posterior surface of humerus; medial head – 1/3 posterior surface of humerus
Insertion: olecranon process of ulna
Action: extends forearm at elbow

MUSCLES OF THE BACK

Trapezius
Position: diamond-shaped muscles extending from occipital bone to thoracic region
Origin: occipital bone, T1–12 thoracic vertebra and C7
Insertion: clavicle, acromion process and spine of scapula
Action: elevates and braces shoulders
rotates scapula
extends and bends neck laterally

Subscapularis
Position: back of scapula
Origin: subscapular fossa of scapula
Insertion: lesser tubercle of the humerus
Action: medially rotates humerus assists to stabilize shoulder joint

Levator scapula
Position: back of neck
Origin: transverse processes of upper 4 cervical vertebra
Insertion: medial border of scapula
Action: elevates scapula

Deltoid
Position: lies over shoulder
Origin: clavicle, spine and acromion process of scapula
Insertion: deltoid tuberosity of humerus
Action: extends and laterally rotates humerus
medial rotation of humerus forwards
abducts humerus

Serratus anterior
Position: upper lateral trunk, over ribs
Origin: upper eight ribs
Insertion: anterior aspect of medial border of scapula
Action: fixes scapula
assists to raise arm upwards above head

Supraspinatus
Position: top edge of scapula
Origin: supraspinous fossa of scapula
Insertion: greater tubercle of the humerus
Action: abducts humerus at shoulder
stabilizes shoulder

Infraspinatus
Position: over scapula
Origin: infraspinous fossa of scapula
Insertion: greater tubercle of humerus
Action: laterally rotates humerus at shoulder
assists to stabilize shoulder joint

Rhomboids (minor and major)
Position: between top of shoulder blades
Origin: C7 and T, T2–5 vertebra
Insertion: medial border of scapula/medial end of scapula
Action: braces shoulder
rotates scapula
fixes the head and neck

Teres major
Position: across lower part of scapula
Origin: inferior angle of scapula
Insertion: medial border of intertubercular groove of humerus
Action: draws arm backwards
medially rotates humerus
adducts humerus
stabilizes shoulder joint

Teres minor
Position: outer portion of scapula
Origin: lateral border of scapula
Insertion: greater tubercle of humerus
Action: lateral rotation of humerus at shoulder
stabilizes shoulder joint

Caraco-brachialis
Position: clavicle along inner part of arm at top
Origin: coracoid process of scapula
Insertion: middle 1/3 medial aspect of humerus
Action: flexes arm at shoulder

MUSCLES OF THE CHEST

Pectoralis major
Position: front of chest
Origin: dual; medial 1/2 of anterior surface of clavicle, sternum and anterior surface of costal cartilage of true ribs
Insertion: bicepital groove of humerus
Action: anterior adduction of humerus medially rotates humerus draws arm across chest

Pectoralis minor
Position: front of chest
Origin: superior surface of 3rd–5th ribs
Insertion: coracoid process of scapula
Action: pulls scapula inferiorly (shoulders down) pulls scapula anteriorly (shoulder forward) forward reach assists to elevate ribs rotation of scapula

Muscles of the trunk

External obliques
Position: forms sides of abdomen
Origin: lower 8 ribs
Insertion: anterior part of iliac crest and linea alba through a broad aponeurosis
Action: compresses abdomen is important for posture pulls pelvis upwards increases intra-abdominal pressure, assists in childbirth aids defecation assists in movement of the spine forward and lateral flexion rotation of trunk

Internal obliques
Position: sides of abdomen
Origin: outer 2/3 of inguinal ligament and 2/3 of anterior of anterior iliac crest, lumbodorsal fascia
Insertion: costal cartilage of lower 3/4 of ribs 7, 8, 9, 10 and by aponeurosis into pubic crest to linea alba; fuses with external obliques and transversalis
Action: see external obliques

Transversalis
Position: forms wall of abdomen
Origin: inguinal ligament, anterior iliac crest, lumbo-dorsal fascia and inner side of costal cartilage of lower 6 ribs
Insertion: by aponeurosis into crest of pubis and linea alba, upper 3/4 of aponeurosis
Action: see external obliques

Rectus abdominis
Position: anterior wall of abdomen
Origin: pubic bone and symphysis pubis
Insertion: xiphoid process of sternum, costal cartilage 5–7 ribs,
Action: assists in flexes trunk when pelvis is fixed draws pelvis anteriorly

Diaphragm
Position: dome-shaped muscle forming a partition between the thorax and abdomen
Origin: lower circumference of thorax to last 5 costal cartilages of the ribs, T12, lumbar 1–3 and sternum
Insertion: fibres converge to a central tendon
Action: assists with inspiration by enlarging the thorax (to 4th intercostals space on right and 5th on left) aids all expulsive actions due to deepened breath

Intercostals (internal and external)
Position: superior/inferior border of rib in intercostals space
Origin: inferior superior border of rib
Insertion: inferior superior border of rib
Action: external muscles elevates ribs so that forced respiration takes place internal muscle depresses ribs and aids forced respiration

MUSCLES OF THE BACK AND TRUNK

Quadratus lumborum
Position: fills space between the oblique muscles and vertebrae, forms part of posterior wall
Origin: iliac crest
Insertion: 12th rib, L1–4 vertebrae
Action: laterally flexes lumbar spine when pelvis is fixed extends spine singularly abducts trunk maintains pelvis in locomotion, assists in inspiration by fixing 12th rib

Erector spinae
Position: deep groove either side of the vertebrae
Origin: either side of spine, back of sacrum and iliac crest
Insertion: many overlapping attachments on vertebrae and adjacent ribs
Action: extends spine maintains posture of the trunk singularly abducts and rotates trunk

Iliacus
Position: crosses front of groin
Origin: inner surface of iliac fossa, iliac crest
Insertion: lesser trochanter of femur
Action: bends trunk and pelvis forward (e.g. sitting up from lying) flexes thigh lateral rotation of thigh

Psoas
Position: crosses front of groin
Origin: transverse processes and bodies of T12–L 5
Insertion: pubic bone femur
Action: flexes thigh assists in abduction and lateral rotation of thigh forward and side flexion of spine

Latissimus dorsi
Position: crosses back from lumbar region to the shoulder
Origin: iliac crest, lower 3 or 4 ribs, spines of lower 6 thoracic,
Insertion: bicepital groove of humerus
Action: extends humerus adducts humerus medial rotation of humerus

Gluteus maximus
Position: crosses back of hip forming the buttock
Origin: crest and posterior surface of ilium, posterior surface of sacrum and coccyx, aponeurosis of erector spinae
Insertion: gluteal tuberosity of femur, iliotibial tract
Action: extends thigh laterally rotates thigh raises trunk from stooping and seated position abduction of thigh

Gluteus medius
Position: lies beneath maximus
Origin: lateral surface of iliac crest, gluteal line
Insertion: greater trochanter of femur
Action: abducts thigh medially rotates thigh stabilizes position of the pelvis on femurs

Gluteus minimus
Position: lies beneath maximus
Origin: outer surface of iliac crest
Insertion: greater trochanter of femur
Action: abducts thigh rotates thigh medially stabilizes position of the pelvis on femurs

MUSCLES OF THE LEG

Anterior aspect

Sartorius
Position: across the front of the quadriceps
Origin: anterior iliac
Insertion: upper part of medial shaft of tibia
Action: abducts thigh
flexes leg at knee and thigh at hip
lateral rotation of thigh

Quadriceps
Group of 4 muscles form the front of the thigh. Rectus femoris crosses both the hip and knee joint, the other 3 only act on the knee joint.

Rectus femoris
Position: front of thigh crosses hip joint
Origin: iliac spine, above acetabulum of pelvic bone
Insertion: base of patella
Action: flexes thigh
extends leg at knee

Vastus intermedius
Position: front of thigh
Origin: upper 2/3 shaft of femur
Insertion: lateral border of patella lateral condyle of patella
Action: extends leg at knee

Vastus lateralis
Position: front of thigh
Origin: great trochanter and gluteal tuberosity of femur
Insertion: lateral border of patella
Action: extends leg at knee

Vastus medialis
Position: front of thigh
Origin: medial lip of linea aspera medial supracondylar line of femur
Insertion: medial border of patella
Action: extends leg at knee

Adductors of the leg

Adductor magnus
Position: inner thigh
Origin: inferior ramus of pubis and ischial tuberosity
Insertion: gluteal tuberosity, medial subracondylar line of femur
Action: adduction at the hip
flexion of hip
medial rotation of thigh
assists hamstrings in extension of hip

Adductor longus
Position: upper inner thigh
Origin: symphysis pubis
Insertion: middle 1/3 linea aspera of femur
Action: adducts thigh
flexion of hip
medial rotation of thigh

Adductor brevis
Position: upper inner thigh
Origin: body and inferior ramus of pubis (behind longus)
Insertion: upper part of linea aspera of femur
Action: see adductor longus

Pectineus
Position: across pubis and hip
Origin: pubis
Insertion: line between lesser trochanter and linea aspera of femur
Action: flexes thigh
adduction of thigh

Gracilis
Position: inner thigh, across groin
Origin: body and lower ridge of pubis, ramus of ischium
Insertion: medial shaft of tibia just below the condyle
Action: adducts thigh
flexes hip
medial rotation of the hip

Muscles of the lower leg

Peroneal muscles (longus and brevis)
Position: outer side of leg
Origin: lower 2/3 lateral side of fibula
Insertion: medial cuneiform and base of 1st and 3rd metatarsal /5th metatarsal
Action: everts foot
plantar flexion
role in limiting inversion

MUSCLES OF THE LEG (cont'd)

Abductors of the leg

Tensor fascia latae
Position: upper part of outer thigh
Origin: anterior part of outer lip of iliac crest and anterior superior iliac spine
Insertion: iliotibial tract, 1/3 of the way down inside thigh, lateral condyle of tibia
Action: flexes thigh
 abducts hip
 medial rotation of thigh
 helps extend knee

Posterior aspect

Hamstrings: Group of three muscles found on the back of the thigh

Biceps femoris
Position: back of thigh
Origin: ischial tuberosity, lateral lip of linea aspera of femur
Insertion: head of fibula and lateral tuberosity of tibia
Action: flexes knee
 extends thigh at hip
 lateral rotation of flexed knee

Semitendonisus
Position: back of thigh
Origin: ischial tuberosity
Insertion: upper part of medial surface shaft of tibia
Action: medial rotation of thigh
 helps raise trunk from stooping by pulling pelvis backwards
 flexes leg at knee
 extends thigh

Semimembranosus
Position: back of thigh
Origin: ischial tuberosity of pelvic bone
Insertion: posterior part of medial condyle of tibia
Action: medial rotation of flexed knee
 helps raise trunk from stooping by pulling pelvis backwards

Anterior lower leg

Tibialis anterior
Position: running outside of tibia
Origin: upper 2/3 of lateral surface shaft of tibia, membrane between fibula and tibia
Insertion: base of 1st metatarsal and under surface of medial cuneiform
Action: inverts foot
 dorsi flexes foot
 helps to support longitudinal arch

Posterior lower leg

Gastrocnemius
Position: forms calf
Origin: 2 heads, just above each femoral condyle
Insertion: forms a broad aponeurosis which unites with soleus to form the tendon calcaneus inserting into posterior surface of calcaneus
Action: plantar flexes foot
 flexes knee

Soleus
Position: lies under gastrocnemius
Origin: upper 1/4 posterior surface shaft of fibula and middle 1/3 medial border of tibia
Insertion: tendon calcaneous
Action: plantar flexes foot
 plays role in balance

Flexors of the toes

- flexor digitorum brevis
- flexor digitorum accessories
- lumbricals
- flexor hallucis brevis
- flexor digiti minimi brevis

Position: lower leg and foot
Origin: posterior surface of tibia
Insertion: base and tendons of the distal phalanges
Action: flexes toes

Extensors of the toes

- extensor digitorum brevis
- extensor digitorum longus
- extensor hallucis longus

Position: lower leg and foot
Origin: front of upper surface of calcaneous
Insertion: 4 tendons to base of metatarsals/distal phalanges, medial cuneiform
Action: extends toes
 dorsi flexion of ankle

Index

abduction 440
accounts/accountant 433
acid 18
acid mantle 44, 440
acne rosacea 54, 440
acne vulgaris 54, 440
actin 440
active transport 18, 440
acupressure (shiatsu) 196–7
acute 440
Addison's disease 440
adduction 440
adenoids 74, 440
adipose tissue 440
adrenalin 440
adrenals 113
adrenocorticotrophic hormone (ACTH) 440
after care 141, 142–5
agranulocytes 64, 441
AIDS (acquired immune deficiency syndrome) 75, 440
aknylosing spondylitis 440
albinism 49–50, 440
aldosterone 440
aliphatic compound 440
allergen 440
allergy 76, 440
alopecia 440
alveoli 93
amenorrhoea 440
anaemia 70
anaesthesia 108, 440
anagen 440
analgesic 440
anaphrodisiac 440
anatomical positions 38
androgen 440
angina 69
angioma 50, 440
anion 440
ankylosing spondylitis 84
anterior 440
anti-depressant 441
anti-diuretic hormone 441
anti-histamine 441

anti-inflammatory 441
anti-microbial 441
anti-rheumatic 441
anti-spasmodic 441
anti-toxic 441
anti-viral 441
antibody (immunoglobin) 440
antigen 441
antioxidant 441
antiseptic 441
anxiety 105–6, 441
aorta 441
aperitive 441
aphrodisiac 441
apocrine gland 441
appendicular skeleton 441
appendix 441
areolar tissue 41
aromatherapy
    after care 238–40
    clinical 225–30
    definition 220
    essential oils 220–2
    history 220
    physiology 222
    routine 231
    safety issues 223–5
    sequence 231–8
    suitability for treatment 224
    using crystals 370–1
aromatic compounds 441
arthritis 83, 441
associated neurone 441
asthma 94, 441
atherosclerosis 68, 441
atom 15, 441
atomic number 441
ATP (adenosine triphosphate) 441
atrophy 58, 441
auto-immune disorder 76, 441
axial skeleton 441
ayurveda 34–6, 441

B-lymphocytes 441
bacteria 53, 441
bacterical 441

balsamic 441
basal metabolic rate 441
basil 244–5
basophils 441
benign growth 441
benzoin 245–6
bergamot 246
black pepper 247
blackheads (comedones) 49
blood 61–2, 64–5, 184
blood pressure 65–6, 69–70, 441
blue nail 58
body fat 177
body massage
    adaptations 210–14
    after care 210
    history 199
    inter-event 213
    mediums 200–1
    muscle stretching/energizing 207–8
    post-event 213
    posture and stance 201–2
    pre-event 212–13
    pre-heating treatments 214–18
    preparation 199–202
    remedial 214
    routine 202–7
    sequence and timing 202
    stretch and release 208–9
    see also massage techniques
body shapes 171
boils (furuncles) 54, 441
bonding 441
brain 102–3
breast 120
brittle nails (*fragitalitas ungium*) 58
bromhidrosis 50, 441
bronchi 92
bronchitis 94, 441
bruise 50, 441
bunion (halux vulgus) 85, 441
burnt out 345–8
bursa 441
bursitis 85, 441
business planning 431–2

cajeput 248
callus 442
callus skin 53
cancellous bone 442
cancer 42, 442
candida albicans (moniliasis/thrush) 99,
  117–18, 442
capillaries 442
capsular ligament 442
capsulitis 90, 442
carbohydrates 147–8
carbuncle 54, 442
carcinoma 442
carminative 442
carpal tunnel syndrome 107–8, 442
cartilage 442
catagen 442
cation 442
cedarwood 248–9
cells 39, 42
cellulite 50, 442
central nervous system 442
cephalic 442
cerebrospinal fluid (CSF) 442
cerebrum 102, 442
chakras 30–3, 368–70
  see also colour therapy
chamomile 249–50
chemical
  bonds 16–17
  reaction 16–17, 442
  sterilization 10–11
chilblain 70
chloasma (melasma) 49, 442
cholagogue 442
choleretic 442
cholesterol 153–4
chronic 442
chyme 442
cicatrisant 442
circulatory system 66–71
circumduction 442
clary sage 251
client care
  after care/advice 141–5
  consultation techniques 134–6
  contra indications 137–41
  counselling skills 131–2
  first impressions 124–5
  interpersonal skills 125–30
  preparing for treatment 133–4
  protecting yourself 132–3
co-enzyme 442
coconut oil 228
coeliac disease 97–8, 442
cognition 442
colitis 98, 442
collagen 45
colour therapy
  after care advice 385
  ascertaining colour needs 379–80
  aura energy/reading 379
  aura-soma 379
  client treatment 377–8
  colour breathing 377
  Colour Me Beautiful 378
  colours used 381–5
  consultation 376
  contra indications 385

electromagnetic spectrum 374–5
  environmental 380–1
  history 374
  illumination therapy 378–9
  main uses 375–6
  material and swatches 378
  self-treatment 377
  visualization and meditation 376
comedones (blackheads) 49, 442
communication 126
  non-verbal 126–7
  verbal 127–30
compact bone 442
compounds 15–16, 18, 442
conjunctivitis 109, 442
connective tissue 442
consultation 134–6, 225
contra indications 137
  general 137
  nutritional therapy 165–6
  seeking professional guidance 138–9
  specific area 137–8
  what you need to know 139–40
contraceptive pill 119–20
Control of Substances Hazardous to
  Health (COSHH) Regulations
  (1999) 4–5
cordial 442
coriander 252
corn 53, 442
corneum 447
cortex 114
counselling 131–2
covalent bonding 442
creams 228–9
Crohn's disease 442
crystal therapy 358–60, 371
crystals
  basic set 363–6
  chakra balancing 368–70
  choosing 360–1
  cleansing 361
  definition 358–9
  energizing 362
  knowing 367–8
  life force energy 359
  male and female 362–3
  self-treatment 367–8
  storing 361
  types 366–7
  using with other therapies 370–1
Cushing's syndrome 442
cypress 252–3
cystitis/urethritis 117, 442
cytoplasm 39, 442

dandruff (pityriasis simplex) 60
debility 442
deodorant 442
depression 106, 442
depurative 442
dermatitis (eczema) 51
dermis 45–6, 442
desquamation 44, 442
diabetes 116
diabetes mellitus 443
diaphysis 443
diastolic blood pressure 443
diffusion 18, 443

digestion 186
digestive system 95, 443
  accessory organs 97
  alimentary canal/gastrointestinal
    tract 95–6
  disorders/diseases 97–9
dipole 443
disabled clients 211
disease 443
distal 443
diuretic 443
diverticular disease 98, 443
dorsal 443
dorsiflexion 443
dowager's hump 175
dysmenorrhoea 443

ear candling
  after care advice 394
  anatomy 393–5
  contra actions 388
  contra indications 388
  healing properties 389
  history 388
  manufacture/composition of candles
    389
  medical terms 396–7
  otoscope 389–90
  physical/psychological
    benefits/effects 390
  treatment 390–3
eccrine gland 443
eczema (dermatitis) 51, 443
effleurage 186–8
elastic tissue 41
elastin 45
elderly clients 211
Electricity at Work Regulations
  (1989) 5
electron 443
elements 15, 443
embolism 67–8, 443
emmenagogue 443
emulsifier 443
endocrine system 111–12
  disorders/diseases 116
  feedback mechanisms 112
  glands and their hormones 112–15
endometriosis 121–2, 443
endoplasmic reticulum 39, 443
energy field 33–4
enzymes 154–5, 443
ephilide 49, 443
epidermis 44–5, 443
epilepsy 106–7, 443
epiphyses 443
epithelial tissue 443
erythema 62, 443
erythrocytes 64, 443
essential oils 220
  categories 244
  chemotypes 243
  classification 241–3
  directory 244–81
  harmony 244
  home treatment/other uses 239–40
  how they work 222
  methods of extraction 221–2
  patch testing 224

pre-blended 225
preparation/blending 229–30
purchase/storage 223–4
selecting a carrier 226–9
selecting for treatment 229–30
synergy 244
toxicity 224
eucalyptus 253–4
euphoric 443
eversion 443
excretion 443
exercise 33–4
expectorant 443
expiration 443
extension 443
eye 108–9

facial, holistic see holistic facial
facilitated diffusion 443
fascia 443
fat cells 40
fats 150–4
febrifugal 443
feet 80, 82
    aromatherapy 236
    body massage 203–4
    condition of nail and skin 324
    movement 38
    odour 325
    oedema 325
    posture and bone structure 323–4
    puffiness/swelling 324
    reflexology 320–38
    Reiki 415
    shape/size 324
    skin colour 325
    temperature 325
fennel 254–5
fibroblasts 40
fire fighting 7–8
first aid box 449–52
flat back 175
flexion 443
follicle stimulating hormone (FSH) 443
folliculitis 55, 443
fracture 83, 443
frankincense 255–6
free radicals 443
fribrous tissue 41
frictions 189–90
functional group 443
fungi 54, 443
fungicidal 444

gall bladder 97
genito-urinary system 185, 444
    disorders/diseases 117–18
    renal/urinary system 116–17
    reproductive organs 118–22
geranium oil 256–7
ginger 257–8
glucagon 444
glucocorticoids 444
glue ear 396
glycolysis 444
golgi body (golgi apparatus) 39, 444
gout 84, 444
Graafian follicle 444
granulocytes 64, 444

grapefruit 258–9
grommets 396
growth hormone 444

haemorrhage 66, 444
hair 59–61
hammer toes 91
hand 79–80
    aromatherapy 238
    body massage 204–5
    movement 38
    personal hygiene 12
    reflexology 338–9
hangnails 58
Haversian system 77, 444
hay fever 94, 444
head lice (pediculosis capititis) 60
health and safety
    duties/responsibilities 9–12
    legislation 2–9
Health and Safety (Display Screen
        Equipment) Regulations
        (1999) 8
Health and Safety (First Aid)
        Regulations (1981) 5–6
Health and Safety (Information for
        Employees) Regulations
        (1989) 9
heart 61, 68–9
heart attack (myocardial infarcation)
        69, 444
heat therapy 214–18
heparin 444
hepatic 444
hepatitis 99, 444
herpes simplex (cold sore) 55, 444
herpes zoster (shingles) 55, 444
hirsutism 60, 444
histamine 444
HIV (human immunodeficiency virus)
        75, 444
hives (urticaria) 52–3
Hodgkin's disease 75, 444
holistic facial
    adaptation 299–300
    after care/further treatments 301–2
    basic face reading 291–2
    cleansing 292–4
    contra actions 301
    definition 284
    masks 300–1
    massage 294–5
    massage sequence 297–9
    preparation 288–90
    skin analysis 290–1
    skin care products 286–8
    skin types 284–5
    toning 294
    treatment 284
    treatment records 302
homeostasis 41, 444
homeostatic 444
hormones 112–15, 444
hot stone massage
    after care advice 424
    care of stones 420
    cold marine stones 419
    contra actions 421
    contra indications 420–1

history 418
hot basalt 418–19
importance of grounding 421
standard set 419–20
treatment 422–4
hyaline cartilage 444
hydrogen 18, 444
hydrolat/hydrosol 229
hydroxyl group 444
hyper-extended knees 176
hyperaemic 444
hyperhydrosis 51–2, 444
hypertension 69–70, 444
hypertensors 444
hyperthryoidism 444
hypertrichosis 60–1, 444
hypertrophy of nail (onychauzis) 58
hypnotic 444
hypodermis see subcutaneous layer
hypomenorrhoea 444
hypotension 69, 444
hypotensors 444
hypothalamus 102, 444
hypothyroidism 444

ileum 444
immune-stimulant 444
impetigo 55, 444
Indian head massage
    adapting to different individuals
        314–15
    after care 315
    contra indications 304
    history 304
    length/frequency of treatment 307
    oils used 306–7
    physical benefits 305
    preparation 304–5
    psychological benefits 306
    routine 307–12
    using crystals 371
infection, preventing 10–11
inferior 444
inflammatory bowel disease (IBD) 98
infra red treatment 218
ingrowing nails (onychopcryptosis)
        58–9
inorganic compound 444
insertion 444
inspiration 445
insulin 445
integumentary system
    hair 59–61
    nail 57–9
    skin 43–7
        conditions, disorders, diseases
            47–56
intermolecular forces 17–18
interpersonal skills 125
    communication skills 126
    non-verbal communication (NVC)
        126–7
    personal presentation 126
    verbal 127–30
interstitial cell stimulating hormone
        445
inversion 445
involuntary muscle 445
ionic bonding 445

ions 445
irritable bowel syndrome (IBS) 98–9, 445
ischaemic heart disease 445
isomer 445
isoprene unit 445
isotopes 445

jasmine absolute 259–60
joints 81–2, 445
jojoba oil 228
juniper berry oil 260–1

kapha types 35
keratin 445
keratinization 44, 445
keratinocyte 44, 445
kidneys 116–17
kinetic theory 18
knock knees (tibial torsion) 176
kyphosis 174–5

larynx 92
lateral 445
lateral flexion 445
lavender oil 261–2
laxative 445
lecithin 153
lemon 262–3
lemongrass 263–4
lentigines 445
lentigo 49
leuconychia 58
leukaemia 67, 445
leukocytes 64, 445
ligament 445
limbic system 102, 445
liver 97
London force 445
lordosis 175
lungs 93
lunula 445
lupus erythematosus 42
lupus erythmatosus 445
luteinizing hormone (LH) 445
lymph 445
lymphatic circulation 184
lymphatic massage 195–6
lymphatic/immune system 71
    disorders/diseases 75–6
    lymph/tissue fluid 71–4
    organs associated with system 74–5
lymphocytes 445

macromolecule 445
macrophages 40
macule 49, 445
male clients 211–12, 300
Management of Health and Safety at
        Work Regulations (1999) 2–3
mandarin 264–5
Manual Handling Operations
        Regulations (1992) 8
marjoram 265–6
marketing 434–9
marma therapy 36
masks 300–1
massage techniques
    additional 192–3
    advanced treatment 193–4

benefits/effects 184–6
    classic 186–92
    other therapies 194–7
    preparation 192
    see also body massage
mast cells 40
matrix 445
ME (myalgic encephalitis) 445
medial 445
medical oedema 70–1
meditation 350–2
medulla 114
melanin 45, 445
melanocyte 445
melasma (chloasma) 49
melissa 266
meninges 103, 445
menopause 120, 445
menorrhagia 445
menstrual cycle 118–19, 445
meridians 21–3
    bladder 26
    central and governing 29–30
    gall bladder 28
    heart 25–6
    kidney 26–7
    large intestine 24
    liver 28–9
    lung 23
    pericardium/circulation 27
    small intestine 25
    spleen/pancreas 25
    stomach 24
    triple warmer 27–8
metabolic pathways 445
metabolism 41–2, 445
metasthetic 445
migraine 104–5, 445
milia 48, 445
minerals 160–1, 164
mitochondria 39, 445
mitosis 45, 445
molecules 15, 18, 446
moles (naevus) 48, 445
monocytes 446
motor nerve 446
motor point 446
multiple sclerosis (MS) 105, 446
muscle energizing techniques (MET)
        207–8
muscle stretching techniques (MST)
        207–8
muscles 184–5, 454–60
muscular system
    disorders 90–1
    functions 85
    major muscles 88–9
    muscle contraction 87
    muscle fatigue 87, 446
    muscle soreness 90
    muscle strain 90
    muscle tissue 41
    muscle tone 87, 177, 446
    tendons 87
    types 85–7
myalgic encephalitis (ME) 75–6
myocardial infarction 446
myofibrils 446
myosin 446
myrrh 267

nail 57–9
nail bed 57, 446
nail plate 57, 446
neroli (orange blossom) 268
nervine 446
nervous system 100, 186
    autonomic 104
    central 102–3
    disorders/diseases 104–8
    nerve cell/neurone 100
    peripheral 103–4
    transmission of impulses 101
nervous tissue 41
neuromuscular techniques (NMT)
        193–4
neurones 101, 446
neutron 446
neutrophils 446
niaouli 268–9
noradrenaline 446
nose 91–2
nucleolus 446
nucleus 39, 446
nutrition
    anti-nutrients 154–6
    balanced diet 164
    consultation 165
    contra indications 165–6
    macro-nutrients 147–54
    micro-nutrients 156–64
    weight parameters 166–7

oedema 325, 446
oestrogen 446
olfactory bulb 446
olfactory epithelium 446
olfactory system 110–11
oligomenorrhoea 446
onychomycosis 446
orange 269
organic compound 446
organs 41, 446
origin 446
oscillator 446
osmosis 18, 446
osteoarthritis 83, 446
osteomalacia 83
osteoporosis 83, 446
otitis media 396
otoscope 389–90
oxytocin 446

pacemaker 68, 446
palmar 446
palmarosa 270
palpation 170
pancreas 97, 114–15
papillary layer 446
paraffin wax 217
paranasal sinuses 396
parasite 53–4, 446
parasiticidal 446
parasympathetic nervous system 104, 446
parathormone 446
parathyroid gland 113
Parkinson's disease 105, 446
paronychia 59, 446
patchouli 270–1
pathogen 446

pelvic girdle 80
pelvic tilt 174
peppermint 271–2
perforated eardrum 396
peripheral nervous system 446
personal hygiene/appearance 12–13
Personal Protective Equipment at
        Work (PPE) Regulations
        (1992) 4
petitgrain 273
petrissage 188–9
pH scale 18, 446
phagocytosis 447
pharynx 92
pine (Scotch) 273–4
pineal gland 113
pitta types 35
pituitary gland 112
Pityriasis simplex 447
plantar 447
plantar flexion 447
plasma 40, 64, 447
platelets 64, 447
polar covalent bond 447
polymers 447
posterior 447
posture 170
    centre of gravity 172
    faults/weaknesses 173–8
    good 172–3
    mechanism 172
    muscular condition 178
    poor 173
    re-education of 173
    reflex 172
    simple exercises 179–81
pre-menstrual syndrome (PMS) 121,
        447
pregnancy 121, 211
premises
    choosing 426
        buying salon with client base
            429–30
        going mobile 427–8
        partnerships 426–7
        renting time in a clinic 428–9
        working from home 427
        working with someone else 426
progesterone 447
pronation 447
prone 447
proteins 148–50
protons 447
protruding abdomen 176
Provision of Use of Work Equipment
        Regulations (PUWER) (1998)
        8–9
proximal 447
psoriasis 52, 447
puberty 118, 447
pubic lice (pediculosis pubis) 60
pulmonary 447
pulse 62
pulse rate 447

Raynaud's disease 70
reflex action 447
reflexology
    benefits/effects 317–18
    contra indications 323

cross reflexes/related areas 320
    definition 317
    feet
        after care 338
        completion of treatment 337
        contra actions 337
        hygiene 338
        mapping of 320–1
        meridians of 321
        pressure techniques 327
        reading 323–5
        reflex point 327
        relaxation massage 336
        signs of imbalance 318
        treatment adaptations 337
        treatment procedures 328–36
        warm-up massage 326
        zone system 319–20
    hands 338–9
    history 317
    preparation 321–3
    referral area 320
    sensations during treatment
        318–19
    treatment 325
    using crystals 370
refracted 447
Reiki
    benefits/effects 399–400
    causes of dis-harmony/dis-ease
        413–16
    contra actions 403
    contra indications 402–3
    definition 399
    intent 399
    meaning of symbols 412–13
    precepts 400
    principles 400
    self-healing 403–4
    three degrees of the Usui 401–2
    treatment 404–11
    understanding attunements 401–2
    using with other treatments 413
relaxation 350
renal system 116–17
repetitive strain injury (RSI) 91
Reporting of Injuries, Diseases and
        Dangerous Occurrences
        Regulations (RIDDOR) (1995)
        6–8
reproductive organs 118–22
respiratory system 91–4, 186
reticular layer 447
rheumatism 447
rheumatoid arthritis 44, 83
ridged nails 58
risk assessment 2–3
rose 274–5
rosemary 275–6
rosewood 276–7
rotation 447
rubefacient 447

salon
    atmosphere 124–5
    security 11–12
sandalwood (East Indian) 277–8
sarcoma 447
sauna 215–16
scabies 56, 447

sciatica 107, 447
scoliosis 174
sebaceous cyst (wen) 52
sebaceous gland 447
seborrhoea 52, 447
sebum 447
sedative 447
sensory nerve 447
serotinin 447
sex glands 113, 115
shiatsu (acupressure) 196–7
shingles (herpes zoster) 55, 444
shoulder girdle 79
skeletal muscle 447
skeletal system 185
    bone tissue 76–7
    conditions, disorders, diseases 83–5
    skeleton 78–82
skin 185
    analysis 290–1
    breaks in surface 47
    colour 177–8
    conditions, disorders, diseases
        177–8
        caused by change in circulation
            50
        changes in pigmentation 49–50
        common blemishes 48–9
        common disorders 50–3
        common lesions 47–8
        infections 53–6
    dermis 45–6
    different skins 47
    epidermis 44–5
    fluid-filled lesions 48
    functions 43–4
    hypodermis or subcutaneous
        layer 47
    scar tissue 48
    shape 48
    superficial healing 46–7
    texture 47
    types 284–5
skin care products 286–8
skull 78
smooth muscle 447
solute 447
solvent 447
somatic nervous system 103–4
spasticity 90
special senses 108–11
spider naevus 50, 447
spine 78–9
spleen 74–5
split nails (lamellar dystrophy) 58
spondylosis 84
sprain 90, 447
staphylococci 447
steam baths/rooms 216
stimulant 447
stock 432–3
stomachic 447
strain 447
stratum 447
stratum corneum 44
stratum germinatum 45, 447
stratum granulosum 44, 448
stratum lucidum 44, 448
stratum spinosum 44–5, 448
streptococci 448

stress 115
   causes 343–4
   chemical and nutritional 342–3, 344
   definition 342
   emotional 342, 344
   environmental 342, 343
   managing 349–56
   reducing 348–9
   response 345–8
   symptoms 344
striated muscle 448
stroke 68, 448
subcutaneous layer 448
sudiferous gland 448
sudorific 448
superior 448
supination 448
supine 448
sweat 46
sympathetic nervous system 104, 448
synapse 448
synaptic cleft 448
synovial joint 448
systolic blood pressure 448

T-lymphocytes 448
tapotement/percussion 190–1
tea tree/ti-tree 278
telangiectasia 50, 448
telogen 448
tendonitis 90
tendons 448
testosterone 448
thalamus 102, 448

thermal auricular therapy *see* ear
   candling
thermal masks 217
thombophlebitis 448
thoracic duct 448
thorax 79, 448
thrombocytes 64, 448
thrombophlebitis 67
thrombosis 67, 448
thrush 99, 117–18, 442, 448
thyme (white/common) 279–80
thymosin 448
thymus 74, 115, 448
thyroid gland 113
thyroid stimulating hormone (TSH)
   448
thyroxin 448
time management 433–4
tinea 56, 448
tinea ungulum 59
tinnitus 397
tissue fluid 448
tissues 40–2, 448
tonic 448
trace elements 160, 161–4
trachea 92
treatment 133–6, 141
tumour 448

ultra violet (UV) radiation 10
urethritis 448
urinary system *see* genito-urinary system
urticaria (hives) 52–3, 448
uterine 448

valency 448
varicose veins 67, 448
vascular naevus 50
vata types 35
vegetable/base oils 226–9
veins 448
vena cava 448
venules 448
verrucae 55–6, 448
vertigo 396
vetivert (vetiver) 280
vibrations 191–2
virus 53, 448
vitamins 156
   fat-soluble 157–9
   water-soluble 159–60
vitiligo 49, 448
voluntary muscle *see* skeletal muscle
vulnerary 448

warts 55–6, 448
water 155–6
weight 166–7
wen (sebaceous cyst) 52
whiplash 91
white corpuscles 64
winged scapulae 176
Workplace (Health, Safety and Welfare)
   Regulations (1992) 3–4

yin/yang 21
ylang yang 281
yoga 354–6